Clinics in Developmental Medicine Nos. 41/42

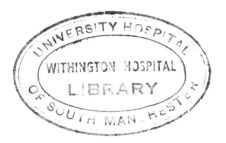

Acute Hemiplegias and Hemisyndromes in Childhood

by
WERNER ISLER

Preface to English Edition by
Hans Zellweger

Translation by E. H. Burrows

1971

Spastics International Medical Publications

LONDON: William Heinemann Medical Books Ltd.

PHILADELPHIA: J. B. Lippincott Co.

ISBN 0 433 35450 X

Printed in England at THE LAVENHAM PRESS LTD., Lavenham, Suffolk.

ACKNOWLEDGEMENTS

The author thanks his teachers, Prof. Hugo Krayenbühl, Prof. Guido Fanconi and Prof. Andrea Prader for their constant encouragement and assistance. The generosity of Prof. Josef Wellauer enabled the author to perform numerous angiograms. Particular thanks are due to the Medical Photographer Mr. Otto Brunner, his secretary Miss Erika Walti, the artist Mr. Walter Adank, and the senior secretary Miss Elsbeth Dudler.

Contents

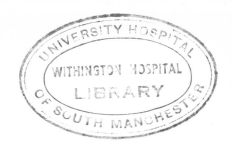

Preface

New methods and new techniques often lead to discoveries in the fields of the medical sciences. Discoveries may also follow when established methods find a wider range of indications, be it when applied to other disease conditions or to other populations. Werner Isler's monograph represents an impressive illustration of this.

Cerebral angiography and pneumoencephalography have been known for more than four decades, but technical difficulties have prevented their wider application to the young and, notably, to those who are in an acute and critical emergency state. This is especially true for the percutaneous method of cerebral angiography. The author of this monograph combines a training in neurosurgical techniques with a wide experience in Pediatric Neurology. By perfecting his techniques, he has reduced and even minimized the hazards associated with cerebral contrast studies. Nevertheless, he does not dismiss lightly the objection that carotid angiography, for instance, represents a risk that may well aggravate the patients' condition. However, 'in the hands of an experienced operator, and with the use of general anaesthesia administered by a competent anaesthetist, angiography can be approached without serious misgivings even in children with acute and severe hemisyndromes.' The author's dexterity has allowed him to repeat contrast studies even after short intervals. In so doing he has been able to disclose the dynamics of main vascular processes. The development of a mycotic aneurysm, the rapid recanalisation after thrombotic arterial occlusions, the extent of post-convulsive edema of a cerebral hemisphere have been *ad oculos* demonstrated.

A number of detailed case histories, accompanied by excellent photographs and schematic illustrations, enrich the book and add to its value. The monograph discloses many new insights into the multifarious etiopathogenetic mechanisms underlying acute hemiplegias and hemisyndromes in childhood. Its English translation may give it the wide distribution it deserves on this side of the Atlantic.

Iowa City, Iowa,   *Hans Zellweger*
Summer 1971

Foreword

Acute hemiplegias in childhood are by no means rare and they involve the paediatrician and paediatric neurosurgeon to the same extent. No simple explanation can be given of their aetiology and pathogenesis, and treatment is difficult and only partially successful. Thus there is an urgent need for an up-to-date and straightforward description of the symptoms which, despite their uniformity, signify so much, and of experience of the various methods employed at present in diagnosis, prognosis, prophylaxis and treatment.

Nothnagel, in 1879, pointed out that cerebral haemorrhage has been the subject of intense medical thought for centuries and that the word 'apoplexy' carries a clinical connotation only, without describing a morbid anatomical entity. In the last 40 years fundamental new concepts have been developed, not only in the pathogenesis of cerebral haemorrhage, but also concerning affections of the cerebral vessels. These new concepts are largely attributable to the development of cerebral angiography which has also made possible the development of present-day cerebral and vascular operative techniques.

Dr. Isler, our paediatric neurologist, has concerned himself actively with the problem of acute hemiplegias in childhood for many years. This monograph reflects his wide personal experience on the basis of 116 cases, most of whom have been followed up for many years. He shows that precise clinical neurological examination is essential, but that neuroradiological methods must also be used, since they explain the aetiology in the vast majority of cases. He indicates, quite correctly, that neuroradiological methods of examination are indispensable for the elaboration of the clinical findings and that only by these methods is it possible to demonstrate the dynamic course of such processes as cerebral oedema, the appearance of mycotic and dissecting aneurysms, spontaneous thrombolysis and progressive thrombosis.

As the author so convincingly demonstrates, the hemiplegia is only one of the symptoms of an organic disease which usually affects the total personality of the child. Behind the relative uniformity of the acute hemisyndrome, there is a surprisingly wide aetiological variety (on the basis of the case histories, 24 different causes are discussed in this monograph), as well as a surprisingly dynamic pattern of pathogenic mechanisms. Much of this information is vital to prognosis and treatment.

The monograph reads well and is superbly documented. Dr. Isler has provided, thanks to his large case material and his fluent knowledge of the relevant world literature, an authoritative differential diagnosis of hemiplegia in childhood that will stand the test of time.

Zurich, January 1969

Prof. Andrea Prader
Prof. Hugo Krayenbühl

iii

Introduction

The stimulus for this monograph was the description of 'acute infantile hemiplegia of obscure origin' introduced by F. R. Ford in his standard work 'Diseases of the Nervous System in Infancy, Childhood, and Adolescence'. As a result of modern neuroradiological methods of investigation, the pathogenesis of a proportion of these cases can now be explained. In particular, cerebral angiography, while demonstrating many expected and many disappointing findings, sometimes provides surprising results. Serial angiography may give significant insight into a dynamic pattern. On the other hand, many problems remain unanswered, particularly concerning the aetiology. New knowledge is bound to accrue from modern developments in cerebral vascular surgery, e.g. biopsy in vessel replacement.

The aim of any treatment is elimination of the cause. Unfortunately, there are no promising signs in this particular field, so it is all the more important to attempt to restrict brain damage as much as possible by the application of significant symptomatic treatment. This is the main reason for presenting this detailed review of the numerous causes of acute hemiplegias and hemisyndromes in childhood.

Acute hemiplegia is by no means rare in childhood. Unfortunately, it usually presents as an illness with a dramatic onset, a severe course and permanent physical and mental deficits. The purpose of this work is to provide as broad as possible an insight into the pathogenic aspects and to study the late effects, as well as to explore ways and means of preventing brain damage or of keeping it to a minimum.

The study comprises 116 cases: 98 from the Department of Paediatrics, University of Zurich; 15 from the Department of Neurosurgery, University of Zurich; and 3 from elsewhere. All except 7 cases were observed and the vast majority followed up personally by the author.

The classification into 24 categories was made on the basis of the angiographic or clinical findings. Eighty-two cases are described in detail, and the clinical courses of the remaining 34 are shown in the Table of Cases (see page 193). The criteria for inclusion in the series rested upon a reasonably broad basis, following the guide lines of Mac Keith at the Clevedon Symposium (1962): hemiplegia (hemiparesis) persisting for longer than one week, of sudden onset, without obvious cause, in children or infants over the age of one month who had previously appeared to be neurologically healthy. The Clevedon study group also came to the conclusion that an age limit is not justifiable. The author has included a number of patients in whom the acute hemisyndrome rapidly regressed. The period of transition from transient to permanent and severe deficits due to a similar pathogenic mechanism is often very brief.

Speculation on the pathogenesis began in the middle of the 19th century. According to Freud (1897), cerebral affections in children were generally considered to be the result of an intra-uterine encephalitis or agenesis. Cotard (1868), a pupil of Charcot, attributed the morbid anatomical findings in infantile cerebral hemiplegia to disturbances of the cerebral blood vessels. In the same year, Benedikt referred to the rôle of acute infectious diseases in the causation of cerebral palsy. Kundrat (1882), in a pathological study, differentiated between congenital porencephalic changes and those occurring postnatally; he sought to attribute the cause to a circulatory disturbance. Von Strümpell (1885) postulated that poliomyelitis could produce a true polioencephalitis; this view, which was accepted for a long time, was later proved to be incorrect. Jendrassik and Marie (1885) recorded a study of two cases of acute hemiplegia in children with histologically proven changes in the blood vessels attributable to an infectious disease. Freud (1897), in a detailed monograph, sought to classify all forms of infantile cerebral palsy, congenital and acquired. In one half of the cases of acquired cerebral palsy the causes were infectious diseases, vascular disturbances, trauma and fright (epilepsy!); the causes in the other cases remained unknown. Freud cited a number of cases of vascular changes demonstrated at autopsy, such as middle cerebral occlusion through embolism or thrombosis or cerebral haemorrhage (Gowers 1888, Lovett 1888, Osler 1889). Since Freud's monograph, some case reports but very few extensive studies have been published. Taylor (1905), on the basis of a review of 42 cases of spontaneous infantile hemiplegia in which previous infectious diseases were ruled out, stressed the importance of vascular lesions in the aetiology.

Ford and Schaffer (1927), in one of the most valuable papers, reported 16 cases (some observed personally and the others extracted from the literature) in which spontaneous and para-infectious vascular occlusions were verified at autopsy. Wyllie (1948), in his presidential address to The Royal Society of Medicine, quoted cases of spontaneous acute hemiplegia in children, in whom 'acute toxic encephalopathy' was demonstrated at autopsy. Grinker and Stone (1928) described the morbid anatomical appearances of this disease entity, which is characterised by oedema, congestion and ganglion cell necrosis, progressing to foci of softening and endothelial proliferation of the smaller vessels without inflammatory changes. Another morbid anatomical form, known as 'haemorrhagic encephalitis' (Wernicke 1881, von Strümpell 1890, Alpers 1928, Baker 1935, Hurst 1941), is characterised by perivascular necrosis and haemorrhage. Only occasionally is this picture seen, e.g. after scarlet fever, in acute hemiplegias of childhood. Another histologically typical form is 'perivenous encephalomyelitis' with demyelination and glial proliferation around smaller veins of the white matter. This finding is particularly common in measles and post-vaccinal encephalitis. Its allergic nature has been postulated by Glanzmann (1927), van Bogaert (1932) and Pette (1942).

Zimmerman (1938) investigated a group of children who had died from infectious diseases accompanied by epileptic convulsions, and in whom a clinical diagnosis of encephalitis was made. This finding was not confirmed: indeed, the appearance of elective ischaemic ganglion cell necrosis corresponded closely to the description of Spielmeyer (1927) and Scholz (1951) of post-convulsive cerebral damage.

The introduction of cerebral angiography into clinical practice by Moniz (1927), represented a great advance, but many years elapsed before it made any inroads into paediatric practice. Nowadays angiography is an indispensible aid in the elucidation of many cases of 'acute infantile hemiplegia of obscure origin'.

PART I

Vascular Malformations

CHAPTER 1

Arteriovenous Malformations

These angiomas are now accepted to be *congenital malformations* (Padget 1956, Hamby 1958). They are not to be confused with arteriovenous fistulae which are caused by traumatic rupture of a large artery into a vein (*e.g.* internal carotid artery into the cavernous sinus). The angioma consists of a tangle of blood vessels with feeding and draining vessels which are usually enlarged and tortuous; the normal capillary bed is missing. As a result of the numerous shunts, the veins contain oxygenated blood. The blood supply to the surrounding cerebral tissues may be affected by the enormously accelerated circulation. Potter (1955) aptly named these arteriovenous aneurysms 'parasites of the circulation'. If the shunt volume is very large, the heart may be affected (dilatation, acute failure).

The site of predilection is in the territory of the middle cerebral artery, although branches of the anterior or posterior cerebral arteries may sometimes be involved; occasionally they represent the only source of supply. More rarely, angiomas occur in the region of the cerebellum. In nine of the ten cases in this series the angioma was supratentorial and in only one (CASE 6) was it infratentorial. Usually, the angioma presents a broad-faced subpial bed with a pyramid of tissue projecting into the cerebral parenchyma for a varying distance. In most of the cases in this series, however, it was situated deep within the substance of the brain.

In spite of the congenital nature of the lesion, it usually presents clinically in the second or third decade of life. Cases in infants are very rare indeed (Harper and Vyse 1953, Clément *et al.* 1954, Schultz and Huston 1956, Ford 1966). The age distribution of the patients in this series was 6-14 years.

According to the literature, arteriovenous malformations occur twice as frequently in males as in females. The 10 cases in this series were made up of 6 boys and 4 girls.

The clinical picture is either that of an intracranial haemorrhage (intracerebral or subarachnoid) or epileptic attacks. Most cases described in the literature have presented with focal epilepsy. According to Ford (1966), haemorrhage from an angioma is uncommon. However, the author's experience indicates the contrary in childhood, since 9 of the 10 cases presented with symptoms of apoplectiform cerebral or subarachnoid haemorrhage, in one case concurrently with epileptic seizures (CASE 1). Only one child (CASE 9), who has been followed up for 10 years, has so far escaped intracranial haemorrhage and continues to experience only focal epileptic attacks. The combination of epilepsy and recurrent subarachnoid or cerebral haemorrhage is almost always caused by an arteriovenous aneurysm (Olivecrona 1950).

The author's case material confirms the general experience that the clinical symptoms of haemorrhage and epilepsy bear no relation to the size of the angioma or whether it is situated on the surface or in the depths of the brain. However, the

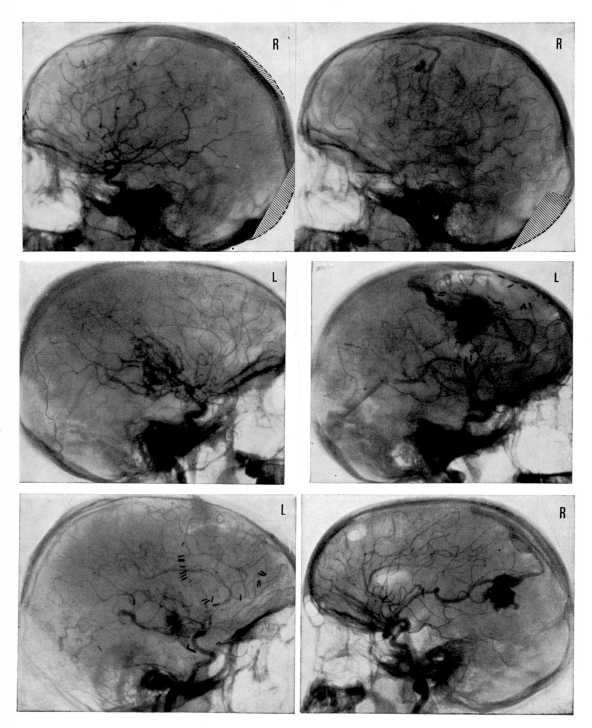

4

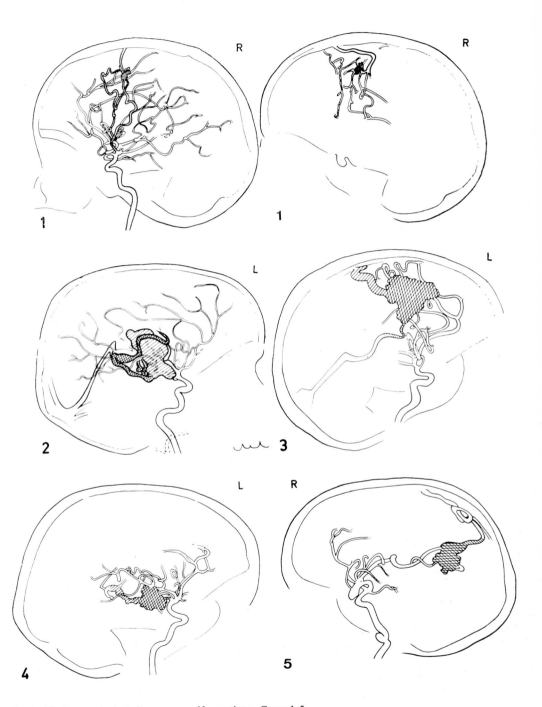

Fig. 1a (*facing page*). Arteriovenous malformations. Cases 1-5.
Fig. 1b (*above*). Line drawings of Fig. 1a.

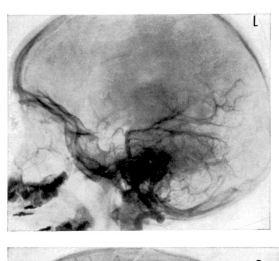
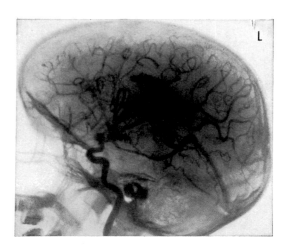
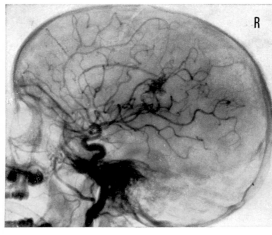
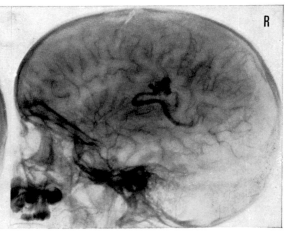
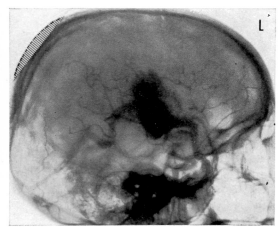
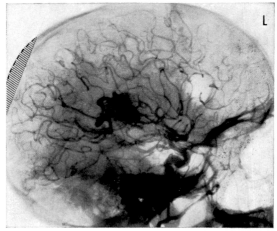

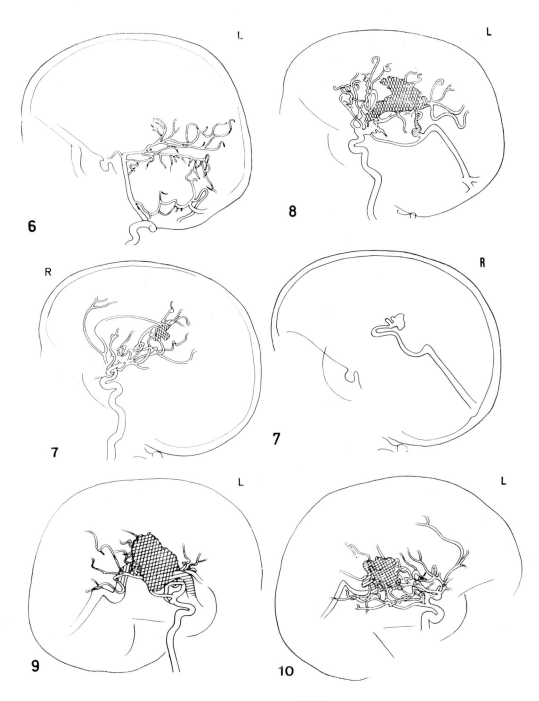

Fig. 1*a* (*facing page*). Arteriovenous malformations. Cases 6-10.
Fig. 1*b* (*above*). Line drawing of Fig. 1*a*.

topographic situation markedly affects the frequency of seizures: angiomas situated centrally or in the parietal region trigger off far more epileptic attacks than angiomas in other locations (Tönnis 1957). Focal seizures or sensory signs may arise from areas of hypoxic tissue distant from the angioma, as a result of an altered circulation caused by a suction effect of the arteriovenous aneurysm on the normal cerebral arteries (Krayenbühl and Yasargil 1958).

The diagnosis can be proved only by angiography. Murmurs over the skull synchronous with the pulse are considered unreliable: they were absent in at least a quarter of the cases described in the literature. It should be pointed out that similar murmurs occasionally occur in children with hydrocephalus or space-occupying intracranial processes, and sometimes also occur in perfectly normal children. It should also be noted that arteriovenous aneurysms draining into the deep mid-line veins (e.g. the vein of Galen) may produce an internal hydrocephalus, due to stenosis of the sylvian aqueduct caused by giant dilatation of these veins (Russell and Nevin 1940, Litvak et al. 1960, Poppen and Avman 1960, Shealy and LeMay 1964). Rarely, paralysis of vertical gaze (Parinaud's syndrome) may be encountered, as in CASE 2 in this series, presumably through pressure or circulatory disturbances affecting the anterior quadrigeminal bodies (excess drainage through the vein of Galen). According to Krayenbühl and Yasargil (1958), cranial nerve lesions are found virtually only with infratentorial angiomas.

No causal relationship appears to have been proved between the rupture of the aneurysm and physical exertion. Of the 9 cases who presented with intracranial haemorrhage, 2 gave a history of the onset occurring during sleep, 3 after waking up, 3 during the day unassociated with any specific effort, and 1 two hours after a very minor head injury.

Arteriovenous aneurysms show a tendency to result in recurrent haemorrhage, in which the risk of irreversible severe neurological deficit or even fatal massive haemorrhage is considerable. Unfortunately, many types of arteriovenous angioma are inoperable, either because of their extent or depth, or because of their situation in functionally vital parts of the brain. In such cases it is sometimes possible to carry out palliative operations (elimination of feeding vessels). Under ideal conditions, the vascular malformation can be radically resected. More hazardous operative measures are justifiable in the presence of severe neurological deficits resulting from cerebral haemorrhage. Other therapeutic measures such as X-irradiation are no longer used.

The cases reported here present many examples of the problems of operative treatment. In two (CASES 1 and 6) it was possible to resect radically the aneurysms responsible for the intracranial haemorrhage, with highly satisfactory results. In CASE 3, severe recurrent haemorrhage occurred 4½ years after partial excision, followed by an irreversible hemiplegia, and radical operation was therefore undertaken. CASES 2 and 4 had inoperable angiomas and suffered recurrent haemorrhages with severe brain damage; the supplying vessels were therefore ligated intracranially—with success. In CASE 8, the internal carotid artery was ligated following irreversible hemiplegia, and observation over 16 years revealed no evidence of recurrent haemorrhage. In CASE 7, extirpation of a small paraventricular vascular mass proved extremely difficult and the child developed an irreversible hemiplegia during the operation. CASE 10 presented with an apoplectiform hemiplegic cerebral haemorrhage from an inoperable angioma, and survived two subsequent attacks of subarachnoid haemorrhage without deepening the residual paralysis. CASE 5 died two days after a massive intracerebral haemorrhage from a circumscribed subpial angioma. CASE 9 was a patient who had suffered for over 10 years exclusively from focal epileptic attacks, no haemorrhage having occurred from the large, deep-seated angioma.

In 7 of these 10 cases the presenting clinical feature of the arteriovenous malformation was apoplectiform cerebral haemorrhage with hemiplegia and, in one child, a fatal outcome two days after the attack. Three cases presented with recurrent subarachnoid haemorrhage, one with ventricular bleeding, and only one case presented with focal epileptic attacks without bleeding. In only one child (CASE 1) was the intracranial haemorrhage accompanied by tonic and clonic convulsions, and then on the side opposite to the hemiplegia. Three children developed symptomatic epilepsy after a long interval following their operative treatment. The clinical course in the 10 cases in this series is shown in the Table of Cases (page 195).

Although arteriovenous malformations are an infrequent cause of acute hemiplegia, in about half the cases they lead to severe and irreversible deficits.

CASE 1

The patient, a boy aged 12 years and 8 months, suffered a sudden rupture of a previously asymptomatic subpial arteriovenous aneurysm in the central area of the right hemisphere. He described the event subjectively as 'blood flowing into the head' and then lapsed immediately into unconsciousness. There was faulty localisation because of the symptoms of status epilepticus with attacks localised strictly on the same side as the haemorrhage. This particular presentation was explained by assuming that generalised epileptic attacks were in fact occurring, but that the affected hemisphere was obstructed by the massive haemorrhage, resulting in the complete flaccid hemiplegia and the absence of response to the epileptic discharges. The typical signs of massive subarachnoid haemorrhage (ventricular rupture) with severe neck rigidity became noticeable only after the initial deep unconsciousness had regressed.

The abnormal vascular mass was demonstrated by right carotid angiography (Figs. 1 and 2); it was also found to receive a blood supply from the left carotid artery through the anterior communicating artery. The massive intracerebral haemorrhage with ventricular rupture could be explained as arising from the subpial vascular mass itself, probably from a supplying or draining intracerebral artery.

The widespread recovery within a few months of operation, with persistence of only a light spastic hemiparesis of the distal part of the upper limb and no significant organic psychosyndrome, is remarkable. Despite early EEG evidence of focal epileptic activity in the cerebral cortex, with prophylactic medical treatment it was $2\frac{1}{2}$ years before the first isolated focal attacks — one of which resulted in a dreamy state — were observed. Following alteration of the medication the patient has been symptom-free for eight months. He is at present successfully completing his fourth year as an apprentice machine fitter.

9

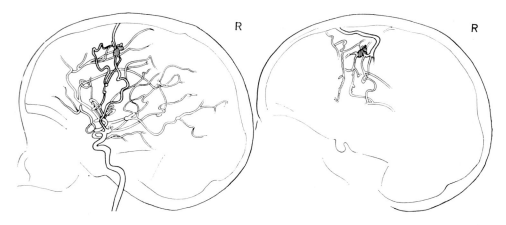

Fig. 2. Arteriovenous malformation of the anterior opercular artery. Line drawings (Case 1).

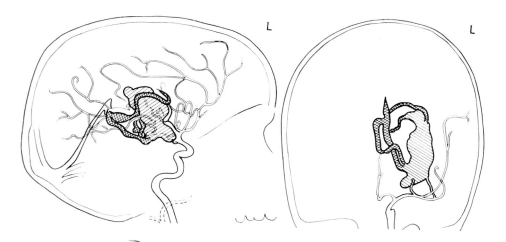

Fig. 3. Arteriovenous malformation of a middle cerebral artery with major drainage into the internal cerebral vein. Line drawings (Case 2).

CASE 2

A large arteriovenous malformation in the depths of the left hemisphere (Figs. 1 and 3) presented with an apoplectiform onset in a 13-year-old girl. The almost total sensory and motor hemiplegia regressed considerably over the course of weeks, but a residual spastic hemiparesis, with severe deficit of fine hand movements and a definite organic psychosyndrome, remained. Parinaud's syndrome, which was present initially, could be attributed to pressure on the anterior quadrigeminal bodies by an enlarged vein of Galen. Eight and a half months after the first attack, the patient suffered a second haemorrhage, again apoplectiform in nature and without epileptic features. On this occasion a severe sensory and motor hemiparesis persisted, as well

10

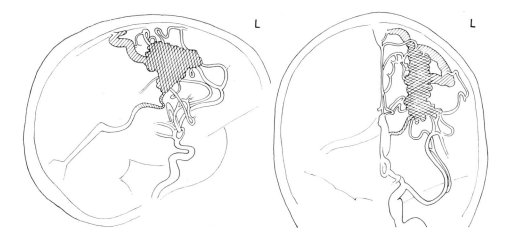

Fig. 4. Arteriovenous malformation involving the pericallosal, callosal marginal and anterior opercular arteries. Line drawings (Case 3).

as a right complete homonymous hemianopia, a partial motor aphasia and a marked organic psychosyndrome.

The clinical course was arrested after ligation of some of the feeding arteries of the malformation. Despite the presence in the EEG of focal and generalised epilepsy potentials, no attacks have occurred during a follow-up of two years—presumably as a result of the permanent anticonvulsant treatment.

CASE 3

A 12-year-old boy who was previously healthy had an attack of cerebral and subarachnoid haemorrhage from an arteriovenous aneurysm (Figs. 1 and 4). An initial paralysis of the right arm and a speech disturbance improved in the course of about 10 days. Carotid angiography revealed the extent of the malformation which was subtotally removed $6\frac{1}{2}$ weeks after the haemorrhage. The patient made a remarkably rapid recovery and was discharged without neurological deficit.

Four and a half years later he experienced a more massive haemorrhage, with more complete paralysis of the right arm. Repeat angiography revealed a further large arteriovenous aneurysm which was totally resected. Post-operatively there was no change in the neurological deficit, but severe mental disturbances now supervened. One and a half years later a deterioration in the neurological picture occurred, when the patient began to experience epileptiform seizures. Sometimes these attacks were focal, sometimes generalised, and they could not be satisfactorily suppressed by medical treatment. Thirteen years after the first attack a very marked organic psychosyndrome was present, as well as severe spastic paralysis of the right arm and a partial motor aphasia. Despite these disabilities, the patient continues to work as a labourer.

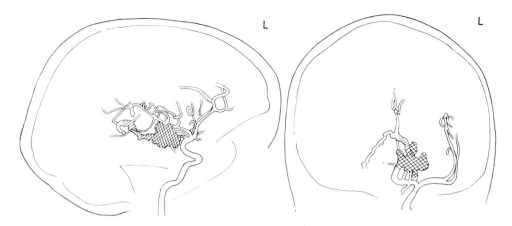

Fig. 5. Arteriovenous malformation of a posterior communicating artery. Line drawings (Case 4).

CASE 4

This 10-year-old boy suffered recurrent attacks of subarachnoid haemorrhage, and, following a cerebral haemorrhage, was unconscious for 10 days; he was left with a severe hemiplegia. The cause was shown angiographically to be an arteriovenous aneurysm of the left posterior communicating artery (Figs. 1 and 5). Operative ligation of two arteries 8 months later failed to exclude the aneurysm. A follow-up angiogram 6 months later revealed that it was being supplied by branches of the anterior cerebral artery. The moderate hemiparesis was unaffected by the operation.

CASE 5

The patient, a boy aged 9 years and 8 months, suffered an apoplectiform insult from a ruptured arteriovenous aneurysm (Figs. 1 and 6), with haemorrhage into the white matter, but without penetration into the subarachnoid space or the ventricular system. Clinical manifestations of the attack included sudden severe headache, vomiting, collapse and progressive drowsiness. In the course of 24 hours a progressive flaccid right hemiplegia and left third nerve palsy developed. Death followed after an illness of $1\frac{1}{2}$ days duration.

During the diagnostic investigations the EEG was misleading in that it produced evidence of a disturbance in the contralateral hemisphere (*viz.* widespread epileptogenic foci), as well as demonstrating severe disturbances with depression in the affected side. This picture prompted thoughts of a toxic or inflammatory encephalopathy rather than an intracerebral haemorrhage. Valuable hours were lost performing an air study, which, in retrospect, was contra-indicated and which undoubtedly played a decisive part in the fatal outcome.

A significant feature was the fact that, despite the marked epileptic cerebral activity demonstrated on the EEG, no clinical attacks occurred.

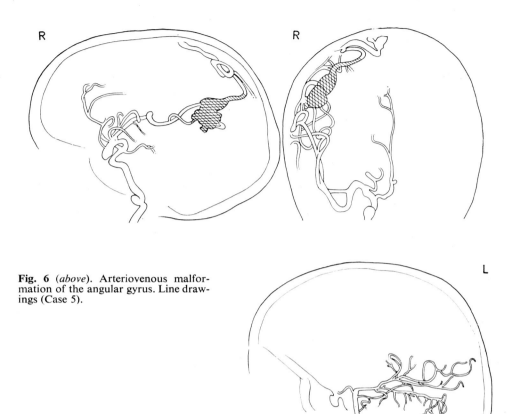

Fig. 6 (*above*). Arteriovenous malformation of the angular gyrus. Line drawings (Case 5).

Fig. 7 (*right*). Arteriovenous malformation of a posterior inferior cerebellar artery. Line drawing (Case 6).

CASE 6

The patient, a 6-year-old boy, suffered his first attack of subarachnoid haemorrhage 2 hours after a minor head injury, with recurrences at intervals of 1 and 3 weeks. The cause was demonstrated on vertebral angiography to be an arteriovenous aneurysm of the left posterior inferior cerebellar artery (Figs. 1 and 7), which was surgically removed 7 weeks after the first haemorrhage; the nature of the lesion was confirmed by histological examination. As a result of the third, clinically most severe haemorrhage, the patient developed signs of raised intracranial pressure. The only localising sign clinically was an inconstant nystagmus. Post-operative recovery was slow but eventually, after many weeks, the patient's condition was satisfactory. However, he was left with an ataxic gait, weakness in the legs (marked muscular hypotonia) and a nystagmus.

The fate of this child was decided by an iatrogenic dissecting aneurysm which is discussed on page 67.

CASE 7

The patient, an 8½-year-old girl in good health, experienced without warning a ventricular haemorrhage due to an arteriovenous aneurysm (Figs. 1 and 8); there was no neurological deficit and the patient made a comparatively rapid recovery. Operative removal of the vascular mass was extremely difficult, and the patient was left with a severe spastic hemiplegia and a marked organic psychosyndrome. EEG heralded the development of severe symptomatic epilepsy. It was possible by means of anticonvulsant treatment to suppress clinical attacks for 3 years. Their onset was associated with severe intellectual deterioration, and within 4 years the patient was a complete invalid.

CASE 8

The patient, a 10-year-old girl, experienced without warning an apoplectiform attack with complete motor and sensory hemiplegia and global aphasia, due to haemorrhage from an extensive arteriovenous aneurysm in the left cerebral hemisphere (Figs. 1 and 9). The internal carotid artery was ligated on the 6th day. After initial satisfactory progress, the patient's condition remained stationary despite 15 months of intensive physiotherapeutic rehabilitation. Sixteen years later a severe spastic hemiplegia including a functionally useless upper extremity remains, with a marked disturbance of gait, severe disturbances of superficial and deep sensibility, an obvious difficulty in finding words, and a moderate intellectual deterioration. She has been well integrated socially, and is able to live a fairly independent life as an unskilled worker. A noteworthy feature is the absence of epileptic seizures for over 15 years.

CASE 9

Focal epileptic attacks occurred in this girl from the age of 14½ years, due to a massive arteriovenous aneurysm in the left insular region (Figs. 1 and 10). No neurological deficit remained. Freedom from attacks followed commencement of anticonvulsant therapy (length of case history: 10 years).

The noteworthy feature in this case is the absence so far of any haemorrhage.

CASE 10

An arteriovenous aneurysm in the left thalamus (Figs. 1 and 11) was silent until the patient was 13 years old, when he experienced a right hemiplegia of sudden onset without subarachnoid haemorrhage. The hemiplegia was of the classical type, with a centrifugal distribution and involving the arm most severely. Apart from the motor deficit, slight disturbances of superficial sensibility over the affected side of the body were also present. The hemiplegia regressed incompletely in the course of months.

Two years later the patient experienced an attack of subarachnoid haemorrhage, which caused slight deepening of the hemiparesis; this was followed after a further 6 weeks by a second attack. His intellectual ability was not significantly affected. The hemiparesis has remained, but no epileptic seizures have occurred (length of case history: 8 years).

For more detailed reports of CASES *1-10 see pages 207-215*

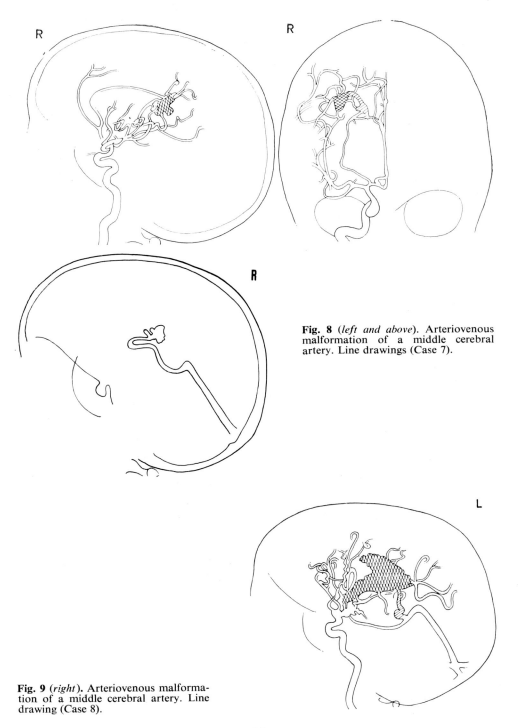

Fig. 8 (*left and above*). Arteriovenous malformation of a middle cerebral artery. Line drawings (Case 7).

Fig. 9 (*right*). Arteriovenous malformation of a middle cerebral artery. Line drawing (Case 8).

15

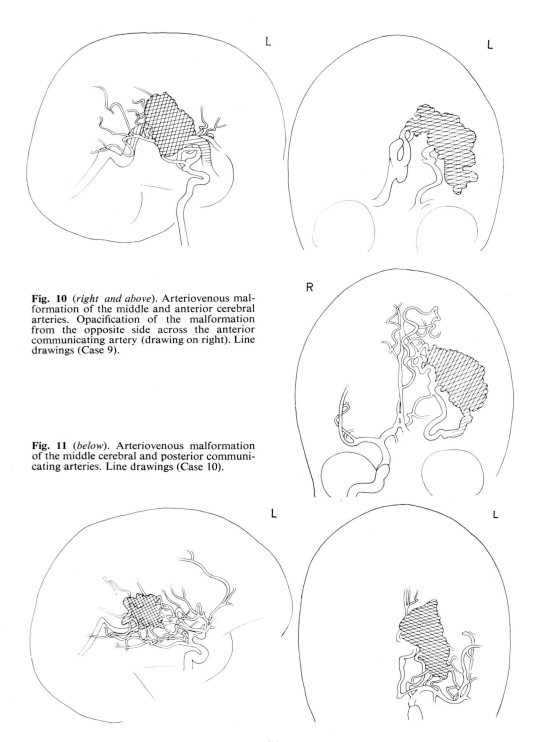

Fig. 10 (*right and above*). Arteriovenous malformation of the middle and anterior cerebral arteries. Opacification of the malformation from the opposite side across the anterior communicating artery (drawing on right). Line drawings (Case 9).

Fig. 11 (*below*). Arteriovenous malformation of the middle cerebral and posterior communicating arteries. Line drawings (Case 10).

CHAPTER 2

Saccular Arterial Aneurysm

— Only congenital aneurysms are considered under this heading, *i.e.* the types arising from a defect in the tunica media. For the acquired types of saccular arterial aneurysms see page 39. In comparison with arteriovenous malformations, saccular arterial aneurysms are clinically far less frequently seen in children. Out of a series of 1125 verified cases, McDonald and Korb (1939) found only 2.5 per cent of the subjects to be under the age of 15 years, and Krayenbühl and Yasargil (1958) found only 2.25 per cent out of 276 cases. The literature contains only a few reports of ruptured saccular aneurysms in neonates or infants (Newcomb and Munns 1949, Krayenbühl and Yasargil 1958, Jane 1961, Jones and Shearburn 1961). The age of predilection is the third to fifth decades, thus involving an older category of patients compared with arteriovenous aneurysms. Males and females are equally often affected.

— The sites of predilection of aneurysm formation are at the sites of branching on the circle of Willis, most commonly the anterior communicating artery, then the origin of the middle cerebral artery or its sylvian branches. Other sites are far more rarely involved.

— Clinically, saccular aneurysms usually present as apoplectiform attacks of subarachnoid haemorrhage with the well-known symptoms of sudden severe headache, combined with vomiting, meningism and loss of consciousness. When there is profound loss of consciousness, the neck stiffness is absent. The cerebrospinal fluid (CSF), which is under increased pressure, is usually uniformly blood-stained, and clears after a distinct xanthochromic phase. A fever of varying severity is usually observed, which is caused by resorption of blood or stimulation of the central temperature regulation centres.

A ruptured saccular aneurysm may occasionally present the picture of a cerebral haemorrhage, and produce an acute hemiplegia when the jet of arterial blood ploughs through the cerebral tissues. Misleading lateralising signs may be encountered if the jet of blood penetrates the contralateral hemisphere. Matson (1965) reported 13 cases of arterial aneurysms in children, 5 of which were accompanied by intracerebral haematoma; only 1 showed a subarachnoid haemorrhage.

Recurrent haemorrhages, which are often fatal, are unfortunately very common.

Angiography is essential for diagnosis. However, a negative result in cases of classical subarachnoid haemorrhage by no means excludes the presence of a saccular aneurysm. It may go undetected through its small size or through spontaneous thrombosis or the presence of vascular spasm in the vicinity, or it may lie in a vascular territory not examined (*e.g.* the vertebro-basilar system). Hofer (1966) quoted 250 cases of subarachnoid haemorrhage with negative angiographic findings; Laitinen (1964, quoted by Matson 1965) could demonstrate saccular aneurysms in only 9 of 35 children with leptomeningeal haemorrhage; and McKissock and Paine (1959) reported an incidence of 50 per cent of unexplained cases in a series of 781 patients.

Occasionally, a ruptured aneurysm may burst entirely into the brain substance, without subarachnoid haemorrhage, *e.g.* in CASE 11 in this series. In these circumstances, angiography is necessary to explain the complex clinical picture.

The less common paretic or paralytic type of aneurysm should be mentioned, which may present with or without subarachnoid haemorrhage. Here the aneurysm sac, through an increase in size or through haemorrhage, exerts pressure upon adjacent cranial nerves. Typical results of this are a unilateral third nerve palsy (aneurysm situated on the posterior communicating artery) or syndromes of ocular muscle paralysis and trigeminal damage (aneurysm situated on the internal carotid artery in the cavernous sinus).

Of the author's two cases, one (CASE 12) showed a typical course. A few weeks after a recurrent attack of subarachnoid haemorrhage in response to a minor head injury, a spontaneous apoplectiform recurrent haemorrhage occurred, which left the patient hemiplegic. In another patient (CASE 11), a complex picture of incomplete symptoms indicated a recurrent subarachnoid haemorrhage, at times associated with unusual hemichoreatic hyperkinesia. It is remarkable that these extrapyramidal 'attacks' arose from homolateral haemorrhage into the temporal lobe and the insular part of the hemisphere. In both patients carotid angiography demonstrated the aneurysm (Figs. 12 and 13).

Surgical treatment plays an important part in cases of haemorrhage because of the high mortality rate. In the case material of the Department of Neurosurgery, University of Zurich, over 40 per cent of all cases die, and more than half of these are never operated upon. Ideally the neck of the saccular aneurysm should be directly ligated, but it is also possible to strengthen the weak wall of the aneurysm with special compounds or—if it is in the right place—by ligation of the internal carotid artery. According to Matson (1965) the surgical results of direct attack on aneurysms are better in children than in adults. Matson considers the chance of an early recurrent haemorrhage in children to be very small, and recommends that the operation should be delayed until the acute phase has passed. Nevertheless, both cases in the author's series presented with recurrent haemorrhages within a few weeks. CASE 11 has experienced no recurrence for over 15 years after wrapping of the aneurysm sac with muscle fibres, and CASE 12 for over 18 years after ligation of the internal carotid artery. The course of both these patients may be studied in Table of Cases (see page 195).

The saccular arterial aneurysm is a rare cause of acute hemiplegia in childhood. Prompt diagnosis is necessary if the risk of fatal recurrent haemorrhage at any time is to be averted by operative treatment. The association of saccular aneurysms with stenosis of the aortic isthmus (coarctation, see page 62), with cystic kidney, with fibro-muscular hypoplasia (see page 47), as well as with aplasia of cerebral arteries (see page 104), is well known.

CASE 11

Diagnosis in this 15-year-old girl was very difficult. She presented with a history of several attacks (all occurring within a few weeks and all of sudden onset) of head-

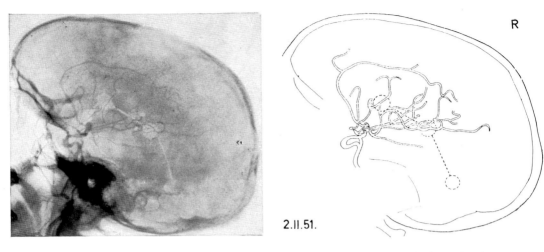

Fig. 12. Saccular aneurysm of a middle cerebral artery. Spastic cerebral arteries, in particular the parietal opercular artery (Case 11).

ache, vomiting and loss of consciousness, accompanied by a marked right-sided extrapyramidal hemisyndrome.

EEG and ventriculography showed the presence of a right temporal lobe lesion, and craniotomy revealed considerable oedema of the temporal lobe. It was the carotid angiogram that demonstrated the cause, namely a saccular aneurysm of the middle cerebral artery (Fig. 12). A misleading feature was the association of homolateral extrapyramidal signs with this aneurysmal haemorrhage into the right temporal lobe.

As a result of permanent damage to the hemisphere, the patient developed a very active temporal lobe epilepsy with typical psychomotor attacks. After 15 years she has been left with a partial homonymous hemianopia and a moderate psycho-organic syndrome.

A significant feature of the case was the absence of neck stiffness, despite repeated haemorrhages from the aneurysm; presumably they were all directed into the temporal lobe and none penetrated into the subarachnoid space.

CASE 12

At the age of 12 years, this boy experienced two attacks of subarachnoid haemorrhage within 3 weeks of each other. Following the second attack, he remained in a coma for several days and was left with a flaccid right hemiplegia.

Angiography revealed a saccular aneurysm on the internal carotid artery (Fig. 13). All three carotid vessels were ligated in the neck one day after the second haemorrhage, and a gradual recovery occurred. With time, the total hemiplegia and aphasia regressed almost completely, and the patient became symptom free.

Follow-up examination $2\frac{1}{2}$ years later revealed a residual expressive facial palsy and difficulty with writing. Eighteen years later a slight disturbance of sensation is still present in the right hand, but motor and intellectual functions are unimpaired.

19

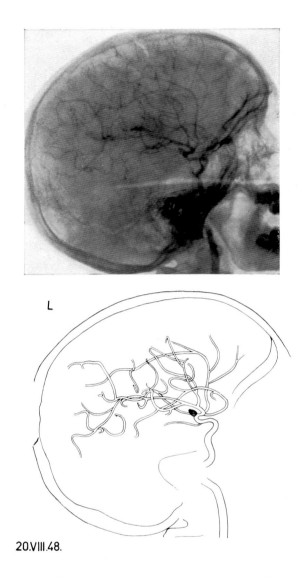

L

20.VIII.48.

Fig. 13. Saccular aneurysm of an internal carotid artery (Case 12).

For more detailed reports of CASES *11 and 12 see pages 217-218*

CHAPTER 3

Cerebral Venous Aneurysm

Intracranial angiomas involving only the veins are rarely encountered in child-hood. The transitional link between racemose arteriovenous aneurysms and cavernous angiomas is not well defined. Cerebral venous aneurysms are not visualised in the angiogram before the venous phase, in contrast to true arteriovenous malformations. According to Ford (1966) these lesions may present clinically during infancy or early childhood, while true arteriovenous malformations usually appear only in the second decade or later. The clinical picture is dominated by focal epileptic attacks, and apoplectiform hemiplegia is not uncommon. In a number of cases a naevus vasculosus is present on the face as well.

In the author's series there were 3 cases (CASES 13-15), with the clinical onset between 9 months and $2\frac{1}{2}$ years. All three children presented with apoplectiform hemiplegia, one without epilepsy, and two with convulsions immediately after the onset of the hemiplegia. All 3 patients had vascular naevi in the skin of the face on the same side as the intracerebral venous angioma. Thus they could be classified as examples of a *neurocutaneous syndrome* (*phakomatosis*).

Poser and Taveras (1957) as well as Thieffry *et al.* (1961) regarded cases with analogous cerebral venous anomalies and facial naevi as examples of the Sturge-Weber syndrome. Two features are essential for the diagnosis of this disease: a vascular naevus on one half of the face, particularly on the forehead and upper lid, and focal or generalised epileptic attacks. In a proportion of cases the 'tram-line' calcification in the affected cerebral hemisphere—often described as pathognomonic of the condition—is absent, even beyond 12 years (Poser and Taveras 1957, Peterman *et al.* 1958, Thieffry *et al.* 1961, Ford 1966). Calcification showing identical radiological appearances may be observed in other diseases such as gliomas, encephalitis or cerebral venous thrombosis (Lindgren 1939, Metzger 1950, Thieffry *et al.* 1961), so that it can no longer be regarded as pathognomonic of the Sturge-Weber syndrome. Other typical but non-essential features of this syndrome are oligophrenia and congenital glaucoma. None of the author's 3 cases has so far exhibited either glaucoma or intracerebral calcification. CASE 13 has shown a completely normal mental develop-ment over the past 5 years, CASE 15 a definite debility over $6\frac{1}{2}$ years. In CASE 14 the mental development was arrested at the age of onset of the disease (9 months) and remained static. Pneumoencephalography revealed a progressive unilateral hemi-spherical atrophy. This case merits particular attention since the intracerebral venous angioma went undetected in a routine 3-picture serial angiogram. The vascular mass opacified very late, about 10 seconds after the injection of contrast medium into the carotid artery, and long after maximum opacification of the cortical veins (Fig. 15).

In view of the considerable variability in the clinical picture of the Sturge-Weber syndrome, the 3 cases described here must be classified as atypical. The clinical course of these cases is given in the Table of Cases (see page 196).

The Sturge-Weber syndrome is closely related to the Bonnet-Dechaume-Blanc syndrome (identical with the Wyburn-Mason syndrome), in which unilateral arteriovenous aneurysms in the vicinity of the di- and mesencephalon are associated with similar lesions in the retina.

CASE 13

This boy exhibited a congenital vascular malformation, with a naevus vasculosus on the left forehead and an angiographically demonstrable extensive venous anomaly of the left hemisphere (Fig. 14a). Up to the age of 1 year the child developed normally. Following an acute upper respiratory infection, unilateral status epilepticus developed on the right side, and an initially flaccid hemiplegia gave way to a spastic one.

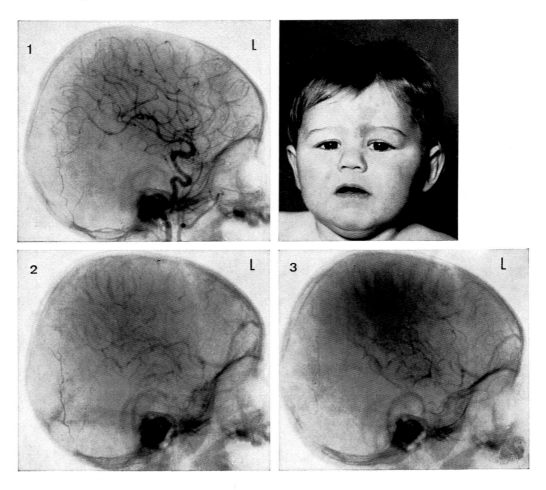

Fig. 14a. Neurocutaneous syndrome. Malformation of deep cerebral veins (phases 2 and 3 of the serial carotid angiogram) homolateral to a vascular naevus in the skin of the forehead slightly left of mid-line (Case 13).

22

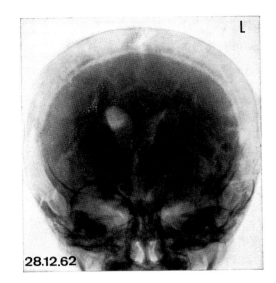

Fig. 14*b* (*right*). Slight displacement of the ventricular system to the right side (? oedema of the left hemisphere) (Case 13).

In the acute stage EEG revealed depressed activity over the affected hemisphere, but a subsequent tracing was normal. Pneumoencephalography 9 days after the attack revealed slight displacement of the ventricular system to the right side, with a somewhat widened right lateral ventricle and a deeply situated body of the left lateral ventricle. This finding was interpreted as evidence of unilateral cerebral oedema, for, if it was the result of displacement caused by the venous anomaly, the relative enlargement of the contralateral ventricle would be difficult to explain (Figs. 14*a* and *b*).

It is significant that, up to the present time, *i.e.* the age of 4½ years, the child has shown a normal mental development despite the cerebral damage. Regular anticonvulsant therapy has suppressed all epileptic attacks.

CASE 14

This boy was born with multiple cutaneous capillary haemangiomas on both sides of the upper half of the body, and at the age of 3-4 years presented with new deposits over the right arm and leg. Development was completely normal up to the 9th month of life, when suddenly and without warning the patient exhibited severe status epilepticus with right-sided convulsions, followed by a flaccid hemiplegia; the paralysis was permanent in the arm, but that in the face and right leg regressed. Following the convulsion, all psychomotor development virtually ceased, and the paralysed arm became underdeveloped.

The cause of the hemiconvulsions was demonstrated angiographically to be a venous malformation in the depths of the left cerebral hemisphere. The lesion was nearly missed on routine serial angiographic studies because it appeared very late, about 10 seconds after the contrast injection (Fig. 15). A second venous anomaly was demonstrated in the opposite hemisphere by right carotid angiography, but no functional significance could be attached to it.

23

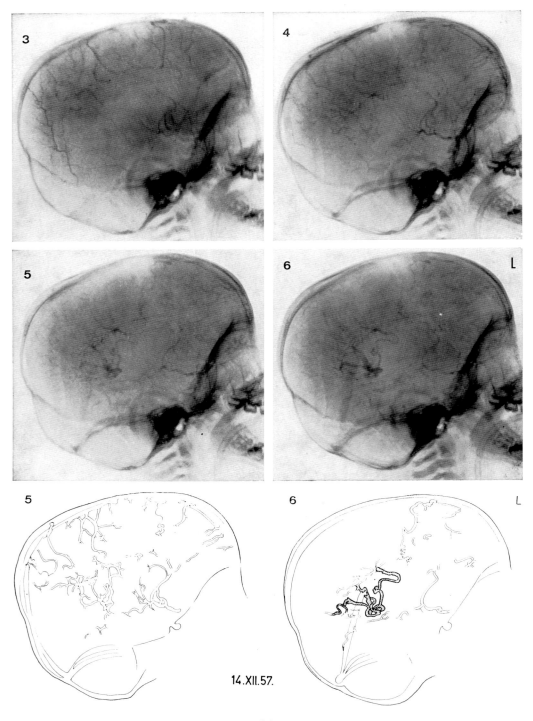

14.XII.57.

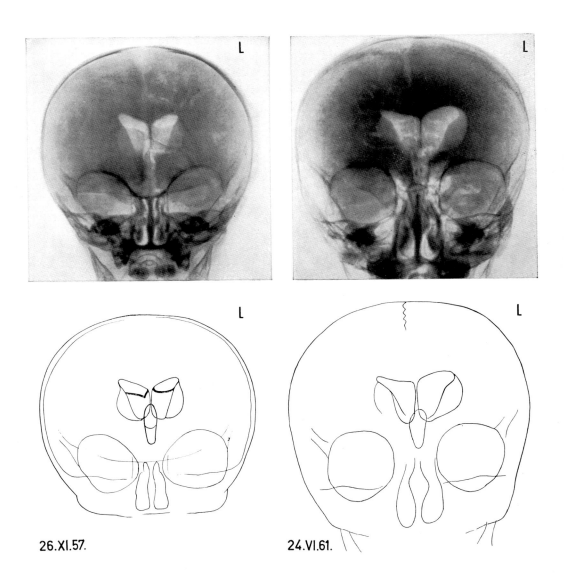

26.XI.57.   24.VI.61.

This page:

Fig. 16. Neurocutaneous syndrome. Progressive atrophy of the left cerebral hemisphere, on the same side as the cerebral venous malformation (Case 14).

Facing Page:

Fig. 15a (*top four pictures*). Neurocutaneous syndrome. Malformation of the deep cerebral veins, with multiple vascular naevi in the skin of the forehead and cheek. A venous angioma was demonstrated extremely late in the serial angiogram (about 10 seconds after contrast injection, phase 5) (Case 14).

Fig. 15b (*lower pictures*). Line drawings of Fig. 15a.

The question of whether the permanent flaccid paralysis of the right arm was a result of damage to the brain during the status epilepticus, or of a disturbance of normal cerebral perfusion due to the malformation, cannot be answered with any measure of proof. Epileptogenic cerebral damage was assumed to be the principal mechanism, since before the onset of the status epilepticus the child had shown a normal development, whereas afterwards development had completely ceased. Moreover, at this juncture the ventricular system showed symmetrical and scarcely dilated appearances.

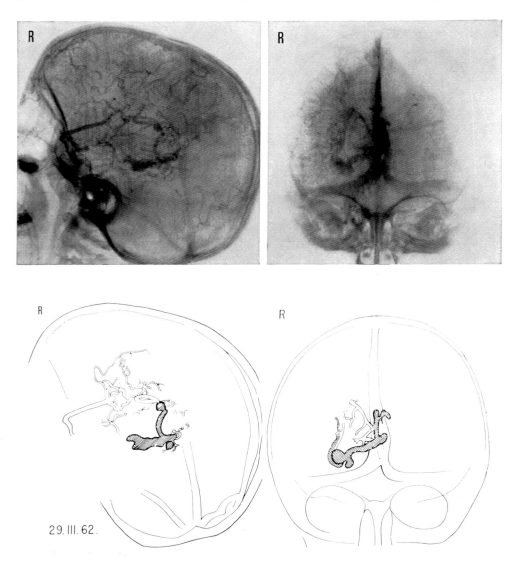

Fig. 17a. Neurocutaneous syndrome. Malformation of the deep cerebral veins on the same side as a vascular naevus in the skin of the forehead (Fig. 17b) (Case 15).

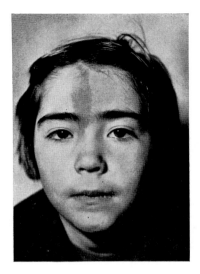 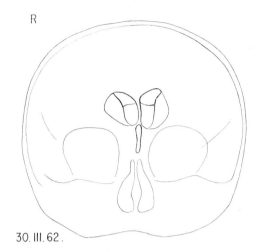

30. III. 62.

Fig. 17b. Vascular naevus in the skin of the forehead to the right of mid-line. Pneumo-encephalography (line drawing) revealed no evidence of hemispherical atrophy (Case 15).

An interesting feature is the central atrophy of the left hemisphere: in the pneumoencephalogram of 26 November 1957 the upper thalamic contour on the left side (*i.e.* the side of the extensive malformation) lay at a higher level than that on the right side, while $3\frac{1}{2}$ years later the left thalamus was shown to be markedly atrophic (Fig. 16). It is assumed that the absence of spasticity in the paralysed extremity could be explained by this finding.

This case illustrates that inadequate serial angiography may result in significant vascular lesions being missed.

CASE 15

This girl, who was born with a capillary haemangioma of the forehead, developed normally up to the age of 2 years and 4 months. She then became suddenly hemiplegic; it was not clear whether an epileptic attack preceded this. During the first 2 days of the acute hemisyndrome, the patient experienced focal seizures on the affected side. Angiography revealed the presence of a large venous malformation in the depths of the right hemisphere, on the same side as the cutaneous haemangioma (Fig. 17a). The hemiplegia disappeared almost completely within two weeks. One year later the patient developed a therapy-resistant epilepsy, which initially had a focal character (weakness of the left leg and turning of the head to the left side) but later became more generalised and was accompanied by a progressive organic psychosyndrome. The epileptic phenomena correlated well with the EEG findings. Eighteen months after the onset of the acute severe hemiplegia, the patient experienced a transient paralysis of the left leg without epileptic features.

For more detailed reports of CASES *13-15 see pages 218-221*

CHAPTER 4

Dissecting Aneurysm

Dissecting aneurysms may be congenital, due to a defect in the wall of the artery, or secondary to arterial diseases (medial degeneration, syphilis) or trauma. Both varieties are extremely rare causes of acute or chronic disturbances of cerebral function in childhood. Only 4 cases could be found in the literature. The first description was that of Norman and Urich (1957) of a fatal case in a 15-year-old boy with a congenital dissecting aneurysm of the middle cerebral artery. This lesion, together with a secondary thrombosis, had resulted in an acute hemiplegia with epileptic attacks at the age of 6 months. Wolman (1959) demonstrated a similar malformation in a hemispherectomy specimen, and reported that in this case the lesion had been present before birth. The same author described a dissecting aneurysm in the terminal segment of the internal carotid artery in a young boy who died of an occluding thrombosis. Wisoff and Rothballer (1961) reported similar findings in an 11-year-old negro girl. Scott *et al.* (1960) discussed, on the basis of an adult case and 15 cases from the literature, the pathogenesis of dissecting aneurysms. They regarded the particular structure of the cerebral arteries (absence of external elastic membrane, paucity of elastic fibres in the media, poorly developed adventitia), combined with sudden changes in the blood pressure, as the principal cause of intramural haematomas dissecting along natural tissue layers of the wall.

Two cases of histologically verified dissecting aneurysm were present in the author's series. One patient (CASE 30) had a history of trauma, and this case is described on page 66. In the other patient (CASE 16), homocystinuria was present. This inborn error of metabolism was first described by Field *et al.* and Gerritsen *et al.* in 1962. In some respects, the picture it presents resembles that of Marfan's syndrome. Gibson *et al.* (1964) reported highly interesting autopsy findings in a 7-year-old boy with homocystinuria: there were extensive changes in the blood vessels with evidence of intimal fibrosis, splitting of the elastic fibres and fusiform aneurysms in muscular arteries, and also of recent and old thrombi in the superior sagittal sinus and in the vicinity of an infarcted cerebral hemisphere. Similar changes were also seen in the arteries of another patient. The histological findings in CASE 16 closely resemble those described by Gibson *et al.* (1964).

The angiographic appearances of dissecting aneurysms are described on page 66.

CASE 16

This boy presented with a disease similar to Marfan's syndrome (arachnodactyly, dolichocephaly, ectopia of the lens). At the age of 7 years and 2 months he experienced a sudden progressive hemiparesis leading to complete hemiplegia. During the previous 9 months he had suffered from acute episodic attacks of headache, sometimes accompanied by vomiting and fever, and once by transient weakness of the legs. The specific

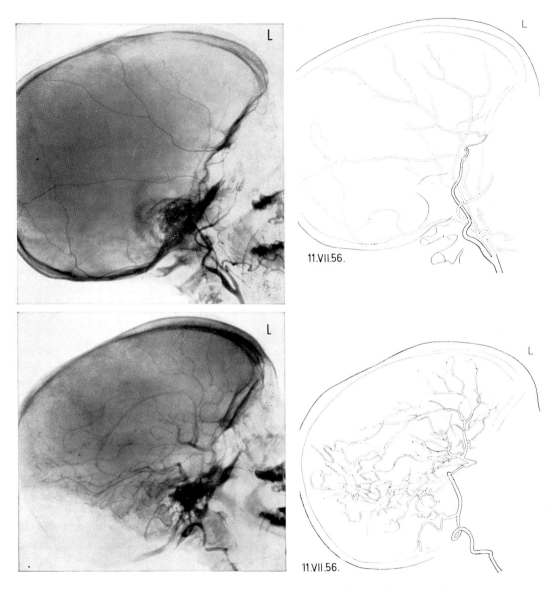

11.VII.56.

11.VII.56.

Fig. 18. Thrombotic dissecting aneurysm of the internal carotid artery in a case of homocystinuria. *Above:* carotid angiogram showing progressive narrowing of the internal carotid lumen, with interruption of the contrast column at the level of origin of the ophthalmic artery. *Below:* vertebral angiogram showing retrograde collateral opacification of the anterior and middle cerebral arteries through the posterior communicating artery (Case 16).

cause of these attacks, which were presumably due to cerebral disturbances, was not clear. The acute hemiplegia was undoubtedly the result of a thrombosis in the distal segment of the internal carotid artery, which was demonstrated angiographically (Fig. 18). This occlusion almost certainly developed secondary to the dissecting aneurysm which was demonstrated histologically (Fig. 19). The pathogenesis of the dissecting aneurysm itself was not clear, but it was unassociated with the effects of carotid angiography—the site of puncture of the common carotid artery and the intact wall of the internal carotid artery at its origin were demonstrated histologically (Fig. 19). The immediate cause of death must, however, be attributed to the left carotid and vertebral angiography. It must be assumed that the presence of the contrast medium in a cerebral circulation made precarious by venous thrombosis, precipitated the massive cerebral oedema and tonsillar herniation. It is not clear when the thrombosis of the cerebral veins and the left cavernous sinus occurred. The clinical picture of bilateral pyramidal disturbances suggests that the venous thrombosis was already present when the angiograms were made.

This child was originally diagnosed as a case of Marfan's syndrome. However, on the basis of the diagnosis of homocystinuria in his older sister in 1966, it must be assumed that he also was suffering from this disease.

For a more detailed report of CASE *16 see page 222*

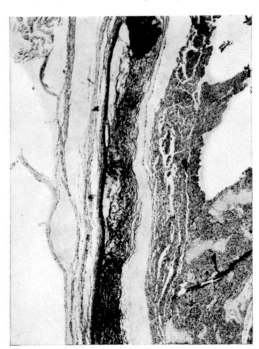 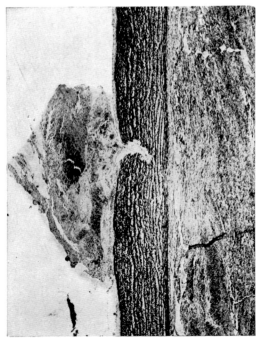

Fig. 19. Dissecting aneurysm in case of homocystinuria (Case 16). *Left:* longitudinal section of the left internal carotid artery showing mural dissection. *Right:* longitudinal section of the common carotid artery with the wall intact around the site of puncture. Magnification 25x. (Institute of Pathology, University of Zurich).

CHAPTER 5

Cerebral Microangioma

After dealing with intracranial arterial and venous malformations, the group of capillary anomalies remains to be discussed. Classification according to the nature of the blood vessel is arbitrary, since combinations and transitional forms are very frequent. For discussion of mycotic cerebral microaneurysms, see page 39.

Margolis *et al.* (1951) first classified small angiomatous malformations in a separate group. In recent years there have been a number of reports of cases of spontaneous cerebral haemorrhage, in which small angiomas have been demonstrated histologically or angiographically (Crawford and Russell 1956, Lazorthes 1956, Gerlach and Jensen 1961, Krayenbühl and Yasargil 1958, Bailey and Woodard 1959, McDonald 1959, Margolis *et al.* 1961, Jensen *et al.* 1963, Krayenbühl and Siegfried 1964, Krayenbühl and Siebenmann 1965, Walter 1965, and Walter and Schütte 1965).

Clinically, microangiomas in children and adolescents characteristically produce spontaneous apoplectiform cerebral haemorrhage or—with recurrent small haemorrhages, which are common—a picture of a space-occupying intracranial process. If the lesion is superficial, signs of subarachnoid haemorrhage may occur as well. Occasionally focal or generalised seizures are present.

The angioma may remain invisible on routine angiography. Occasionally, a circumscribed area of poor contrast opacification may be picked out by careful study. Rapid serial angiography producing many pictures of the arterial and capillary phases gives a better yield of positive results. Histological examination confirms the minuteness of the malformation relative to the patient's clinical pictures, and careful examination of the wall of the haematoma is necessary for its identification.

Four patients in the author's series showed characteristic findings. One (CASE 17) experienced a sudden attack of subarachnoid haemorrhage some weeks after an episode of headaches, followed by signs of raised intracranial pressure and discrete unilateral deficit. The angiographic appearances merely indicated the picture of an intracranial mass lesion. The cause of the cerebral haemorrhage was shown by histological examination to be a small arteriovenous aneurysm. CASE 20 presented with an apoplectiform cerebral haemorrhage associated with a period of headache. Only in CASE 18 was there angiographic evidence of the microangioma (Fig. 21). In this case, also, angiography merely gave evidence of a space-occupying lesion, and a small cavernous angioma was revealed only upon histological examination. In CASE 19 the cause of a subcortical cerebral haemorrhage associated with signs of subarachnoid haemorrhage remained unexplained, both angiographic and histological examinations failing to demonstrate it. The authors surmised, nonetheless, that the cause was a microangioma.

Clinical details of the four cases in this group (*i.e.* CASES 17-20) are given in the Table of Cases on page 196.

31

CASE 17

The patient, a 14-year-old boy in a secondary school, experienced a cerebral haemorrhage from an angioma (Fig. 20) in the white matter of the parieto-occipital part of the right hemisphere. Clinically, he presented with signs of severe intracranial pressure (attacks of headache, vomiting, papilloedema). A notable feature was a left-sided recurrent facial palsy and transient sensory disturbances in the arm. The only clinical finding was a partial hemisyndrome. Complete recovery occurred after operative removal of the vascular malformation and evacuation of the haemorrhage.

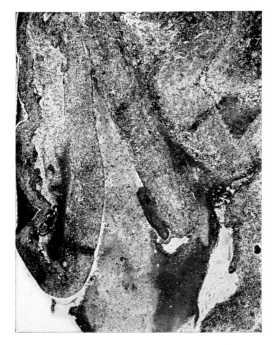

Fig. 20. Cerebral microangioma. Section from vascular mass. Magnification 25x. (Institute of Pathology, University of Zurich) (Case 17).

CASE 18

The patient, a girl of 2 years and 4 months, experienced a left-sided hemiplegia and hemianopia of sudden onset, due to a ruptured microangioma in the depth of the right temporal lobe (Fig. 21). Following removal of the malformation and intensive physiotherapy, the severe hemiparesis persisted. Eleven months after the onset, reduced growth in the length of the left extremities was already apparent.

The dilatation of the contralateral (left) pupil deserves special mention. Fortunately this false lateralising sign was not of importance in this case, because persistence of reaction to pain revealed a unilateral motor deficit. Despite the incomplete coma, no neck rigidity was present, although the latter is usually a prominent sign of non coma-producing subarachnoid haemorrhage. EEG revealed generalised epileptic discharges 4½ months after the onset of the illness and focal discharges 7 months later. However, no seizures have so far appeared with the patient on regular anticonvulsant treatment.

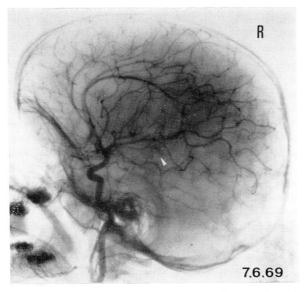

Fig. 21. Microangioma in the mid-temporal region (arrow) (Case 18).

CASE 19

This case presented considerable diagnostic difficulty. The patient, a young girl, presented initially at the age of 5 years and 9 months with fever, vomiting, headache and unusual sensitivity to noise. A cerebrospinal pleocytosis and mild throat infection prompted the suspicion of non-paralytic poliomyelitis.

One week after the onset of the illness and when the temperature was still elevated, a second attack of headache occurred, accompanied by several neurological signs, *viz.* central right facial palsy, a dilated left pupil and a nominal dysphasia; on this occasion no vomiting occurred. The CSF was now shown to be blood-stained and xanthochromic. EEG, interpreted in conjunction with the clinical picture, indicated the presence of a severe diffuse cerebral disturbance with a marked maximum in the left postcentral region, and suspicious left fronto-temporal epilepsy potentials.

Three days later the only true epileptic attack, consisting of clonic right hemi-convulsions, occurred; the child was completely aphasic. Carotid angiography demonstrated a space-occupying lesion, and a subcortical haematoma about the size of a walnut was removed from the left temporal lobe (Fig. 22). After the operation the patient made a satisfactory recovery, but was left with a permanent organic

33

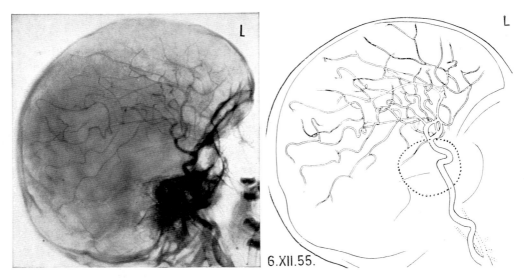

Fig. 22. Spontaneous haemorrhage into the left temporal lobe. Displacement of the cerebral arteries upwards and medially. Site of the haematoma outlined in the line drawing (Case 19).

psychosyndrome of moderate severity, including a weakness of memory and a partial nominal dysphasia.

The cause of the cerebral haemorrhage was not clear. Histologically, the only finding was a healing inflammatory reaction in the marginal tissues of the haematoma. The speculated causes included haemorrhage from a small vascular malformation (aneurysm, angioma) or a haemorrhage from an inflammatory focus. (With a case history extending over 8 years, a tumour could almost certainly be excluded.) Against an inflammatory cause was the absence of changes in the blood characteristic of inflammation (erythrocyte sedimentation rate (ESR), white cell total and differential counts were all normal). The febrile state was interpreted as damage to the centre of temperature regulation in the adjacent hypothalamus by perifocal oedema or vascular disturbances; perhaps a resorption fever also played a part.

Six months after the acute cerebral haemorrhage, the patient was re-admitted to hospital with measles encephalitis, diagnosed on the basis of a mild cerebrospinal pleocytosis. During this illness, attacks of anxiety convulsions and optic hallucinations were observed, which pointed to epileptic discharges from the left temporal lobe. It was therefore concluded that the case was not one of measles encephalitis but, rather, that the patient was in a post-epileptic state following a seizure that had not been observed.

Follow-up EEG $5\frac{1}{2}$ years later revealed an epileptic focus in the left temporal lobe. In 1963 ($7\frac{1}{2}$ years after the cerebral haemorrhage) further attacks occurred, characterised by unusual sensations in the head, which appeared to be clinical manifestations of epileptic discharges—a diagnosis confirmed by their disappearance with phenobarbitone therapy.

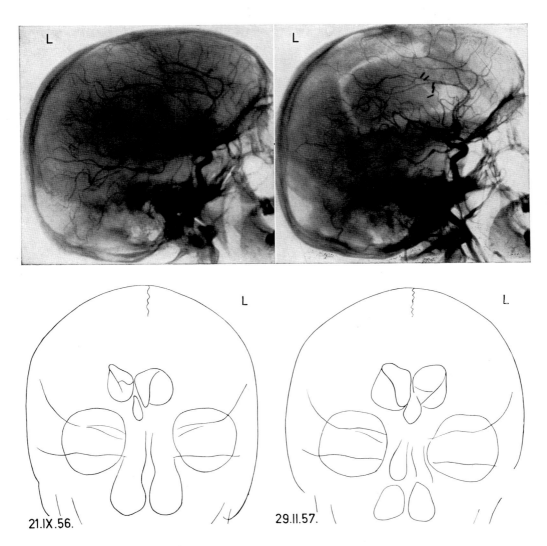

Fig. 23. Cerebral microangioma. Spontaneous haemorrhage into the white matter of the left cerebral hemisphere. *Top left:* carotid angiogram made before operative removal of the haematoma, showing marked splaying of the insular arteries and depression of the middle cerebral artery. The microangioma cannot be seen. *Top right:* carotid angiogram made after operative removal of the haematoma, showing normal appearances. *Bottom left:* line drawing of pneumoencephalogram made before operation, showing displacement of the ventricular system to the right side by the haematoma. *Bottom right:* line drawing of pneumoencephalogram made after operative removal of the haematoma, showing slight displacement of the ventricular system to the left side (Case 20).

CASE 20

This girl experienced, at the age of 16 years, after several weeks of headache, an apoplectiform right hemiplegia with motor aphasia, caused by cerebral haemorrhage from a cavernous angioma. After operative removal of the haematoma, a moderately severe spastic weakness remained, which mainly involved only the arm. The speech disturbance disappeared completely. Two further epileptic attacks occurred, 4 and 8 months later. Anticonvulsant therapy was then commenced but abandoned after 2 years. In the 7 succeeding years, the patient has been symptom-free (Figs. 23 and 24).

For more detailed reports of CASES *17-20 see pages 224-226.*

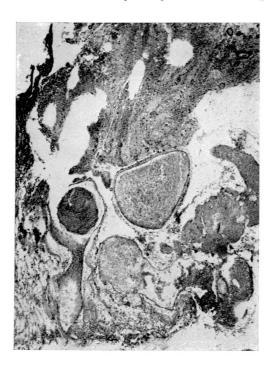

Fig. 24. Cerebral microangioma. Section from a cavernous vascular mass. Magnification 25x. (Institute of Pathology, University of Zurich) (Case 20).

PART II

Arterial Occlusions

CHAPTER 6

Focal Arteritis

The aetiological rôle of infectious illnesses in producing severe damage in the arterial walls with secondary brain damage was discussed by Ford and Schaffer (1927) in their original paper on acquired hemiplegia in children. Litchfield (1938) was able to demonstrate inflammatory infiltrate in the adventitia and media of the cavernous part of the internal carotid artery, in an 11-month-old boy who died from carotid thrombosis following a retropharyngeal abscess.

The condition of focal arteritis with secondary thrombosis has been recognised in life only since the introduction of cerebral angiography and its application in children. Pouyanne *et al.* (1957) described the case of a 12-year-old boy with cervical lymph nodes adherent to a thrombosed internal carotid artery; Rocand, Perrot and co-workers (cited by Rocand 1961) reported the case of an 11-year-old girl with carotid occlusion at the level of an operatively verified adenopathy; Bickerstaff (1964) demonstrated, with early angiography, irregular indentations of the internal carotid lumen in 4 children with acute hemiplegia following upper respiratory tract infections; Adler (1965) described a similar case. Shillito (1964) reported further similar cases and referred particularly to one case in which inflammatory involvement of the internal carotid at the skull base was observed at autopsy.

Mycotic aneurysms occurring with bacterial endocarditis are a special form of focal arteritis. They arise as a result of septic emboli which lead to inflammatory luminal damage, notably in the distal segments of the cerebral arteries—in contrast to the situation of congenital saccular aneurysms. Bell and Butler (1968) reported two cases in children with acute hemiparesis. In one case the aneurysm ruptured, and was excised and confirmed histologically. In the other the diagnosis was made angiographically (multiple aneurysms with arterial occlusion). A noteworthy observation made by these authors is the fact that mycotic aneurysms tend to rupture late, many months after antibiotic cure of the bacterial endocarditis. The association of acute neurological signs with congenital or rheumatic heart disease must always raise the suspicion of septic embolism with arterial occlusion, mycotic aneurysm or cerebral abscess.

There are two cases in the author's series, in neither of which is there any doubt of the inflammatory pathogenesis of the carotid occlusion. In the first patient (CASE 21), a 2½-year-old girl, hemiseizures and hemiplegia occurred following tonsillitis with very marked cervical lymph node enlargement. Angiography demonstrated significant narrowing of the internal carotid artery at the level of the adenopathy. Follow-up angiography 1 year later revealed an extensive ballooning of the artery at this level, which was considered to be a mycotic aneurysm. In the other patient (CASE 22), a carotid thrombosis developed during a severe attack of scarlatiniform stomatopharyngitis with lymph node enlargement on the side of the thrombosis.

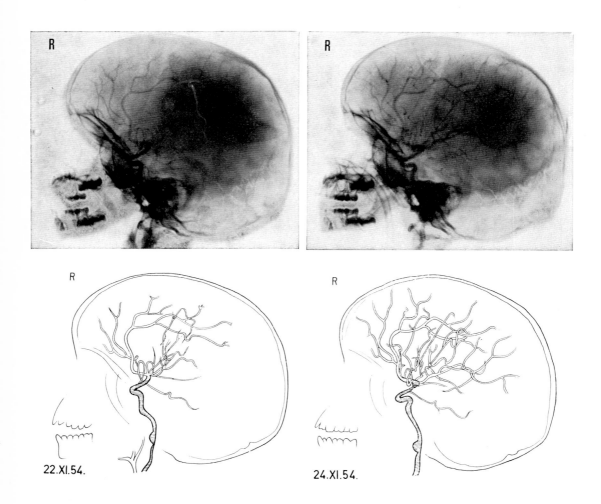

Fig. 25*a*. Focal arteritis in a case of lymphadenitis. *Left:* carotid angiogram showing a cuff of stenosis of the internal carotid artery in the upper cervical region, with localized out-pouching of the arterial walls just distal to it. Spasm of middle cerebral branches. *Right:* follow-up angiogram made 2 days later. Localised out-pouching of the internal carotid walls unaltered; however, the lumen at all levels has reverted to normal calibre. Excellent opacification of the middle cerebral artery (Case 21).

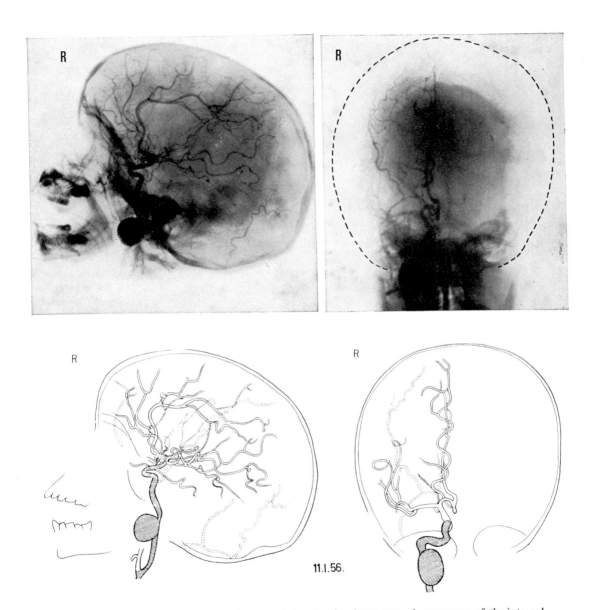

Fig. 25b. Follow-up angiogram made 1 year later showing large mycotic aneurysm of the internal carotid artery at the site of the out-pouching. (Case 21).

41

The clinical course of these two cases is given in the Table of Cases on page 196.

The author believes that focal inflammatory lesions of the arterial wall are far more commonly the cause of para- or post-infectious carotid thrombosis than has hitherto been accepted. Five further cases of arterial occlusion occurring during, or as a result of, an acute infectious illness are described on pages 93-102, and similar cases in the literature are reviewed. It is possible that these cases belong in the group discussed here.

Angiography is essential in explaining the association between local inflammatory processes and arterial thromboses, and should be carried out not only as early as possible but also as part of the follow-up examination. Bickerstaff (1964) considers bilateral angiography for the purposes of comparison, as well as subsequent follow-up angiography, to be essential in such cases.

Further clarification of the aetiology of 'spontaneous' arterial occlusion is to be expected from progress in vascular microsurgery. Nowadays, it seems possible to by-pass occluded arteries and to examine histologically the affected segment (Yasargil 1971, personal communication).

CASE 21

The patient, a girl aged 2 years and 4 months, experienced a sudden severe haemorrhage from the throat one week after a mild infection with enlarged lymph nodes at the right angle of the jaw. A few hours later tonic and clonic unilateral convulsions occurred, with an apoplectiform flaccid weakness of the left side of the body. The vascular origin of this hemiplegia was convincingly confirmed by angiographic examination. The initial angiogram revealed a severe narrowing of the internal carotid artery immediately proximal to its point of entry into the carotid canal of the skull base, with an area of out-pouching of the arterial wall just distal to it (Figs. 25a and 26). This finding was confirmed by repeat angiography two days later. Somewhat surprisingly, one year later a large saccular aneurysm was demonstrated at the site of the out-pouching on the internal carotid artery (Figs. 25b and 26). It was assumed that the aneurysm had arisen as a result of inflammatory damage to the arterial wall (arteritis), which itself had resulted from the acute lymphadenitis at the right angle of the jaw. The apoplectiform insult one week later was considered to represent an acute disturbance of the cerebral circulation, resulting from an arterial spasm. The initial angiogram revealed only a few unusually narrow branches of the middle cerebral vessels, while in the second angiogram, two days later, several large sylvian branches opacified well but the insular arteries remained thin. While the view cannot be refuted that the temporary spasm of the middle cerebral artery could have arisen from the angiogram itself (reaction to puncture of the common carotid artery or to the contrast medium), it seems unlikely in view of the previous presence of an arteritis. The mycotic aneurysm was too far removed from the site of the puncture of the common carotid artery for it to have resulted from direct needle damage. Histological examination of the excised segment of internal carotid artery excluded a dissecting aneurysm resulting from the puncture or sub-intimal contrast injection.

The massive initial haemorrhage is more difficult to explain. Presumably the site of bleeding lay in the region of the fauces, although careful examination failed to

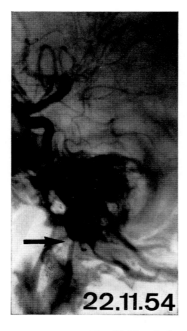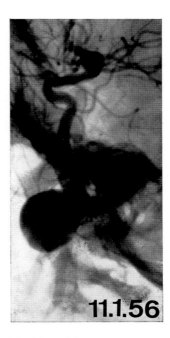

Fig. 26. Detail views from Fig. 25a and b.

reveal it. A mouth wound, *e.g.* a bitten tongue during an unobserved epileptic attack, could be excluded for all practical purposes, since a wound producing so massive a haemorrhage would scarcely have gone unnoticed. There were no indications of oesophageal varices. It is assumed that the source of the haemorrhage was a faucial branch of the external carotid artery, damaged in the same way as the internal carotid artery, and that the haemorrhage followed spasm of the artery. Faucial bleeding from the aneurysmal wall of the internal carotid is thought to be less likely, since no swelling was found at the angle of the jaw, nor was it palpated within the faucial wall.

The pneumoencephalogram demonstrated very clearly the results of acute severe disturbances of arterial perfusion of the right cerebral hemisphere (Fig. 27). The first examination, made one week after the insult, revealed unilateral oedema of the right hemisphere. Subsequent examinations showed the development of massive atrophy of the right hemisphere, which was probably aggravated by carotid ligation.

The spastic hemiparesis was in no way aggravated by carotid ligation. On the contrary, it improved markedly with prolonged intensive physiotherapy. Burr-hole investigation one year later revealed the presence of a cerebral cyst, representing a focus of cerebral softening.

Twelve years after the cerebral insult, a considerable spastic hemiparesis persists. It is most marked in the arm, and there is a mild disturbance of gait and an organic psychosyndrome. A noteworthy feature is the fact that with regular anticonvulsant drug treatment no epileptic attacks have been observed for the past 10 years.

43

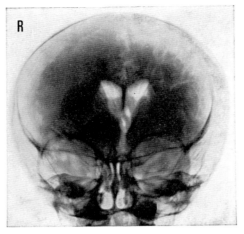
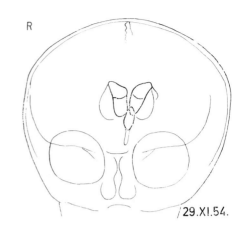

29.XI.54.

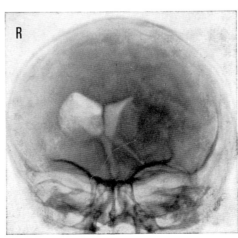
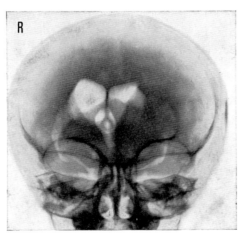
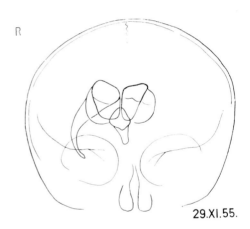

29.XI.55.

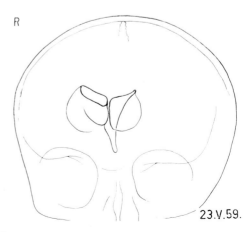

23.V.59.

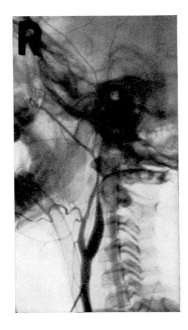
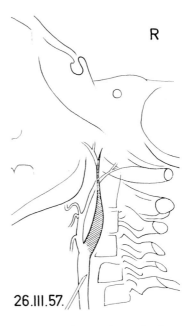

Fig. 28. Inflammatory thrombosis of the internal carotid artery in scarlet fever pharyngitis (Case 22).

CASE 22.

During an attack of scarlet fever complicated by otitis media and haemorrhagic stomatopharyngitis, the patient, a girl aged 10 years and 3 months, developed a progressive flaccid hemiplegia which was complete within 3 days. The cause of the hemiplegia was demonstrated angiographically to be a thrombosis of the internal carotid artery in its extracranial course (Fig. 28). As in CASE 21, a massive haemorrhage from the nasopharynx heralded the arterial occlusion.

The remarkable feature of this case was the regression of the complete flaccid hemiplegia, which had lasted for 3 weeks, shortly after contralateral stellectomy, which was performed after vasodilator medication had proved useless. The operation was performed on the assumption that elimination of sympathetic innervation would lead to an improvement in the cerebral collateral circulation.* The improvement that began within 2 days cannot be taken as definite proof of the value of the operation, since experience in many cases has shown that spontaneous regression of a flaccid

---

*Case published by Hürzeler, D. (1959) 'Stellektomie bei Carotisthrombose mit Hemiplegie.' Pract. oto-rhino-laryng. (Basel) 21, 168.

Facing Page: **Fig. 27.** *Top:* displacement of the ventricular system to the right side by oedema of the right hemisphere during the phase of acute arteritis. *Centre and bottom:* progressive atrophy of the right hemisphere, with displacement of the ventricular system to the right side and enlargement of the right lateral ventricle (Case 21).

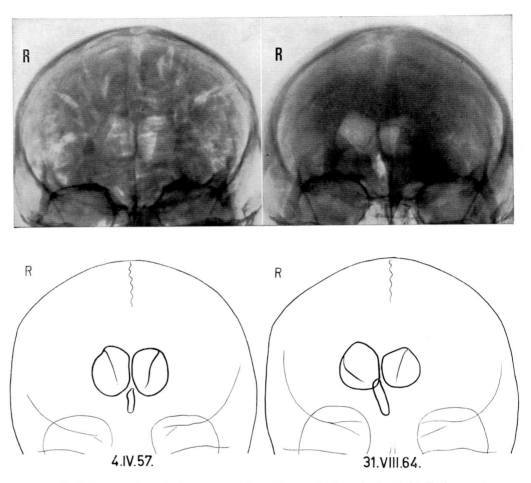

Fig. 29. *Left:* normal ventricular system 12 days after carotid thrombosis. *Right:* displacement of the ventricular system to the right side 7 years later, as a result of hemispherical atrophy (Case 22).

hemiplegia may start after many weeks, without operations on the sympathetic nervous system. Nevertheless, it was assumed in this patient that the operation resulted in an improved collateral circulation, leading to a corresponding functional recovery in the affected area. However, the further course showed this collateral supply to be inadequate. Pneumoencephalography performed 7 years later revealed the right cerebral hemisphere to be markedly atrophic (Fig. 29). The weakness persisted as a severe spastic hemiparesis. Presumably the marked organic psychosyndrome played a significant part in the poor functional condition of the patient, in that all physiotherapeutic measures came to nought due to very poor patient co-operation.

For more detailed reports of CASES *21 and 22 see pages 227-230.*

Fibromuscular Hyperplasia

— This aetiologically unknown affection is characterised by a dysplasia of the walls of medium-sized and smaller arteries of the muscular type. Most commonly the renal arteries are affected, mainly in women in young adulthood or middle age, with the clinical picture of an ischaemic renal hypertension. The angiographic appearances are characterised by notching and aneurysmal out-pouchings of the arterial lumen so that it resembles a string of pearls—according to Kincaid (1966) the pathognomonic appearance of fibromuscular hyperplasia. McCormack *et al.* (1967) distinguished four different varieties on morbid-anatomical grounds: (1) intimal fibroplasia, (2) medial fibroplasia, usually with mural micro-aneurysms, (3) subadventitial fibroplasia, often with involvement of the external elastic membrane, and (4) genuine fibromuscular hyperplasia with segmental concentric stenosis produced by cuffs of hyperplastic smooth muscle and collagen.

Fibromuscular hyperplasia is rarely observed in other arteries such as the superior mesenteric, coeliac, external iliac and internal carotid. Connett and Lansche (1965) published the first histologically confirmed case of fibromuscular hyperplasia involving the extracranial part of the internal carotid in a 34-year-old woman with acute hemiplegia. Palubinskas and Newton (1965) reported three further cases, diagnosed angiographically, with bilateral involvement of the internal carotid: in one of these three women, histologically-confirmed fibromuscular hyperplasia of the renal arteries was also present. Huber and Fuchs (1967) made the diagnosis on the basis of the characteristic angiographic findings in CASE 23 reported below, and included in their paper two further cases of acute hemiplegia (a 7-year-old girl and a 54-year-old woman). The two children represented the first known cases showing involvement of intracranial arteries (middle cerebral and internal carotid), although neither was confirmed histologically. A noteworthy feature of all the cases of extra-cranial internal carotid involvement reported in the literature is the presence of a loud murmur over the carotid artery synchronous with the pulse. This sign was not present in either of the children with involvement of intracranial arteries.

Andersen (1970) published details of two cases of children with extensive lesions. In one of these, an 8-year-old boy suffering from endocardial fibro-elastosis, the fibromuscular hyperplasia included involvement of both the carotid and the vertebral arteries, in addition to lesions of the renal, mesenteric, hepatic and lumbar arteries.

Palubinskas *et al.* (1966), in a review of 70 cases involving the renal arteries, found an unexpectedly high percentage (8.5 per cent) of patients with saccular cerebral aneurysms. The authors concluded that common aetiological factors were responsible for both arterial dysplasias.

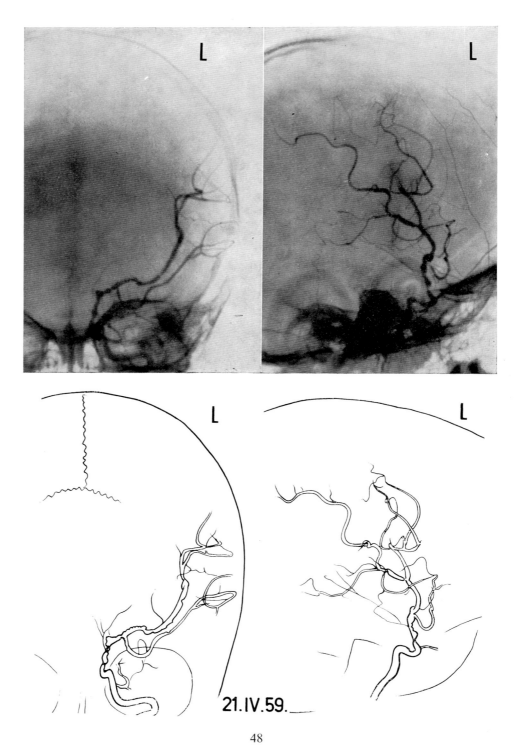

21.IV.59.

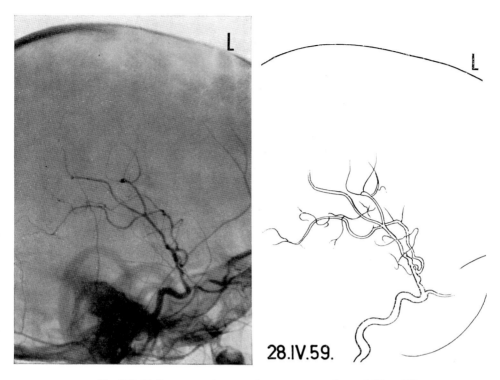

Fig. 30*b*. Follow-up angiogram. Appearances unchanged (Case 23).

CASE 23

The child, a girl aged 2 years and 9 months, fell suddenly unconscious after a two-day period of excessive tiredness. A complete right flaccid hemiplegia and loss of speech were present, but no convulsions were observed. Carotid angiography revealed a 'string of beads' appearance of the terminal part of the internal carotid artery, and non-filling of some branches of the middle cerebral artery (Fig. 30). These appearances were interpreted as being due to an organic vascular lesion, *e.g.* endarteritis, presumably, because of the raised erythrocyte sedimentation rate (ESR), of infectious origin. In 1967 Huber and Fuchs made the diagnosis of fibromuscular hyperplasia in this patient on the basis of the characteristic angiographic changes. Despite intensive physiotherapy, a considerable hemiparesis, including severe loss of function of the hand, remains after $7\frac{1}{2}$ years. No significant organic psychosyndrome has yet appeared. Jacksonian attacks, which commenced 2 years after the insult, have been suppressed with drugs.

For a more detailed report of this case see page 231.

Facing page:　　　　**Fig. 30***a*. Fibromuscular hyperplasia (?). 'String of pearls' appearance in terminal segment of internal carotid and commencement of middle cerebral arteries. (Case 23).

49

CHAPTER 8

Multiple Occlusions with Unusual Net-like Collaterals ('Moyamoya' Disease)

Since 1964, several reports have appeared in the literature, mostly from Japan, which refer to a peculiar cerebrovascular network associated with multiple intra-cranial arterial occlusions. Suzuki and Takaku (1969) coined the term 'Moyamoya' disease (*Moyamoya:* Japanese word indicating something hazy, like a puff of smoke drifting through the air) to describe the appearance of the abnormal net-like col-laterals. Nishimoto and Takeuchi (1968) collected 96 cases, and Kudo (1968, quoted by Suzuki and Takaku) 146 cases from the whole of Japan. Kudo (1968) considered the disease to be confined to Japanese, especially as 3 patients reported in the American literature were also of Japanese extraction (Leeds and Abbott 1965, Weidner *et al.* 1965). Recently, 18 cases have been reported in subjects who were not of Japanese descent (Taveras 1969, Solomon *et al.* 1970, Harwood-Nash *et al.* 1971). In two patients in this series presenting with hemiparetic attacks, the same type of angio-graphic pattern was found (CASES 24 and 25).

At present, more than 150 cases have been described, mostly in young subjects. Of the 96 cases collected by Nishimoto and Takeuchi, 73 had shown the disease before the age of 20 years and 56 before the age of 10 years. Three cases in infancy are reported (Taveras 1969, Solomon *et al.* 1970; CASE 24).

In the younger subjects a female preponderance is present. Of the total of 85 cases aged under 20 years in the literature, 56 have been female and 29 male patients. In adults no significant sex difference appears to exist.

Clinically, the most typical symptoms in the younger patients are a hemiplegia of apoplectiform onset, with or without accompanying epileptic seizures. An intellectual deficit is often present, with, less frequently, speech disorders, headache, hyperkinetic behaviour and cranial nerve involvement (facial nerve). Intracranial haemorrhage—rare in the young patients—is considered to be the most constant symptom in adults. Taveras (1969) stressed the occurrence of spontaneous subdural haematomas due to rupture of transdural anastomotic channels.

Prognosis is surprisingly fair, with only moderate disability and, in some instances, with practically no neurological deficit; however, severe permanent disability or death may occur in children, even without intracranial haemorrhage.

The dynamic processes associated with this disease were observed in the follow-up angiograms of 4 young patients by Suzuki and Takaku (1969). From the serial angiographic appearances, these authors identified six stages of the disease, commenc-ing with a simple narrowing of the carotid bifurcation. Further stages included the development of an extensive collateral network at the base of the brain and, eventually, a reduction and disappearance of these abnormal collaterals. At some point, the occlusion became bilateral, although the time and extent of this process varied.

Taveras (1969) considers that, in most cases, the lesions progress to complete obstruction of nearly all the major arterial channels. In the early stages, a very localised narrowing of the internal carotid artery at its bifurcation may be observed. Then the occlusion spreads to involve the trunk of the anterior and middle cerebral arteries, sometimes also the posterior communicating and proximal posterior cerebral arteries, and finally the basilar artery. He points out that the distal branches of the main cerebral arteries usually remain unaffected. Because the circle of Willis is involved early, and cannot therefore serve as a collateral pathway, unusual sources of collateral supply are found, namely, (1) from perforating branches in the region of the basal ganglia, sometimes through anastomoses between the anterior and posterior choroidal arteries; (2) from leptomeningeal arterial anastomoses (until the basilar artery becomes occluded); and (3) from transdural external-internal carotid anastomoses (rete mirabile). Taveras emphasizes that narrowing of the internal carotid artery is an acquired phenomenon caused by the small volume of blood flowing through it, and not by hypoplasia.

The aetiology of this disease is not known, although three autopsy cases have been reported. Maki and Nakata (1965) described the case of a 9-year-old girl who died of a non-traumatic subdural haematoma. At autopsy, the lumen of the circle of Willis arteries was narrow but patent. Histological examination revealed thickening of the intima, without changes in the media or adventitia, and no inflammatory changes. The vessel walls in the abnormal vascular network were described as resembling those found in the Sturge-Weber syndrome. The autopsy case reported by Kawakita *et al.* (1965) was a 12-year-old girl in whom both internal carotid and both anterior and middle cerebral arteries were almost completely occluded by greyish-black thrombi. Histologically, the appearances were identical to those in the other case. In addition, mild to severe arteriosclerotic lesions were found in the internal, external and common carotid arteries, as well as in some visceral arteries. Pulmonary and visceral tuberculosis was also present. In the third autopsy case, reported by Suzuki *et al.* (1965), the findings within the skull were distorted by an old tuberculous meningitis.

Suzuki and Takaku (1969) considered Moyamoya disease to be an acquired abnormality: trauma or inflammation of the head or neck could perhaps provoke persistent spasm around the carotid bifurcation which might then lead to an organic occlusion producing an abnormal collateral network. They also discussed similarities between this syndrome and the pulseless (Takayasu) disease. Taveras (1969) enumerated various pathogenic factors responsible for intracranial arterial occlusions. He favoured a non-specific inflammatory aetiology or, possibly, an auto-immune reaction, and rejected the theory of an underlying arteriosclerotic lesion or any relationship to pulseless disease.

Taveras holds the view that, in most cases, the arterial lesions develop within a relatively short period—a few weeks to a few months. Once the major intracranial vessels are occluded, the occlusive process ceases to spread further. Occlusions usually involve only the trunk of the middle and anterior cerebral arteries, while the large

51

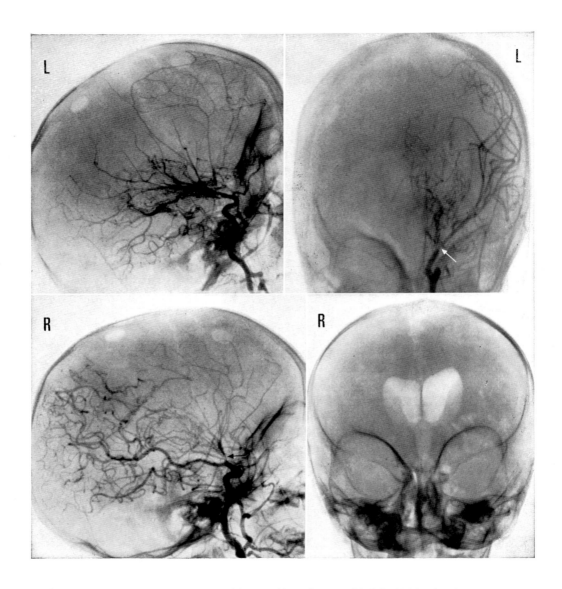

Fig. 31*a.* 'Moyamoya' disease. *Top:* left carotid angiogram (20 July 1965), showing numerous abnormal vessels in the area of distribution of the middle cerebral artery. Narrowing at the origin of the middle cerebral artery (arrow in AP arteriogram). *Bottom left:* right carotid angiogram (13 August 1965), showing narrowing at the origin of the middle cerebral artery (arrow). Unusually large posterior communicating artery. Abnormal blood vessels in parietal region. *Bottom right:* pneumoencephalogram (19 July 1965) showing moderate asymmetrical internal hydrocephalus (Case 24).

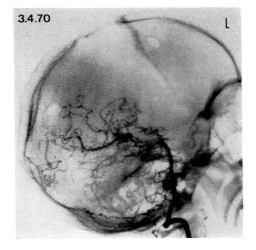

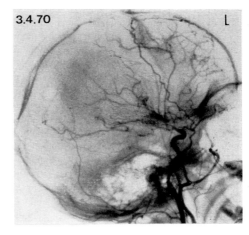

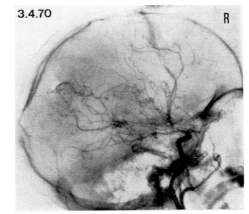

Fig. 31*b*. Follow-up angiograms 4½ years later (Case 24). Increase of collateral supply by transdural anastomoses. Note intact major arterial channels on left vertebral angiogram (top left).

arteries remain patent. Suzuki and Takaku discussed the dynamics of arterial lesions, especially in young patients, on the basis of vertebral angiography in 8 cases. None showed any changes before ramification of the basilar artery.

Because of the prominent vascular network, a congenital anomaly (angiomatosis combined with arterial hypoplasia) was first postulated.

Follow-up studies, including repeat angiography, in the 2 cases in this series revealed several findings which conflict with the views of Taveras and Suzuki and Takaku. In CASE 25, the left internal carotid artery, and the trunk and branches of the middle cerebral artery, still remained patent one year after the onset of the first symptoms (Fig. 32). A rich blood supply to the affected right side from the intact left middle cerebral artery occurred via the anterior communicating artery. This case proved the involvement of the vertebral artery in the occlusive process. It is believed that Taveras correctly interpreted the narrow lumen of the entire left vertebral artery when it was supplying only the posterior inferior cerebellar artery as being the result of reduced blood flow. In CASE 24, follow-up angiograms made 4½ years after the onset of the disease revealed that the abnormality had persisted, only minor differences being shown. This experience conflicts with the rapid angiographic changes described by Suzuki and Takaku in younger patients.

In the author's two cases, mental retardation was present from birth. Suzuki and Takaku found mental retardation in 6 out of 12 cases. The possibility exists of vascular disease acquired *in utero*, with an abnormal vessel network developing during maturation of the vascular system.

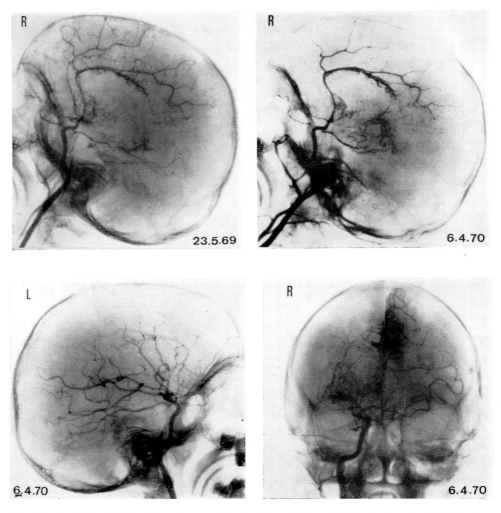

Fig. 32a. *Top left:* right carotid angiogram. Trunk of the middle cerebral artery is occluded. Extensive collateral network through the lenticulostriate, pericallosal and posterior choroidal arteries. *Top right:* repeat angiogram. Increase of collateral flow through posterior choroidal artery. *Bottom left:* normal left carotid angiogram. *Bottom right:* right carotid angiogram. Large supply to the intact left side! (Case 25).

This unusual disease, characterized by multiple occlusions of the arteries arising from the circle of Willis, remains a puzzle. Is the occurrence of multiple arterial occlusions within a few weeks or months consistent with the fact that many cases show only mild transient symptoms, and many only suffer minor residual disability or none at all? Is it possible for so extensive a collateral network to develop within such an unusually short period? Repeat serial angiograms, using a catheter to avoid artefacts, *e.g.* a vascular spasm induced by needle puncture, would be necessary to answer these questions.

CASE 24

This case presented an unusual diagnostic puzzle. At the age of 9 months, the patient, a girl, was involved in a road accident and possibly sustained a head injury. Two days after the accident, an attack of repeated right-sided convulsions occurred, followed by transient hemiparesis. After a 3-week interval of normal behaviour, the child developed a complete right hemiplegia. On EEG a marked depression was present over the left hemisphere, and pneumoencephalography showed some asymmetry of the ventricular system. Bilateral burr-holes—made on suspicion of traumatic subdural haematomata—revealed no abnormalities. Cerebral angiography revealed the presence

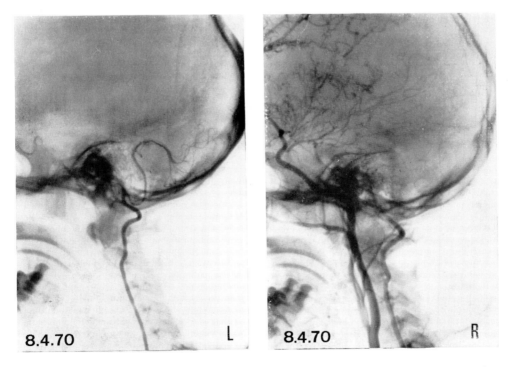

Fig. 32*b*. *Left:* left vertebral angiogram. Occlusion of the artery distal to the origin of the posterior inferior cerebellar artery. Note the thin calibre of the vertebral artery. *Right:* angiography by catheter in the right subclavian artery. Right vertebral and basilar arteries normal. (Case 25).

55

of an extensive collateral network of anastomotic vessels related to multiple stenoses of the trunks of the main intracranial arteries on both sides (Fig. 31a).

Two months later, after almost complete recovery, the patient was again admitted following a sudden hemiplegia on the opposite (left) side. Some weeks later an attack of epileptic convulsions occurred, resulting in further deterioration. Since that time, the child has remained bedridden due to bilateral spastic hemiplegia, and there is evidence of severe mental damage. Follow-up angiography, $4\frac{1}{2}$ years after the onset of the illness, revealed no essential changes in the appearances of the vessels (Fig. 31b).

CASE 25

This moderately retarded girl presented at the age of $6\frac{1}{2}$ years with a transient speech disorder (partial motor aphasia). Three weeks later a left hemiparesis and a focal epileptic seizure suddenly occurred. Full recovery took place within two days. Cerebral angiography revealed abnormal collateral net-like vessels associated with multiple sites of cerebral artery occlusion (in the trunk of right middle cerebral artery, in the main branch of right posterior cerebral artery, and in the left vertebral artery). Follow-up angiography, one year after the occurrence of transient ischaemic symptoms, revealed that only minor changes had taken place. The left internal carotid, left middle and anterior cerebral arteries remained unaffected (Fig. 32).

For more detailed reports of CASES *24 and 25 see pages 232-234.*

CHAPTER 9

Arteriosclerosis

The literature of arteriosclerosis, the disease par excellence of advanced age, is now so large that it is scarcely possible to review it. Increasing interest in the pathogenesis of the disease has nowadays widened speculation so much that even a 'paediatric disease' has been mentioned (Holman 1961, Reisman 1965). Only very rarely in the literature is arteriosclerosis reported as a cause of vascular disturbances in childhood.

Janssen (1957), in a review of arteriosclerosis in childhood, described, on the basis of 115 personal cases and 152 cases taken from the literature, four groups which he classified as follows.

(1) Calcinosis resulting from disturbances of calcium metabolism or from possible dystrophic changes in congenital anomalies of the vascular wall. This type of arteriosclerosis occurs only in the initial years of life.

(2) Arterionecrosis due to a toxic infectious cause or as a result of vitamin D or adrenalin intoxication. This group also consists chiefly of children in the first years of life.

(3) Arteriosclerosis due to malignant hypertension, which affects patients of all ages.

(4) Arteriosclerosis occurring as part of a complex metabolic disturbance. This type does not occur before the twelfth year of life. However, the author reviewed only the aorta, the large arteries and the coronary arteries, not the arteries of the brain.

Stötzer (1960) examined at autopsy the larger arteries (aorta, common carotid and extremity arteries) of 100 children under the age of 13 years, including neonates. Of these, 23 infants showed a dietary-provoked lipidosis of the aorta, and 26 older children an intimal sclerosis. The author viewed the aetiological factor as hypoxia. No evidence of an inflammatory pathogenesis could be found.

Baker and Iannone (1959), in a large investigation of the cerebral vessels, demonstrated the presence of atherosclerotic processes in the larger branches of the circle of Willis, in patients still in the second decade of life, while degenerative fibrous changes were not found in the smaller intracerebral arteries and arterioles before the third decade.

Cochrane and Bowden (1954) introduced their paper on arterial calcification in infancy and childhood with the statement: 'Calcification of the arteries is one of the most important causes of occlusive arterial disease in infancy and childhood'. These authors found marked changes in the internal elastic laminae of large and small arteries, particularly the coronary vessels, in 6 infants who had died of cardiac insufficiency. Similar findings have been reported by van Creveld (1941), Andersen and Schlesinger (1942), Field (1946), Stryker (1946) and Prior and Bergstrom (1948) in infants with renal hyperparathyroidism. In 2 older children with renal diseases,

Cochrane and Bowden found severe secondary arterial lesions, which in one case involved the cerebral vessels as well.

Ford and Schaffer (1927) described, in a 4-year-old boy who died of thrombosis of the middle cerebral artery, intimal plaques and medial degeneration in the cerebral and visceral arteries. The most impressive case is that of Griffioen and Pieterse (1965), namely a 12-year-old boy who died of hypertensive apoplexy, and in whom a severe extensive arteriosclerosis was demonstrated at autopsy. Duffy *et al.* (1957) reported the autopsy findings in a 16-month-old boy with multiple vascular malformations and spontaneous carotid thrombosis, in whom degenerative changes, including calcification, were present in the adventitia. Murphey and Shillito (1959) discussed a 19-month-old child with acute hemiplegia due to carotid occlusion, in whom an induration in the terminal segment of the internal carotid artery was shown at autopsy to be a calcified plaque. Matson (1965) observed atheromatous plaques in the intima during operation on two small children with saccular aneurysms.

Mellick and Phelan (1965) reported an unusual observation in a 4-year-old boy with intermittent hemiplegic attacks and unassociated attacks of unilateral headache following occlusion of the internal carotid artery by an atheromatous plaque at the level of the bifurcation. Carotid angiography revealed a conical occlusion to be present, similar in appearance to CASE 22 (Fig. 28). Insertion of a dacron prosthesis was moderately successful. Unfortunately, no follow-up angiogram was made after the operation.

According to present day knowledge, atherosclerosis and arteriosclerosis play only a minor part in the causation of spontaneous cerebral arterial occlusions in childhood. The vast majority of young patients fortunately survive a thrombotic insult, so it is not known whether 'arteriosclerosis' is the cause of at least some such cases of thrombosis. If this were the case, however, one might expect this generalised disease to produce not merely a single thrombosis in the internal carotid or some other cerebral artery, but, sooner or later, further circulatory disturbances as well. There has been no evidence of this in a number of patients observed over a long period.

In a single child in this series of patients (CASE 26), histologically confirmed arteriosclerotic lesions were demonstrated in the cerebral vessels in association with a spontaneous thrombosis of the carotid artery. This 13-year-old girl, who died in an acute episode, is also the only case in the series in which the internal carotid thrombosis was bilateral.

It is surprising that bilateral thrombosis of the internal carotid artery is compatible not only with life, but with complete fitness for work. Fields *et al.* (1961) described 16 patients aged 45-68 years, of whom 10 survived and 6 were completely fit for work. Atherosclerotic lesions were present in all 16, and in all the occlusion was initially unilateral.

CASE 26

This case of thrombosis of the distal end of the internal carotid artery, proved by angiography (Fig. 33) and at autopsy, presented an unusual course and a surprising histological picture. The patient, a girl of nearly 13 years, after a trivial accident without definite injury to the head, experienced transient slight headache and then,

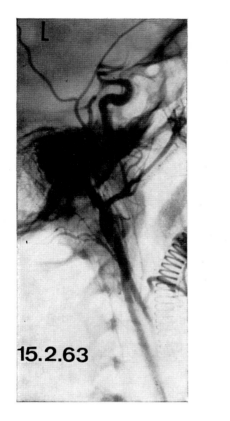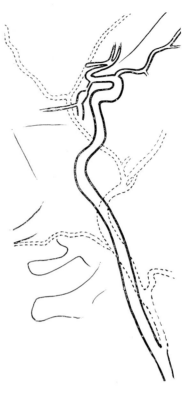

Fig. 33. Spontaneous thrombosis of the internal carotid artery distal to the carotid siphon in arteriosclerosis (Case 26).

after a lucid interval of 1 day, continuous severe headache with vomiting and urinary incontinence; as her condition deteriorated she gradually passed into a deep coma, and finally died. The only lateralising clinical signs (homolateral pupillary dilatation and a contralateral Babinski response) indicated left-sided brain damage. The EEG findings confirmed the lateralisation. Repeat examination before the patient passed into coma revealed no evidence of a hemiparesis. A presumptive clinical diagnosis of acute extradural or subdural haematoma was shown to be incorrect by burr-holes.

At autopsy, bilateral internal carotid thromboses were demonstrated, reflecting the situation at the time of death; at the time of the left carotid angiogram, the left carotid siphon was still patent, and it must have thrombosed further during the 30 hours before death. Since extensive haemorrhagic softening was demonstrated only in the left cerebral hemisphere, the thrombotic occlusion in the right internal carotid artery must have developed at a considerably later stage—and the macroscopic appearances of the thrombus at autopsy supported this. Alternatively, an unusually efficient collateral circulation must have developed from the basilar artery via the

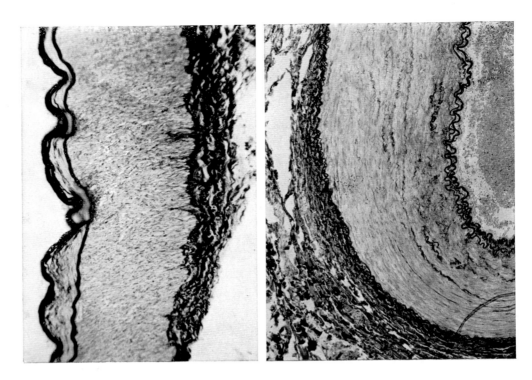

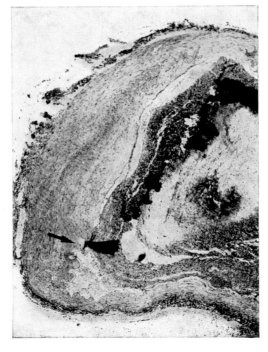

Fig. 34a (*above*). Arteriosclerosis of the internal carotid artery. *Left:* thickening of the intima. *Right:* splitting and fragmentation of elastic fibres of the media (Institute of Pathology, University of Zurich) (Case 26).

Fig. 34b (*left*). Splitting of the internal elastic lamina (arrow) and the tunica media. Intimal proliferation. Thrombus. (Institute of Pathology, University of Zurich) (Case 26).

posterior communicating artery. In this respect, the left cerebral hemisphere was at a disadvantage, due to the hyperplastic nature of the proximal part of the posterior cerebral artery between its origin in the basilar artery and the mouth of its posterior communicating branch. For this reason, a right hemiplegia should have been all the more likely. It is possible that the carotid thrombosis was not completely occluding the artery at the time of onset of the coma, and therefore no hemiplegia occurred.

Histological examination of both thrombosed arteries revealed evidence of a chronic injury to the vessel wall, with relatively acellular intimal plaques, a split internal elastic lamina and small lacerations of the tunica media (Figs. 34a and b). According to the pathologist (Professor E. Uehlinger), these mural defects were compatible with long-standing trauma. No evidence of any inflammatory changes could be observed. The pathologist thought it unlikely that there was any connection with the meningococcal meningitis of infancy.

It seems obvious that these long-standing defects in the arterial wall played a pathogenic rôle in the thrombosis, although it is no longer possible to prove that this interpretation is correct.

For a more detailed report of this case see page 235.

CHAPTER 10

Hypertension

Hypertension in children, as in adults, may lead to acute circulatory disturbances in the brain. The causes of hypertension in childhood are chiefly chronic renal diseases, renal malformations and aortic isthmus stenosis, while essential hypertension, endocrine diseases, (phaeochromocytoma), primary hyperaldosteronism, Cushing's syndrome, the adreno-genital syndrome, hyperparathyroidism or other causes (lead poisoning, cortisone or ACTH treatment) very rarely lead to an acute cerebral incident.

Haggerty *et al.* (1956), in a series of 9 children with essential hypertension, found two, aged $4\frac{1}{2}$ and $7\frac{1}{2}$ years respectively, with convulsions and hemiplegia; the pathogenesis of the cerebral involvement was not investigated in detail. In the case reported by Mymin (1960) with severe aortic isthmus stenosis and pulmonary hypertension, a carotid thrombosis was present. Griffioen and Pieterse (1965) reported the case of a 12-year-old boy with severe hypertension who died following an apoplectiform cerebral haemorrhage—shown at autopsy to be due to an extensive arteriosclerosis.

The association of aortic stenosis with saccular intracranial aneurysms, as well as the combination of such aneurysms with congenital cystic kidney, is well known. No such cases with acute hemiplegia in children are known to the author. Nagant *et al.* (1960) reported the case of a 26-year-old woman with a phaeochromocytoma and severe hypertension who died of a cerebral haemorrhage.

In the author's series there were two instances of acute hemiplegia associated with severe hypertension. In CASE 27 severe renal hypertension, due to aplasia of one kidney and chronic pyelonephritis of the other, was present. In the second patient (CASE 28), a severe aortic isthmus stenosis was the cause. It is noteworthy that in both cases the hypertension was first detected during clinical investigation of the acute hemiplegia, although in both children hypertensive symptoms (headaches, vomiting, nycturia) had been present for several months. Carotid angiography in both children revealed spastic blood vessels, associated in one case with a subarachnoid haemorrhage. Vasospasm is extremely common with subarachnoid haemorrhage, particularly following rupture of saccular aneurysms (Allègre and Vigouroux 1957, Johnson *et al.* 1958, Pool *et al.* 1958, Fletcher *et al.* 1959, Lende 1960, Driesen 1962, Maspes and Marini 1962, Corday *et al.* 1963, du Boulay 1963, Friedenfelt and Lundström 1963). In CASE 27 the vasospasm was directly associated with the hypertension, as was confirmed by the extensive fundal changes.

CASE 27

The patient, a 9-year-old boy, developed within several hours a progressive motor and sensory hemiparesis with homonymous hemianopia. The cause was discovered to be severe renal hypertension associated with aplasia of one kidney

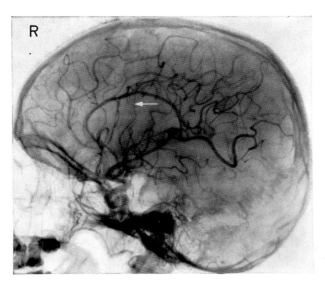

Fig. 35. Renal hypertension. Spastic insular artery (arrow) (Case 27).

and malformation and chronic pyelonephritis of the other. Fundal changes, the angiographic appearances (Fig. 35) and the CSF findings indicated an angiospastic insult to the brain. It was assumed that this insult involved not only ischaemia but also secondary cerebral oedema. In any event, the damage was very extensive and resulted in a neurological deficit, as shown by EEG tracings. A striking feature was the fact that the paralysis developed first in the leg and then spread stepwise to involve the arm and face.

With hypotensive and vasodilator drugs the hemiplegia virtually disappeared within a few weeks. Two years later no neurological deficit remained, and the boy was free from complaints. The persistent hypertension has been satisfactorily controlled with Reserpine.

CASE 28

The patient, a boy aged 13 years, experienced two attacks of subarachnoid haemorrhage, the initial one taking the form of an epileptic attack. These attacks were related aetiologically to the presence of a congenital stenosis of the aortic isthmus, which was producing marked hypertension in the pre-stenotic vascular territory. Although there could be no doubt about the vascular origin of the hemiparesis and motor aphasia, the pathogenic mechanism was not clear. Bilateral carotid angiography showed that the left anterior cerebral artery and its branches were supplied from the right side, and that both anterior cerebral arteries were unusually thin

63

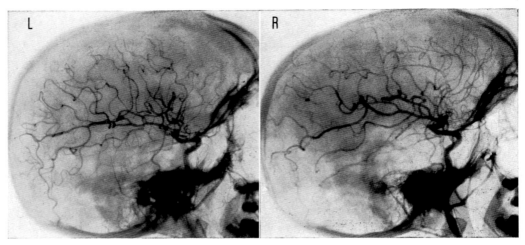

L

R

22. VIII. 63   22. VIII. 63

Fig. 36. Hypertension in aortic isthmus stenosis. Source of haemorrhage not demonstrated. *Left:* left carotid angiogram, showing possible spasm of anterior cerebral artery. *Right:* right carotid angiogram, showing spastic branches of the anterior cerebral artery (Case 28).

(Fig. 36). This finding was interpreted as a spastic reaction to the subarachnoid haemorrhage. Temporary functional impairment of this vessel would explain the paralysis of the leg (through deprivation of the appropriate part of the motor cortex) but not the expressive aphasia, which arises in an area of the brain irrigated by the middle cerebral artery. It was also not possible to observe the site of the haemorrhage angiographically. A significant haemorrhage into Broca's area was considered unlikely in view of the absence of focal signs on the EEG. Complete recovery occurred within 2 years.

For more detailed reports of CASES *27 and 28 see page 237.*

CHAPTER 11

Traumatic Vascular Occlusion

Direct injury to the internal carotid artery with secondary thrombotic occlusion is a known, but very rare, cause of acute hemiplegia in childhood. A typical mechanism of injury is a fall on the face with a pointed object in the mouth, which then perforates the soft palate and damages the internal carotid in the vicinity of the tonsillar fossa (Caldwell 1936, Leriche 1950, Philippides *et al.* 1954, Braudo 1956, Fairburn 1957). The author can add one patient (CASE 29) to the literature.

Another mechanism of injury is described in conjunction with closed neck trauma. Sedzimir (1955) assumed that spasm occurs with secondary thrombosis of the internal carotid artery when it is overdistended at the base of the skull. Clarke *et al.* (1955) regarded post-traumatic thrombosis as the result of intimal damage, due to over-stretching of the internal carotid artery over the transverse process of a cervical vertebra in forced rotation. Boldrey *et al.* (1956) considered that many cases of thrombosis arise from traumatic compression or mechanical tearing of the internal carotid artery over the arch of the atlas. Murphey and Miller (1959), Frantzen *et al.* (1961) and Therkelsen and Hornnes (1963) reported cases of secondary thrombosis following blunt trauma in the vicinity of the neck arteries, also as a result of mechanical compression by a foreign body. Duman and Stephens (1963) described a case of dissecting aneurysm with occlusion of the middle cerebral artery after blunt trauma to the skull. These workers also critically reviewed 3 of the 6 cases reported by Frantzen *et al.* (1961) which also showed occlusion of the middle cerebral artery, and concluded that they were, in fact, cases of traumatic dissecting aneurysm. Jacobsen and Skinhøj (1959) reported a very similar case in an 11-year-old boy. It seems possible that one of the author's patients (CASE 40, see page 90) belongs in this category.

The interval between the injury and the onset of neurological signs merits careful attention. In CASE 29, a 3-year-old boy with a perforating injury of the internal carotid artery in the tonsillar fossa, 14 hours elapsed before the onset of an apoplectiform hemiplegia; in CASE 30, a patient with a traumatic dissecting aneurysm, the interval was $3\frac{1}{2}$ months. In the above-mentioned cases in the literature (16 children aged $1\frac{1}{2}$-16 years), the hemiplegia followed immediately upon the trauma in only two instances, and in the remainder there was a free interval varying from several hours to three days in duration. Mis-diagnosis of intracranial haemorrhage (subdural or extradural haematoma) is a very real possibility. However, the apoplectiform onset of the hemiplegia should make these diagnoses questionable. Angiography is essential in such cases.

In one of the author's patients (CASE 30), a dissecting aneurysm, which had developed after a carotid puncture performed, during attempted angiography, by an inexperienced doctor, provoked an acute hemiplegia only after an interval of $3\frac{1}{2}$

months. At this point, a carotid angiogram showed narrowing of the main trunk of the middle cerebral artery for a 2 cm long segment (Fig. 38), at a distance from the customary site of thrombotic occlusion, namely the mouth of the artery. This angiographic appearance is typical in cases of dissecting aneurysm, and hardly ever occurs in cases of thrombosis. Histological examination confirmed the presence of a dissecting aneurysm. Poppen (1951) diagnosed two cases of dissecting aneurysm on the basis of the angiographic appearances, one of which was confirmed histologically.

Boyd-Wilson (1962), in a review of 900 cases submitted to carotid angiography, found that in one per cent of these cases inner layers of the artery became detached. These detachments accompanied technically complicated carotid punctures and occurred almost exclusively in elderly subjects, particularly arteriosclerotics. Analogous findings were reported by Idbohrn (1951), Sirois *et al.* (1954), Liverud (1958), Fleming and Park (1959), Lepoire *et al.* (1964) and Rajszys and Sabat (1964), as well as by Crawford (1956), on the basis of autopsy findings. Fortunately, in children this complication of carotid angiography appears to be very rare.

CASE 29

The patient, a 3-year-old boy, suffered a perforating injury to the left internal carotid artery in the throat. After a brief initial period of collapse, he exhibited no neurological deficit until 14 hours later, when a flaccid right hemiplegia with complete expressive aphasia appeared. Simultaneously, tonic convulsions of the contralateral extremities commenced, which recurred for 12 hours. The cause was a thrombosis of the internal carotid artery at the base of the skull, which was demonstrated angiographically 8 months later (Fig. 37).

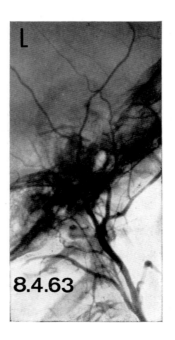

Six months after the carotid injury, epileptic attacks with adversive seizures commenced, which could be largely suppressed with drug treatment.

While the speech disturbance disappeared completely within 6 months, the severe spastic hemiparesis remained, including almost complete loss of function of the hand and a moderate disturbance of gait.

An unusual feature was the presence of hemiconvulsions in the acute phase, restricted to the non-paralysed side of the body. It is assumed that generalised attacks were in fact occurring, but that the ischaemic hemisphere was no longer capable of responding to the epileptic discharges.

Fig. 37. Thrombosis of the internal carotid artery after a perforating throat injury. Carotid angiography: the contrast medium was injected into the common carotid artery, but only the external carotid artery and its branches were opacified (Case 29).

CASE 30

For a discussion of the recurrent subarachnoid haemorrhages from the arterio-venous malformation, see page 13.

Three and a half months after a technically unsuccessful left carotid angiogram, the patient developed a right hemiplegia. A left carotid angiogram at this stage revealed a significant narrowing of the main trunk of the left middle cerebral artery and non-filling of most of its sylvian branches. Following transient improvement, the child died 3½ weeks later, after terminal convulsions and coma. The diagnosis of partial middle cerebral artery thrombosis was shown to be incorrect, in that an extensive dissecting aneurysm of the internal carotid artery was present, which could be shown to be extending into the main branches of the middle cerebral artery. The resulting disturbance of arterial perfusion led to cerebral softening in the left basal ganglia and internal capsule, and this softening appeared compatible with the 3-week-old acute hemiplegia (Figs. 38, 39 and 40).

Pathogenically, it seems highly likely that a sub-intimal contrast injection at the time of the unsuccessful angiogram was responsible for the dissecting aneurysm.

No explanation could be found for the recent softening demonstrated in the right hemisphere, since the vascular system was intact; possibly vasospastic circulatory disturbances played a part.

For more detailed reports of CASES *29 and 30 see pages 238-239.*

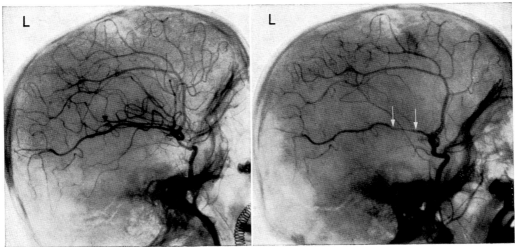

13. X. 58   14. 1. 59

Fig. 38. Traumatic dissecting aneurysm of the internal carotid and middle cerebral arteries following unsuccessful carotid arteriography. *Left:* 3 weeks after failed carotid puncture, only the terminal segment of the internal carotid appeared narrowed. *Right:* follow-up angiogram 3 months later, showing narrowing of a segment of the middle cerebral artery (arrows), as well as defective filling of the insular arteries (Case 30).

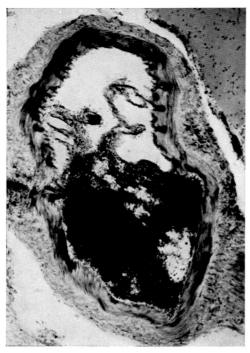

Fig. 39. Traumatic dissecting aneurysm. *Left:* middle cerebral artery, with true lumen above and false lumen below. Magnification 90x. (Case 30).

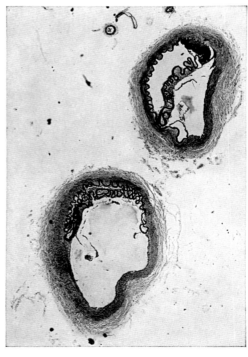

Right: two branches of the middle cerebral artery, showing the false lumen to be considerably larger than the true one. Magnification 30x. (Department of Neurology, University of Zurich) (Case 30).

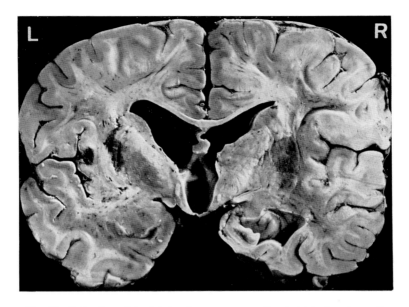

Fig. 40*a*. Softening of the left insular cortex extending into the basal ganglia. Enlargement of the left lateral ventricle and the third ventricle (Case 30).

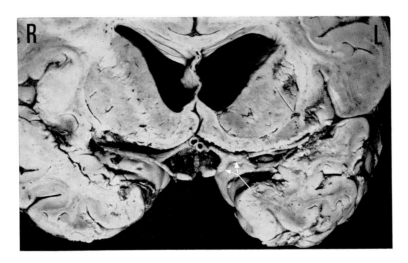

Fig. 40*b*. Coronal section of the brain at the level of the carotid siphon. Terminal segment of left internal carotid and proximal part of left middle cerebral arteries thickened by a thrombotic dissecting aneurysm (arrow). Lumen of both anterior cerebral arteries normally patent (Case 30).

CHAPTER 12

Embolism

Cases of proven cerebral thrombo-embolism causing acute hemiplegia in child-hood are scarce in the literature. While the possibility of thrombo-embolism is always alluded to in descriptions of congenital cyanotic heart disease, specific case reports are rare. On the other hand, septic embolism, the precursor of cerebral abscesses, is well documented. However, cerebral abscesses only infrequently present as cases of acute hemisyndrome (see page 155). For discussion of mycotic cerebral aneurysms in bacterial endocarditis, see page 39.

Gross (1945) described a 13-month-old child with Fallot's tetralogy, in whom an apoplectiform hemiplegia occurred following multiple embolism from a thrombosed ductus arteriosus. Banker (1961), in a review of autopsies carried out on 48 children with cerebral vascular occlusions, found 10 cases of embolism (3 of which were neo-nates) with extensive cerebral infarction, and 38 cases of septic embolism. Richwien and Unger (1966) reported the case of a $13\frac{1}{2}$-year-old boy with Wallenberg's syndrome, resulting from thrombo-embolism of a cerebral blood vessel in the posterior fossa, in the presence of a congenital heart lesion. This child suffered an apoplectiform hemiplegia 11 months later, and died shortly afterwards of cardiopulmonary in-sufficiency. Autopsy revealed thrombi in the left heart, as well as splenic and renal infarcts. Schad (1966) observed 2 small children with severe cyanotic heart disease and acute hemiplegia, in whom the latter was assumed to be the result of embolism. Since a significant polycythaemia is usually present in cases of severe cyanotic heart disease, the increased viscosity of the blood and slowed circulation could provoke an acute thrombotic vascular occlusion and mimic an embolism. No differential diagnosis is possible on clinical grounds.

Post-operative embolisms following operations for congenital heart disease are not considered here. The author has observed isolated cases of this type following correction of aortic isthmus stenosis. One case was published by Geisler *et al.* (1965).

Cerebral arterial embolisms produced by detached tumour particles have been described in two children with myxomas of the left auricle (Gleason 1955, Chao *et al.* 1960). Both cases were only diagnosed at autopsy, although in Chao's case the presence of unusual cells in the peripheral blood prompted the suspicion of an intracardiac myxoma.

An exceptional rarity is echinococcal embolism in the internal carotid artery leading to apoplectiform hemiplegia; a case was described in a youth by Paillas *et al.* (1959).

There were two patients in this series in whom thrombo-embolism was assumed, although in neither was it proved. In one patient (CASE 31), the source of the embolism was believed to be a huge arteriovenous malformation of the lungs, which possessed wide drainage vessels into the left auricle. The second patient (CASE 32) suffered an apoplectiform attack during an episode of acute cardiac decompensation with auricular fibrillation associated with myocarditis. Both cases were only explained subsequently, and in both the diagnosis was a retrospective one.

In a boy with an arteriovenous malformation (CASE 31) carotid angiography performed 2 years after the apoplectiform insult (which had produced a permanent severe hemiparesis) showed completely normal appearances. The question therefore arises of whether an embolic occlusion can disappear. Dalal *et al.* (1965, 1966) reported nine cases, some of which showed severe and permanent neurological deficits. In two, the spontaneous dissolution of thrombotic emboli was demonstrated; in one of these, a 21-year-old man, serial angiography demonstrated disappearance of the emboli within a few days, while the other case was followed up at autopsy. Fisher (1959) observed fragmentation and destruction of emboli ophthalmoscopically in a 54-year-old man with transient monocular blindness. Similar observations were reported by Russell (1961). These highly significant findings prompt critical questions over the efficacy of fibrinolytic therapy in embolic and thrombotic occlusions. In any event, they indicate that a normal angiogram made several days after an apoplectiform insult by no means rules out the diagnosis of embolism (and thrombosis, see CASE 35, page 83).

CASE 31

The patient, at the age of 9 years and 4 months, suffered a complete right hemiplegia and aphasia. Unfortunately, no precise details are available of the findings at that time, although it is known that the patient was treated for a 'meningoencephalitis'. The speech disturbance rapidly regressed, but a severe spastic hemiplegia remained.

Investigation 2 years later revealed the presence of a large arteriovenous malformation in the lungs, with wide drainage into the left auricle. It is assumed that a causal association existed between this vascular malformation and the acute hemiplegia. An embolism could possibly have been responsible although, at the time of angiography prior the chest operation, the great vessels supplying the brain all showed normal appearances. However, it is possible that the embolus could have been driven peripherally and was consequently no longer visible angiographically, or that a thrombolysis had occurred (Figs. 41 and 42).

The initial diagnosis of 'meningoencephalitis' is considered by the author to have been probably incorrect, especially in view of the apoplectiform onset of the total hemiplegia. The same objection can be made to the diagnosis of cerebral abscess.

CASE 32

The patient, a 3-year-old boy, experienced an acute cardiac illness, presumably myocarditis, during the course of an influenzal infection. During convalescence, cardiac failure suddenly occurred, and generalised oedema developed. At the peak of the illness, the patient suffered an apoplectiform insult, which resulted in complete hemiplegia following prolonged coma. The pathogenesis, in retrospect, is somewhat obscure, although there is no doubt of the cardiac origin of the attack. It is possible

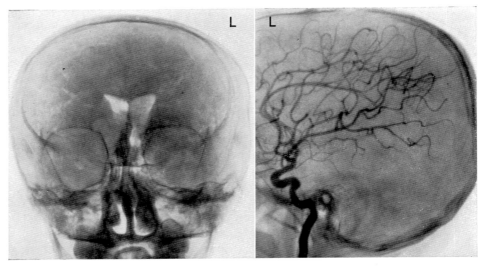

L L

22. II. 66   22. II. 66

Fig. 41. Slight enlargement of the left lateral ventricle and normal left carotid angiogram 2 years after probable embolism in a left-sided cerebral artery (Case 31).

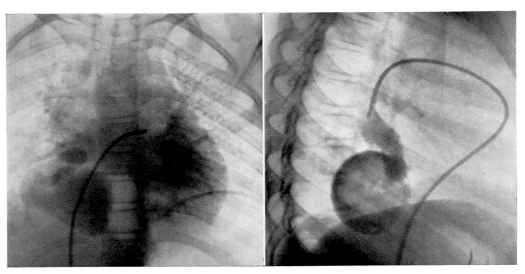

16. II 66

Fig. 42. Extensive arteriovenous malformation of the lungs with large draining vessel into the left auricle (Case 31).

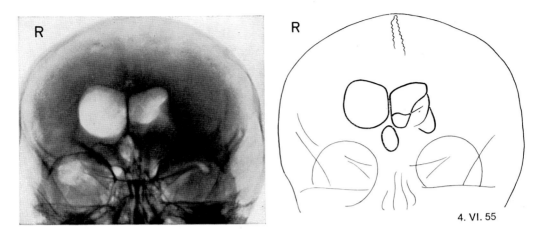

Fig. 43. Atrophy of the right cerebral hemisphere, following acute hemiplegia during cardiac decompensation in myocarditis 3½ years previously (Case 32).

that embolism from auricular fibrillation was the cause—a view supported by the presence 4 months later of recurrent attacks of paroxysmal tachycardia.

The hemiplegia persisted as a severe spastic hemiparesis. Although EEG 3 years later revealed the presence of an active epileptogenic focus, no attacks have been observed in the patient in the course of 15 years.

For more detailed reports of CASES *31 and 32 see page 240.*

CHAPTER 13

Spontaneous Cerebral Arterial Occlusion

Spontaneous occlusion of the cerebral arteries is seen nowadays with increasing frequency, because of the routine angiographic examination of children with acute hemiplegia. Wisoff and Rothballer (1961) reported 2 personal cases and collected 27 from the literature. At least some of these cases exhibited a probable causal condition (Petit-Dutaillis *et al.* 1949: local arteritis; Boldrey 1956: traumatic arterial damage; Ford and Schaffer 1927: generalized arteriosclerosis; Banker 1959: nephrosis in remission; Murphey and Shillito 1959: cervical lymphadenopathy; also 4 cases with dissecting aneurysm). Since that time, a further series of cases has been added: Taveras and Poser (1959), Rocand (1961), Byers and McLean (1962) Rouzaud *et al.* (1962), Silverstein and Hollin (1963), Faris *et al.* (1964), Krayenbühl and Yasargil (1964), Geisler *et al.* (1965), Davie and Coxe (1967), Lehmann *et al.* (1970), Solomon *et al.* (1970) and Harwood-Nash *et al.* (1971).

Twelve children (CASES 34-45) in the author's series showed a spontaneous occlusion in the region of the internal carotid territory or its large branches, and in none of these cases could any definite cause be demonstrated. In 5 children (CASES 41-45) the occlusion occurred during, or in association with, an ordinary febrile illness; in CASE 35 a cardiac defect was possibly the cause, while in CASE 40 a mild head injury may have been responsible.

In this case material, the absence of spontaneous occlusions of unknown aetiology in the cervical part of the internal carotid artery is striking. In all the patients with occlusion in the neck (CASES 16, 21, 22 and 29) a definite aetiology was present. In the literature of spontaneous occlusion, also, the incidence of intracranial occlusions predominates 2-3-fold over extracranial occlusions. Murphey and Shillito (1959) expressed the view, on the basis of personal experience, that some of the cases of cervical internal carotid occlusion observed angiographically are, in fact, cases in which the primary lesion was situated intracranially, and in which the thrombosis extended proximally in the artery. In the following analysis of cases of arterial occlusion observed angiographically or at autopsy from the author's personal series and from the literature, all patients with probable causal diseases have been excluded (*e.g.* significant cervical lymphadenopathy, clinically manifest heart disease, arteriosclerosis, dissecting aneurysm). The case records of some patients are incomplete, accounting for the discrepancy in patient totals when certain specific points are discussed.

No significant age predilection could be demonstrated on the basis of the cases taken from the author's series and those found in the literature; from a total of 48 patients there was an age range from 9 months to 19 years. This finding was true of the healthy patients experiencing a spontaneous arterial occlusion, as well as of those cases of undetermined aetiology occurring during or after a febrile illness.

Similarly, no sex (22 boys, 19 girls) or lateralising (23 left-sided, 22 right-sided occlusions) predilections could be demonstrated.

In 31 of a total of 38 cases the arterial occlusion led to an apoplectiform hemiplegia, which in only 4 was accompanied by initial epileptic seizures (hemi- or generalised). Ten of these cases were from the para- or post-infectious group, and of these only one showed initial epileptic attacks. In the cases of occlusion occurring without accompanying illness (21 cases), the attack was preceded in 5 children by headache, tiredness or vomiting for hours or several days, and, in the case of Rouzaud *et al.* (1962), by behavioural changes lasting 6 weeks. In 7 children the hemiplegia occurred stepwise, in one case following an ordinary infectious disease; the remaining 6 children were perfectly healthy. In none of this group of cases were epileptic convulsions observed.

Extremely interesting findings were demonstrated on follow-up angiography, which was carried out in 9 of the author's 13 patients. In CASE 35, which presented a biphasic pattern of hemiplegia, spontaneous recanalisation of the partially occluded internal carotid artery occurred within two weeks (Figs. 47 and 48). The angiographic changes were even more rapid in CASE 38, in which non-filling of the internal carotid artery at the base of the skull was demonstrated on the day of the apoplectiform insult; two days later the internal carotid opacified to the level of the siphon, and one year later the entire carotid tree opacified, with the exception of the anterior cerebral artery (Figs. 51*a* and *b*). In CASE 45 a partial thrombosis of the middle cerebral artery was demonstrated one week after the onset of the illness, and this appearance was unaltered $3\frac{1}{2}$ weeks later; two follow-up angiograms performed after 6 months revealed opacification of a recanalised anterior insular artery (Fig. 59). Complete recanalisation occurred in CASES 41 and 44. These phenomena are viewed as evidence of spontaneous thrombolysis, analogous to the observations of Dalal *et al.* (1965, 1966).

In contrast to these angiographic observations, CASE 37 presented a picture of progressive thrombosis with complete obstruction at the bifurcation of the internal carotid artery, after initially showing only a partial occlusion of the middle cerebral artery—and, most interesting, this occurred during regression of the severe initial motor deficit!

In the great majority of cases, an occlusion of a major cerebral artery, either permanent or temporary, led to irreversible and severe neurological signs. This was found in 8 of the author's 12 patients, with case histories of 4-20 years duration. A similar finding appeared to be present in CASE 35, although the period of observation in this case is still too short. Only 2 children (CASES 37 and 42) exhibited a near-complete recovery of the motor deficit. Special circumstances were present in CASE 36, which showed an angiographically constant and circumscribed narrowing of the anterior cerebral artery over 16 months ('thromboangiitis obliterans'). This boy had presented clinically with a hemisyndrome, which cleared very rapidly with complete recovery.

The clinical course of these patients is portrayed in the Table of Cases (pages 198-199).

Recovery from the hemiplegia which follows occlusion of a cerebral artery depends on two critical factors: (1) the patency of the lenticulostriate arteries, which supply the internal capsule, and (2) the development of individual and very variable

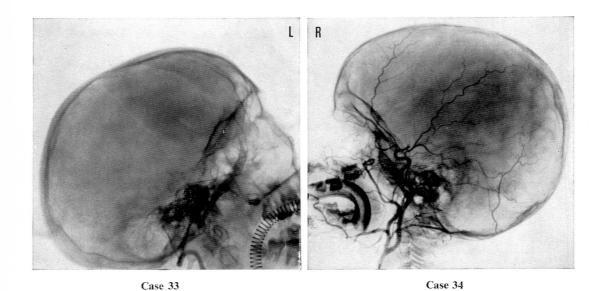

Case 33

Case 34

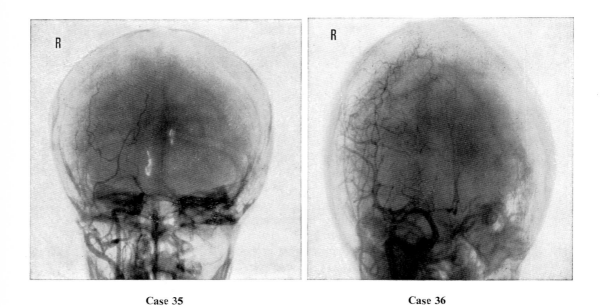

Case 35

Case 36

Fig. 44. Spontaneous occlusion of cerebral arteries (Cases 33-36).

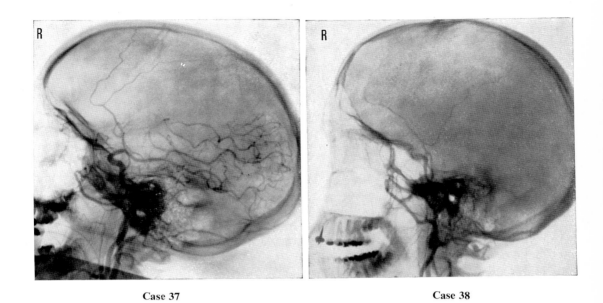

Case 37

Case 38

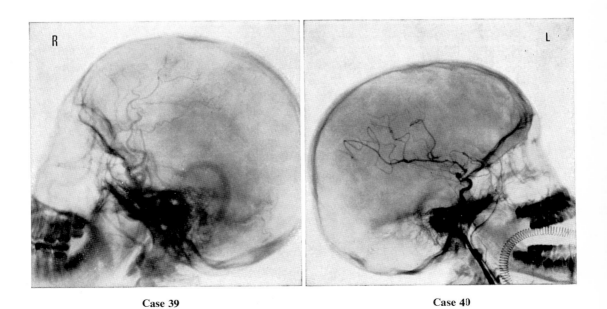

Case 39

Case 40

Fig. 44 (contd.) (Cases 37-40).

paths of collateral circulation. If the middle cerebral artery is occluded in the vicinity of the origin of the lenticulostriate arteries, an irreversible neurological deficit will follow. However, if the occlusion is either distal or proximal to their origin, recovery will depend on the development of a sufficiently prompt and adequate collateral circulation. It is known that only a few critical minutes are available for the deviated bloodstream to prevent parenchymal necrosis. Reactive effects on the general systemic circulation (shock) may catastrophically reduce the functional integrity of an anatomically complete collateral network, as Denny-Brown (1951), Meyer and Denny-Brown (1957), Bernsmeier (1963) and others have expressly shown.

The following examples illustrate the significance of the collateral circulation extremely well by means of angiograms. In CASE 37, an effective collateral circulation developed through the anterior communicating artery from the opposite side, while the thrombotic process itself gradually progressed (Fig. 50). In CASE 42, a rich collateral supply was established through the ipsilateral pericallosal artery (Fig. 56) which, it must be presumed, enabled complete recovery of the ischaemic region to take place. In contrast, however, CASE 43 showed a permanent and complete loss of function, despite the development of a rich collateral supply from the contralateral side (Fig. 57a) similar to that in CASE 37. Surprisingly, the pneumoencephalogram made 15 years later revealed no evidence of hemispherical atrophy (Fig. 57b). This finding, also, was in stark contrast to the severity of the permanent motor and psychomotor deficits. Presumably, occlusion of the lenticulostriate arteries must have been responsible for the persistence of these deficits.

The development of residual epilepsy as a late complication was observed in 4 of the author's 13 patients (CASES 38, 39, 41 and 44). The latent period varied from 1 to 9 years. It is possible that this number will be increased by cases in which the period of observation is still not very long.

Seven of the author's 13 patients exhibited a serious organic psychosyndrome (CASES 34, 39-41, 43-45), mostly those with severe motor deficits. CASES 37 and 38 were exceptional in this respect.

Arterial occlusions in the region of the vertebral or basilar arteries are extremely rare in children. The solitary case (33) in the author's material showed an angiographically confirmed subtotal occlusion of the left vertebral artery with a clinical picture resembling Wallenberg's syndrome. Dooley and Smith (1968) published a case of a 6-year-old boy with occlusion of the basilar artery, marked by an initial episode of hemiparesis and truncal ataxia. Fowler (1962) reported two cases verified at autopsy (aged $1\frac{1}{2}$ and $7\frac{1}{2}$ years), one of which showed an inflammatory thrombosis and the other a thrombosis or embolism. The case described by Richwien and Unger (1966) resulting from embolism is described on page 70. Pribram (1961) reported the absence of opacification of the basilar artery in the presence of well-visualised vertebral arteries in a $2\frac{1}{2}$-year-old girl with a temporal lobe abscess. The angiographic appearance was interpreted as circulatory impairment following the acute intracranial pressure, with tonsillar herniation in the foramen magnum.

In many cases the cause of spontaneous cerebral artery occlusion in children remains completely obscure. Various aetiologies have been suggested in these chapters. It is possible that traumatic, hypoxic, inflammatory or toxic lesions contribute more

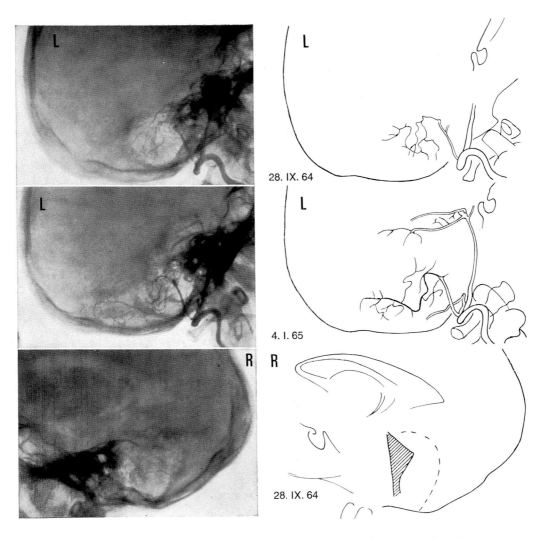

Fig. 45. Wallenberg's syndrome. *Top:* vertebral angiogram, showing interruption of the contrast column at the commencement of the basilar artery. Normal opacification of the posterior inferior cerebellar artery arising proximal to the site of obstruction. *Centre:* follow-up angiogram 6 months later, showing poor opacification of the basilar artery and its branches. *Bottom.* pneumoencephalogram, showing slight enlargement of the lateral ventricles. In the line drawing, the outline of the air is hatched (Case 33).

significantly than has been accepted in the past. Ford and Schaffer (1927) quoted a detailed autopsy investigation by Wiesel (1906) of 300 young patients who had died of various infectious illnesses. In many he found destructive, partly necrotic changes in the three layers of the blood vessels, surprisingly without any inflammatory components. Similar findings were reported by Winkelmann and Eckel (1935). Stötzer (1960) demonstrated intimal fibrosis in 20 out of 100 autopsy cases aged less than 14 years, which in all cases was attributed to hypoxia. It is not unreasonable to suppose that these vascular changes may lead to spontaneous thrombosis.

Sandifer (1962) postulated an allergic pathogenesis in the sense of an anaphylactic vasculitis in cases of idiopathic occlusion of the middle cerebral artery. Pribram (1961) described 11 adult cases with angiographic appearances resembling thrombotic occlusion of the cervical internal carotid, in association with intracranial haemorrhage. In none of these, however, was an anatomical obstruction present, but merely, in the author's view, a massive circulatory disturbance due to the acutely raised intra-cranial pressure. In one case this author was able to demonstrate restitution of the normal intracranial vascular pattern following removal of the raised pressure (ventricular puncture) without involving withdrawal of the carotid needle.

It is perhaps possible, through the application of modern surgical achievements (blood vessel repair, thrombectomy), to demonstrate the aetiology of some cases by means of biopsy. In the small number of surgically treated cases that have been published, it has already been shown that inspection of the carotid artery yields aetiological information (Petit-Dutaillis et al. 1949, Pouyanne et al. 1957, Mellick and Phelan 1965).

Davie and Coxe (1967) reported a case that is significant from the surgical viewpoint. These authors were able to perform a successful thrombectomy within 48 hours of the attack in a 2-year-old boy with acute hemiplegia due to para-infectious thrombosis of the internal carotid in the region of the bifurcation. The actual cause of the occlusion could not be found; it is possible that biopsy would have given an answer. These authors attributed the poor results of thrombectomy reported in the literature to the fact that the operations, although successful, were usually performed too late. The present author shares the view that carotid angiography in acute hemi-plegias should be performed as soon as possible.

CASE 33

This 12-year-old girl suffered from an illness characterised by recurrent bouts of symptoms similar to Wallenberg's syndrome. Vertebral angiography revealed a subtotal occlusion of the left vertebral artery in the vicinity of its point of entry into the skull (Fig. 45). Since on repeat vertebral angiography 3 months later filling of the basilar artery and its branches was also poor, the findings of the initial examination appear to the author to be significant and not attributable to technical artefact. The cause of the occlusion could not be explained.

CASE 34

In this patient, a 2-year-old girl, a flaccid incomplete hemiparesis of sudden onset occurred in the absence of any existing illness. Angiography revealed the cause

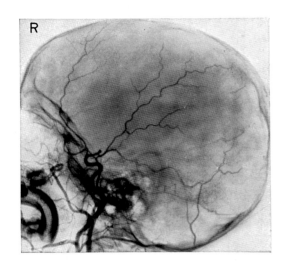

R

Fig. 46. Spontaneous occlusion of the internal carotid artery near its termination. Good opacification of the posterior communicating and posterior cerebral arteries, and also of the ophthalmic artery. In the line drawing, the branches of the external carotid artery are shown as dotted lines (Case 34).

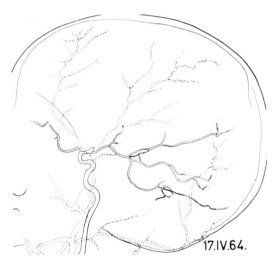

17.IV.64.

to be an occlusion of the carotid artery in the distal part of the siphon (Fig. 46). The pathogenesis could not be explained: there were no causes of embolism apparent, nor any general signs supporting a diagnosis of inflammatory thrombosis (fever, raised sedimentation rate, abnormal blood picture). The history indicated a course involving two attacks, in that, 8 days before the acute insult, the child became suddenly pale and vomited, although she exhibited no obvious cerebral signs. The development of a rapid, albeit incomplete, collateral circulation must be assumed, in view of the incomplete nature of the paralysis; the EEG appearances support this view. A noteworthy feature was the absence of epileptic manifestations, which presumably saved the child from a complete hemiplegia.

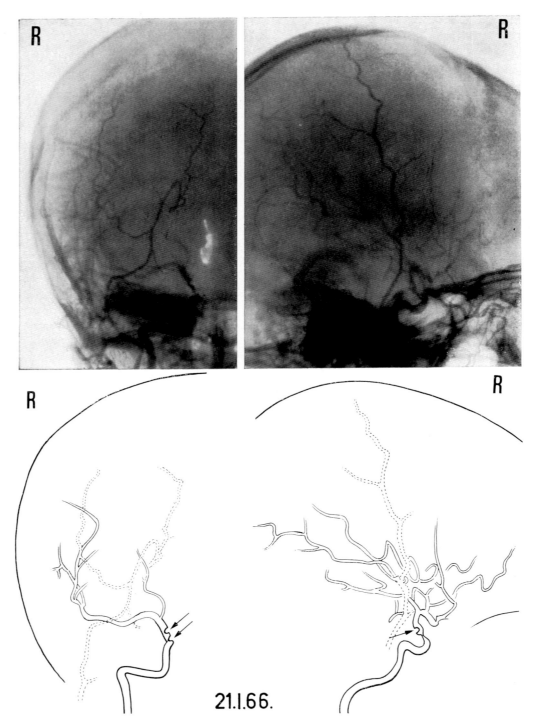

21.I.66.

Follow-up examination $2\frac{1}{4}$ years later revealed the presence of a persistent spastic hemiparesis and an organic psychosyndrome.

CASE 35

The patient, an $11\frac{1}{2}$-year-old girl in perfect health, experienced an acute left motor and sensory hemiplegia in two stepwise attacks. The first attack was apoplectiform and accompanied by a brief period of unconsciousness at the height of extreme physical exertion. The clinical picture (near-complete paralysis of the arm and lower facial muscles, mild paresis of the tongue and leg, and a sensory hemihypaesthesia) corresponded to circulatory deficiency in the vicinity of the middle cerebral artery. During a second attack, 5 days later, and after partial recovery, the entire left side of the body, and in particular the leg, became completely paralysed without loss of consciousness. This event led to the conclusion that the anterior cerebral artery as well as the middle cerebral artery was now involved.

The clinical suspicion of an arterial occlusion was confirmed by carotid angiography on the ninth day of the illness. The terminal part of the internal carotid artery in the distal part of the siphon showed a thread-like narrowing and a cone-shaped indentation of the lumen (Fig. 47). The trunk and main branches of the middle cerebral artery opacified poorly, and the anterior cerebral artery was not seen at all. The site of origin of the anterior cerebral artery from the internal carotid distal to the filling defects was patent and smooth-walled. The left carotid angiogram, performed on the 10th day of the illness (Fig. 48), is of interest as a comparison: not only did the right anterior cerebral artery opacify through the anterior communicating artery, but its occluded proximal part also opacified almost to its site of origin on the internal carotid artery. Thus the occlusion was shown to be complete, and to extend over a narrow segment only, possibly due to segmental spasm or a thrombus.

The arterial occlusion disappeared spontaneously without specific treatment (anticoagulants, vasodilators). Follow-up angiography 2 weeks later revealed good filling of the anterior cerebral artery from the carotid, and excellent opacification of the entire vascular tree; in particular the stenosed area previously demonstrated was now patent and its lumen smooth-walled (Fig. 48).

No indication of the pathogenesis of the arterial occlusion can be given. An association is assumed with the compensated cardiac defect (apparently an obstruction of the left ventricular outflow tract), which was a chance finding. The author assumes that an acute haemodynamic failure occurred in this patient at the height of excessive physical exertion. A critical fall of the cardiac minute volume could have produced spasm with secondary thrombosis in the terminal part of the internal carotid. The second episode of paralysis can be explained as a progression of the thrombotic process, or as a fresh spasm. The angiographic appearances were compatible with the presence of either, or a combination of both. Complete disappearance of thrombi through recanalisation or spontaneous fibrinolysis is a known phenomenon (Dalal et al. 1965, 1966).

Facing page: **Fig. 47.** Partial spontaneous occlusion of the terminal part of the internal carotid artery, with thrombotic narrowing of the lumen (arrows in the line drawing) (Case 35).

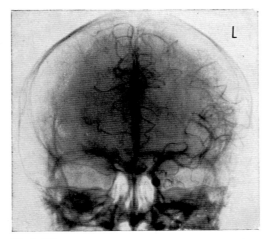

22. I. 66

Fig. 48. *Left:* left carotid angiogram of 22 January 1966. Opacification of the right anterior cerebral artery via the anterior communicating artery (compare Fig. 47).

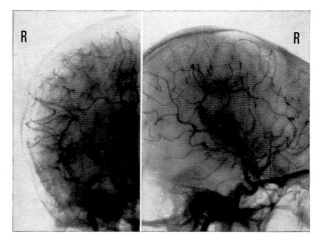

Right: follow-up angiogram two weeks later. Complete recanalisation of the terminal internal carotid (compare Fig. 47) (Case 35).

4. II. 66   4. II. 66

A further aetiological possibility is an embolus, arising from a mural thrombus associated with the cardiac defect. The biphasic course must be ascribed to a second embolism or thrombosis, or spasm. However, emboli rarely occur in the presence of perfect health. Moreover, only a fresh embolus could have been present, since old emboli become organised and are not easily or promptly detached. If an embolus was present it could have been destroyed in the periphery of the vascular tree.

Other pathogenic mechanisms such as cerebral haemorrhage, arteriovenous malformation with secondary thrombosis or spasm, or a primary coagulation disturbance appear to be ruled out on the basis of the clinical picture.

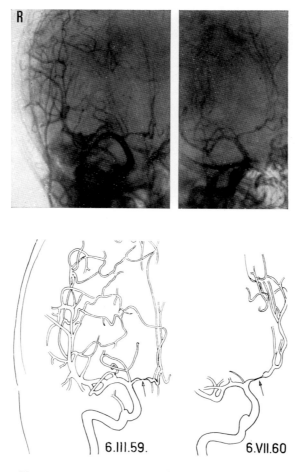

R

6.III.59.   6.VII.60

Fig. 49. Endarteritic narrowing of the proximal part of
the anterior cerebral artery (arrow in line drawings).
Unaltered appearances in follow-up angiogram 16 months
later (Case 36).

CASE 36

The patient, a 14-year-old boy, experienced without warning an apoplectiform
attack with motor and sensory paralysis of the left leg, dysarthria, facial palsy,
unilateral headache and vomiting. Spontaneous and complete recovery of the hemisyndrome occurred within 3 hours. Since then he has been completely free from
symptoms (duration of case history: 7 years).

Carotid angiography revealed the cause to be a partial occlusion of the anterior
cerebral artery, which showed unchanged appearances 16 months later (Fig. 49). It
is presumed that an endarteritic process was involved.

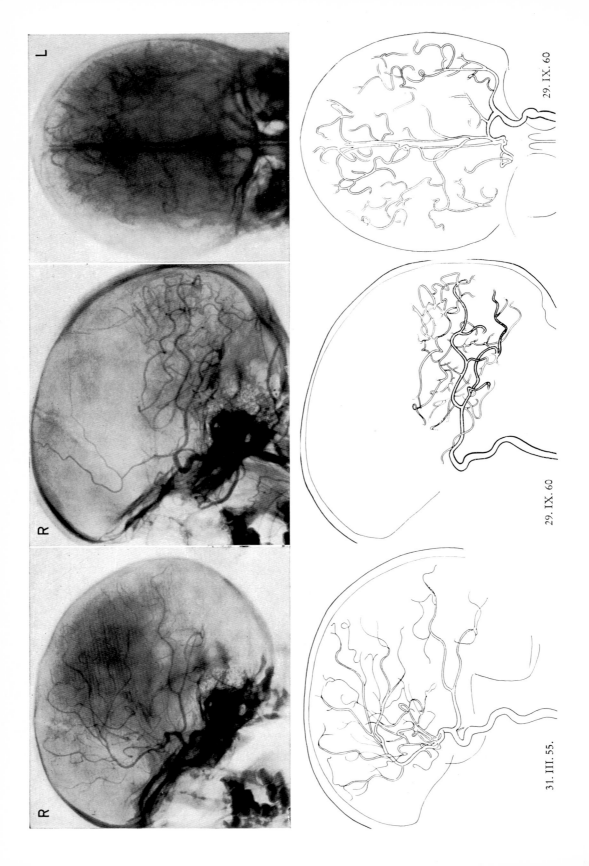

29. IX. 60

29. IX. 60

31. III. 55.

CASE 37

The patient, a perfectly healthy 5-year-old girl, experienced an incomplete left hemiplegia of sudden onset. An initial epileptic attack can in all likelihood be ruled out, since the child at the time of the insult had been left unobserved for less than one minute and was found to be fully conscious after its onset. For two days the position remained stationary, then on the third day the child awakened with a completely paralysed arm; the face and leg remained only partially affected.

Carotid angiography revealed the cause to be a partial occlusion of the middle cerebral artery, with some of its branches receiving a collateral blood supply from the anterior cerebral vessels (Fig. 50).

Over the course of months the neurological deficit improved, but a slight spastic hemiparesis remained, involving the distal part of the arm most severely. Both left extremities showed retardation of growth. A remarkable feature was the absence of a psycho-organic syndrome.

Follow-up carotid angiography 5 years later revealed that the right middle cerebral artery had become totally occluded, its branches receiving a rich collateral blood supply partly from the right posterior cerebral group and partly from the right anterior cerebral vessels which were filling from the left side (Fig. 50).

Thus a progressive thrombosis of the right middle cerebral artery must have taken place during the recovery phase of the hemiparesis. Clearly the collateral circulation over the right hemisphere was adequate to ensure no further deficit.

The cause of the initial middle cerebral artery occlusion remained unexplained. No clinical evidence of embolism could be found. It is possible that an episode of primary arterial spasm led to secondary thrombosis, or perhaps thrombosis was a primary event accompanying a subclinical infection.

Nine and a half years after the insult, the patient experienced an attack of headache and unsteadiness lasting only a few minutes. An EEG then showed epilepsy potentials for the first time, prompting the suspicion of an epileptic equivalent. The child was placed on anticonvulsants, and has remained free from attacks for two years. Recently she passed her final examinations at a high school.

CASE 38

At the age of 14½ years this boy exhibited, suddenly and without previous warning, the apoplectiform onset of a left hemiplegia without epileptic manifestations or loss of consciousness. Eleven days later he experienced a severe recurrence of the hemiparesis which was by that time already regressing. The cause was shown by carotid angiography to be an occlusion of the internal carotid artery. (Fig. 51a). The pathogenesis is not clear. The first angiogram revealed interruption of the contrast column in the internal carotid artery at the level of its entry into the skull base, while repeat examination two days later showed it to be at the distal end of the carotid siphon. Follow-up examination 15 months later revealed completely normal appearances of the middle cerebral vessels, but no filling of the anterior cerebral group. If

Facing page: **Fig. 50.** Progressive spontaneous thrombosis in the intracranial bifurcation area of the internal carotid artery. Rich collateral circulation from the opposite side (right) (Case 37).

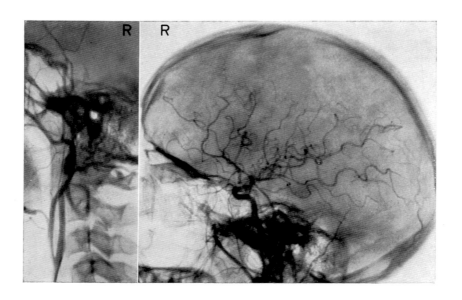

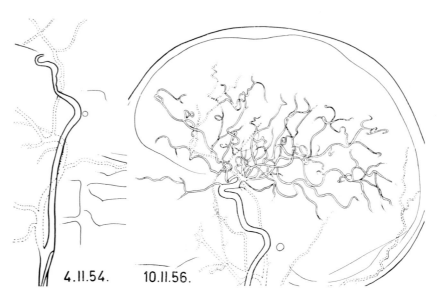

4.II.54.   10.II.56.

Fig. 51a. *Left:* spontaneous occlusion at the carotid siphon. *Right:* follow-up angiogram 15 months later. Complete filling of middle cerebral artery, but anterior cerebral artery not visualised (thrombotic occlusion?) (Case 38).

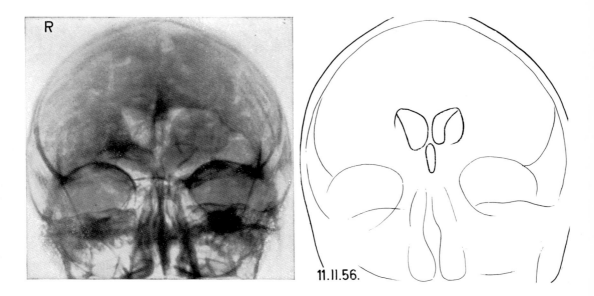

Fig. 51*b*. Pneumoencephalogram 15 months after the insult. No signs of hemispherical atrophy!
(Case 38).

this was a case of thrombosis, then recanalisation had occurred. While the absence of filling of the anterior cerebral artery may be attributed to a permanent thrombosis at its origin, it is possible that its origin was hypoplastic and that the anterior vessels received their supply from the left internal carotid artery via the anterior communicating artery. Unfortunately no answer can be supplied to this problem, since left carotid angiography was not performed. Embolism should also be considered in the pathogenesis, although there were no clinical features in the case history to suggest it. Finally, transient spasm should be discussed: this theory is supported by the two distinct levels of obstruction demonstrated in the first two angiograms made two days apart, and also by the patency of the arterial tree 15 months later (Fig. 51*a*).

As a result of the severe circulatory disturbance, a significant spastic hemiplegia remained present clinically. Despite prolonged physiotherapy, the hand remained useless, but the leg showed some measure of recovery and the patient was left only with a slight limp. Jacksonian epileptic attacks commenced one year after the insult, and these have been successfully controlled by regular drug treatment during the past ten years. A noteworthy feature is the absence of any intellectual deficit, the patient being employed full-time as a bank official after successfully completing a commercial course.

CASE 39

The patient, a healthy 17-year-old boy, suffered without warning an apoplectiform attack which left him hemiplegic; there was no loss of consciousness or evidence of

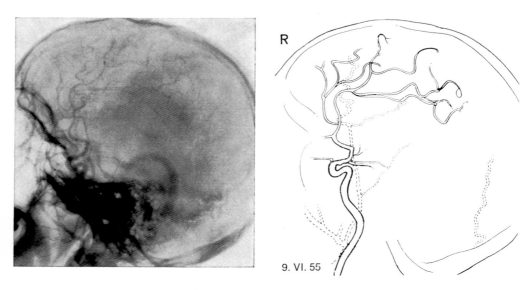

Fig. 52a. Spontaneous occlusion of a middle cerebral artery at its origin (Case 39).

9. VI. 55

R

epilepsy. The cause was shown by carotid angiography to be an occlusion of the middle cerebral artery (Fig. 52a). Pneumoencephalography 3 weeks after the attack revealed a normal ventricular system, but repeat examination 18 months later revealed definite atrophy of the ipsilateral hemisphere (Fig. 52b). One year after the arterial occlusion the patient began to experience epileptiform attacks, which undoubtedly emanated from the atrophic hemisphere. Repeated EEGs over the next 5 years revealed persistent depression over the affected hemisphere but no evidence of epilepsy potentials. A considerable degree of spastic hemiparesis remained, including a functionally useless hand, but only a minor disturbance of gait and an organic psychosyndrome. Length of history: 11 years.

The pathogenesis of the middle cerebral artery occlusion was not clear. No evidence of systemic disease could be demonstrated.

CASE 40

At the age of 9 years, the patient, a girl, suffered an insignificant head injury without definite signs of cerebral concussion. Three weeks later she suddenly developed a complete right hemiplegia with motor aphasia and hemisensory disturbance; there was no loss of consciousness or evidence of epilepsy. The insult was heralded by two days of mild general disturbances consisting of lassitude and sporadic headaches. Carotid angiography revealed a segment of severe stenosis of the middle cerebral artery, with defective filling of the middle cerebral branches, abnormally thin insular arteries and marked extravasation in the left parietal region (Fig. 53). Exploratory craniotomy revealed an extensive area of softening in the white matter of the left hemisphere.

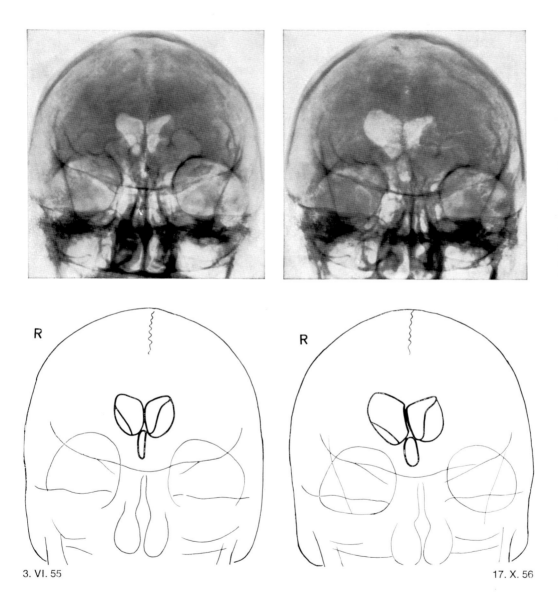

R

R

3. VI. 55

17. X. 56

Fig. 52*b*. *Left:* slight enlargement of the right lateral ventricle 1 month after the arterial occlusion. *Right:* definite atrophy of the right hemisphere 16 months later (Case 39).

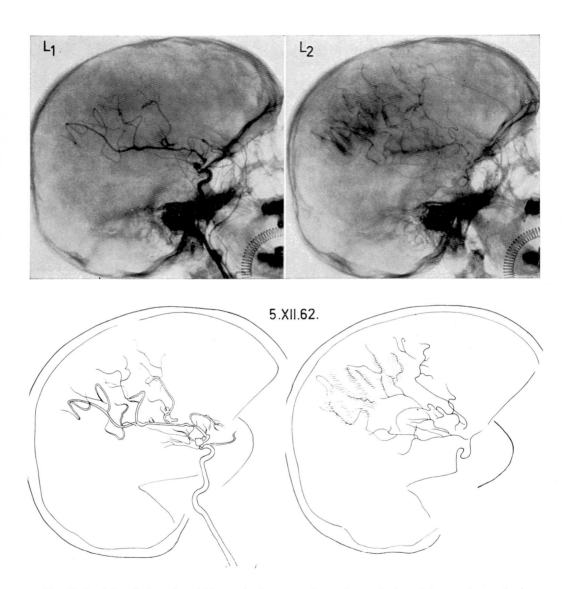

5.XII.62.

Fig. 53. Partial occlusion of a middle cerebral artery and complete occlusion of the anterior cerebral artery. Haemorrhagic softening in the parietal region, shown by irregular contrast opacification (Case 40).

92

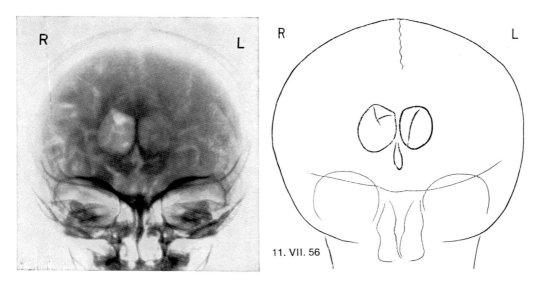

11. VII. 56

Fig. 54a. Pneumoencephalogram 6 weeks after partial occlusion of the right middle cerebral artery in acute myocarditis. Atrophy of the right hemisphere with slight enlargement of the right lateral ventricle and displacement of the ventricular system to the right side (Case 41).

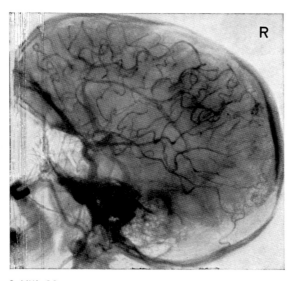

Fig. 54b. Normal carotid angiogram 10 years after partial occlusion of the middle cerebral artery (Case 41).

8. VIII. 66

93

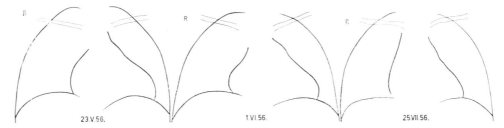

Fig. 55. Line drawings of chest radiographs made during and after recovery in a case of acute myocarditis (Case 41).

There can be no doubt of the vascular cause of the apoplectiform hemiplegia. However, the actual mechanism of provocation of the insult is not clear: it could have been a traumatic dissecting aneurysm, thrombosis or embolism. The irregular angiographic appearances of the arterial lumen prompt consideration of fibromuscular hyperplasia. Primary cerebral haemorrhage, *e.g.* from a microangioma, is considered unlikely. A spontaneous thrombosis is presumed to be the cause, possibly secondary to a traumatic dissecting aneurysm. The absence of clinical evidence of organic heart disease is against an embolism.

Clinically, a severe spastic hemiparesis, with a complete loss of function of the right hand and a moderate disturbance of gait, has remained, and the patient has a definite organic psychosyndrome. No epileptic attacks have been observed in the four years following the insult.

CASE 41

The patient, a girl, experienced at the age of 2 years and 4 months, an apoplectiform left hemiplegia, with a brief loss of consciousness but no convulsion, following a previous febrile upper respiratory tract infection. Carotid angiography revealed the presence of a subtotal occlusion of the right middle cerebral artery (unfortunately the film was lost). Clinical evidence of an acute endomyocarditis was present (Fig. 55). It is not clear whether the intracranial lesion was caused by an embolism or an arterial thrombosis. Follow-up carotid angiography performed 10 years later revealed recanalisation of the occluded branch arteries (Fig. 54b), an outcome compatible with either mechanism: in the case of embolism this would indicate disintegration of the embolus or its passage into a smaller peripheral vessel, and in the case of thrombosis a simple recanalisation.

The hemiparesis remained flaccid for several weeks and was then gradually transformed into a severe spastic state. Another effect of the cerebral ischaemia was an organic psychosyndrome of moderate severity, which led to a marked reduction in the intellectual capacity of the patient.

A remarkable feature of the case is the fact that, despite the lack of prophylactic drug treatment due to parental objection and the presence of epileptic discharges in the EEG, the patient has experienced only one definite attack of epilepsy, which occurred 9 years after the insult.

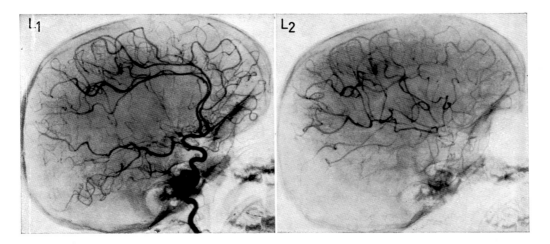

Fig. 56. Post-infectious occlusion of a middle cerebral artery. Rich collateral circulation through branches of the anterior and posterior cerebral arteries (right) (Case 42).

CASE 42

This girl, at the age of 14 months, suffered an acute subtotal flaccid right hemiplegia in the course of a mild cold. The hemiplegia developed stepwise over 24 hours, and at one stage clonic seizures were observed.

Carotid angiography performed 12 days after the onset of the hemiplegia revealed the presence of an occlusion of the middle cerebral artery (Fig. 56). Pneumoencephalography (performed on the sixth day of the illness) revealed a displacement of the ventricular system to the right side, a feature interpreted to indicate the presence of oedema of the left hemisphere. The EEG revealed a massive depression over the corresponding half of the brain.

With regular physiotherapy the child made a remarkable recovery. Five years later only a slight spastic hemiparesis remained, with minimal functional incapacity of the right hand. No intellectual deficit had yet appeared, and the girl started school quite normally soon after her 6th birthday. No epileptic attacks have so far occurred, and no drug treatment has been prescribed.

CASE 43

This girl, at the age of 14 months, exhibited an acute flaccid hemiplegia (which later became spastic), accompanied by a bout of fever which lasted 5 days. The course of events can no longer be precisely reconstructed, since details of the attack were obtained from statements made 15 years later. Carotid angiography revealed a subtotal occlusion of the middle cerebral artery, with retrograde filling of the affected areas by collateral channels from branches of the anterior cerebral artery (Fig. 57a). Pneumoencephalography (Fig. 57b) surprisingly showed no evidence of atrophy of the affected hemisphere, a finding which contrasted with the severity of the spastic

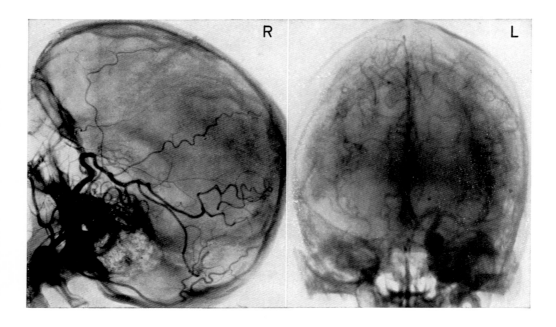

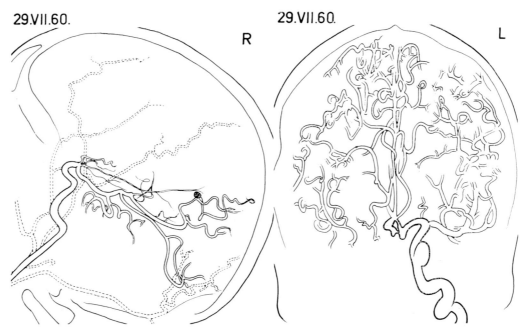

Fig. 57a. Carotid angiogram made 15 years after para-infectious occlusion of the intracranial carotid artery. *Left*: middle and anterior cerebral arteries occluded. Posterior cerebral artery well filled via the posterior communicating artery. Branches of the external carotid are shown as dotted lines in the line drawing. *Right*: rich collateral circulation from the opposite side (Case 43).

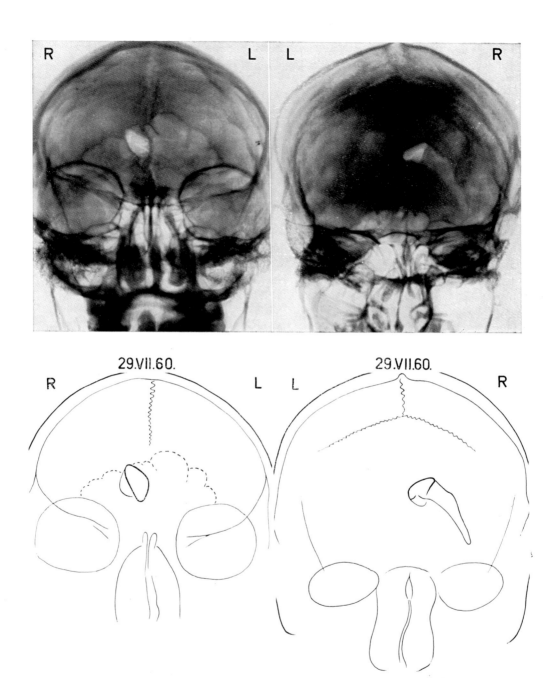

Fig. 57*b*. Pneumoencephalogram made 15 years after the insult. Only the right lateral ventricle, *i.e.* on the side of the arterial occlusion, is filled and appears normal. No signs of hemispherical atrophy! (Case 43).

hemiplegia. It is possible that occlusion of the lenticulostriate arteries prevented recovery from the severe motor deficit, while the rich collateral circulation protected the patient from hemispherical atrophy.

No definite cause can be advanced for the middle cerebral artery occlusion. It is presumed to have been the result of an inflammatory thrombosis.

Case 44

This girl, at the age of 1½ years, experienced an apoplectiform flaccid right hemiplegia with motor aphasia about one week after recovery from pneumonia; there was no loss of consciousness and no accompanying epileptic phenomena. Carotid angiography revealed an occlusion of the middle cerebral artery (Fig. 58a). It seems highly likely that the initial attack resulted in the acute hemiplegia. The lower limb paralysis was initially overlooked and only confirmed subsequently.

The aetiology is presumed to have been a thrombosis of the cerebral artery, associated with the clinically cured pneumonia. The question of embolism must be raised although, in the absence of clinical evidence of a heart defect, this diagnosis must be considered unlikely.

The carotid angiogram demonstrated impressively the development of a collateral circulation, with retrograde filling of the main branches of the occluded middle cerebral artery from the anterior cerebral group. However, this circulation was either functionally inadequate or perhaps developed too late to compensate for the occluded lenticulostriate arteries. A severe spastic hemiparesis remained present, with marked underdevelopment of the affected extremities, particularly the arm. However, the motor aphasia regressed completely (did the centre for speech migrate to the other side?).

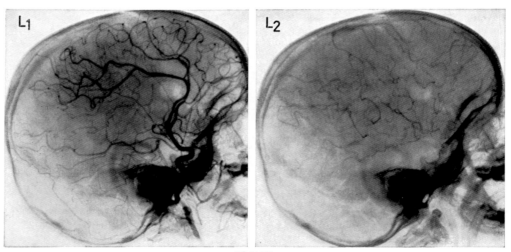

18.II.57

Fig. 58a. Post-infectious occlusion of the middle cerebral artery. *Right:* weak collateral circulation through the ipsilateral pericallosal artery (Case 44).

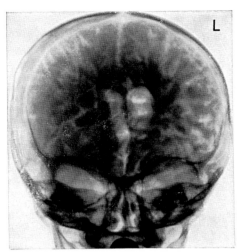

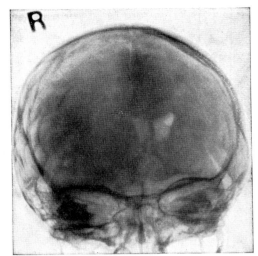

14. II. 57

18. XI. 66

Fig. 58*b*. Progressive hemispherical atrophy. *Left:* pneumoencephalogram 3 weeks after the insult. Enlargement of the left lateral ventricle and displacement of the ventricular system to the left side. *Right:* pneumoencephalogram 10 years later. Massive atrophy of the left hemisphere (Fig. 44).

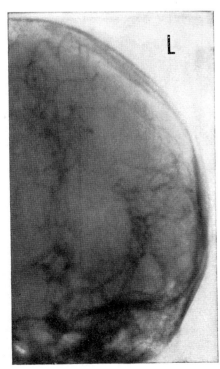

Fig. 58*c*. Follow-up angiogram 10 years after the insult. Recanalisation of the occluded middle cerebral artery (Case 44).

18. XI. 66

99

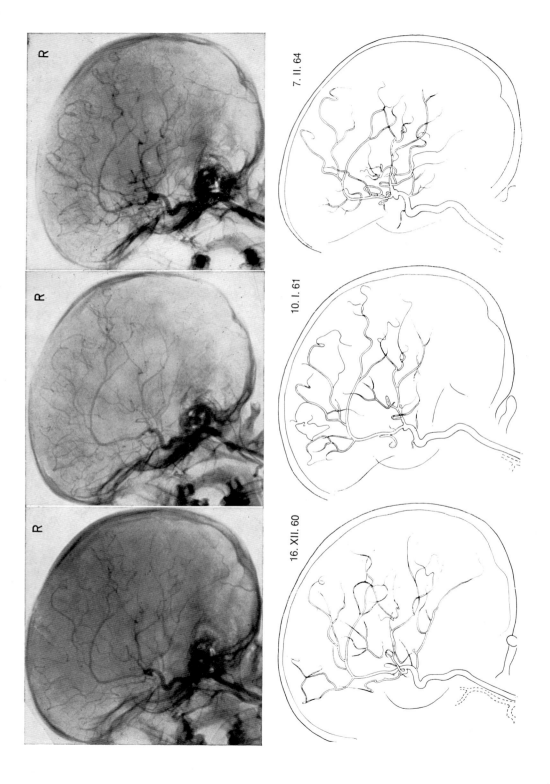

The hemispherical atrophy demonstrated in the pneumoencephalogram (Fig. 58b) made 3 weeks after the insult must be attributed to the acute circulatory disturbance and not to any pre-existing cause.

After a 9-year interval free from attacks, the patient experienced an epileptic hemiseizure for the first time. It may be noted that a routine EEG made two weeks later revealed no epilepsy potentials, and that an epileptogenic focus was revealed only by a sleep tracing.

Carotid angiography performed 9 years after the insult revealed that the occluded middle cerebral artery had recanalised (Fig. 58c). A pneumoencephalogram made 10 years after the insult showed a markedly atrophic ipsilateral hemisphere, but no significant dilatation of the lateral ventricle (Fig. 58b).

Apart from the permanent severe spastic hemiplegia with limb atrophy, a definite unilateral diminution of superficial and deep sensibility was present. It is impossible to judge whether the loss of motor function could have been further minimised, had the parents been more co-operative concerning follow-up physiotherapy. A considerable organic psychosyndrome was present, as reflected by the child's IQ of 62.

CASE 45

The patient, a girl aged 5 years and 3 months, was found lying in the street, unsteady and drowsy and giving confused answers, 1-2 hours after a minor injury with no evidence of brain damage. Three weeks prior to this collapse, she had undergone tonsillectomy and this had been followed by a simple attack of measles; recovery from both was complete. On admission to hospital she had an incomplete flaccid left-sided hemiplegia. An interesting feature was the preservation of active finger movements in the presence of complete paralysis of the proximal muscles of the arm.

Carotid angiography revealed the cause of the acute hemiparesis to be a partial thrombosis of the middle cerebral artery, with retrograde opacification of the opercular and insular arteries (Fig. 59). Follow-up angiography $3\frac{1}{2}$ weeks later revealed identical findings, but 6 months later recanalisation of one of the anterior insular arteries had occurred. A follow-up angiogram made 3 years later revealed no further recanalisation, the posterior insular and the opercular arteries opacifying as before through retrograde channels. Pneumoencephalograms made 7 months and 3 years after the insult revealed a moderate progressive atrophy of the right cerebral hemisphere.

The aetiology of the vascular occlusion is not clear. A mild leucocytosis with a neutrophilia and a shift to the left, as well as a mildly raised ESR, represented no more than a vague indication of an inflammatory thrombosis; thus some connection could have existed with the tonsillectomy 3 weeks previously or with the attack of measles from which the patient had just recovered.

Despite the use of vasodilator treatment (Papaverine), the hemiparesis regressed only partially over the course of weeks, and regular physiotherapy during the

Facing page: Fig. 59. Post-infectious partial occlusion of the middle cerebral artery. *Middle:* findings unchanged one month after the insult. *Right:* recanalisation of one of the formerly occluded insular arteries 3 years later (Case 45).

succeeding $5\frac{1}{2}$ years produced no further improvement. A further result was a definite infantile organic psychosyndrome.

The EEG findings were interesting: in the acute phase immediately after the insult a marked focal depression of cerebral activity was present over the affected hemisphere, which had completely disappeared one month later. The generalised epilepsy noted immediately after the onset appeared to increase in intensity later on. However, no clinical attacks were observed over a period of $5\frac{1}{2}$ years. This result is attributed to the success of prophylactic drug treatment (phenobarbitone).

For more detailed reports of CASES *33-45 see pages 241-255.*

CHAPTER 14

Fetal Cerebral Arterial Occlusions

There is general agreement that the most common cause of hemiplegia or hemiparetic cerebral palsy is brain damage sustained at the time of birth (hypoxaemia, intracranial haemorrhage, mechanical trauma). However, as long ago as 1868 Cotard (and later Kundrat (1882) and others) produced evidence at autopsy of arterial occlusions as the cause of congenital hemiplegia. Eicke (1947) attributed endarteritic cerebral arterial occlusion to fetal meningitis. Bertrand and Bargeton (1955) produced analogous findings and discussed the occurrence not only of endarteritic changes but also of thrombosis or embolism secondary to chronic fetal meningitis.

Clark and Linell (1954) described the case of an infant of short gestation with an internal carotid artery occlusion. The authors assumed the cause to be a paradoxical fetal embolism of necrotic placental tissues. Cocker *et al.* (1965) described two infants with occlusion of the middle cerebral artery, confirmed at autopsy, and attributed pathogenically to an embolism from a fetal placental vein. These authors made the significant observation (supported by van Creveld's coagulation studies in neonates, 1959) that thrombotic or embolic arterial occlusions in the neonatal period are subject to prompt dissolution and recanalisation. It can, therefore, be understood why arterial occlusions are so rarely observed at subsequent autopsy examinations.

Larroche and Amiel (1966) described two additional cases proven at autopsy. In the first of these the middle cerebral artery thrombosis or endarteritis had definitely occurred during intra-uterine life, while in the other a perinatal embolic occlusion of the artery was present, which the authors considered to be an iatrogenic thrombo-embolism from the umbilical vein which had occurred during exchange transfusion. They referred to a report by Farber and Vawter (1964) of a case of fatal pulmonary embolism occurring in association with a fourth exchange transfusion.

In this series the diagnosis of fetal or perinatal cerebral arterial occlusion was made in 3 children on the basis of carotid angiography and pneumoencephalography (CASES 46, 47, 48). These children were aged respectively $3\frac{1}{2}$ months, 4 years and $7\frac{1}{2}$ years at the time of diagnosis. In CASE 47 there can be no doubt that the middle cerebral artery occlusion occurred during fetal life; the child was born a microcephalic. The problem arises in the other 2 children of whether review several years later can justify attributing the arterial occlusion to the fetal or perinatal period. According to Prichard (1964), a congenital cerebral hemiplegia resulting from near-complete absence of cerebral myelinisation above the tentorium in neonates would not be clinically recognisable before the second or third month of life. However, it is difficult to imagine that a complete occlusion of a middle cerebral artery with massive parenchymal necrosis could occur after birth and pass unnoticed.

A noteworthy feature of the 3 cases in this series was the great range of clinical deficits. CASE 46 showed the least deficit, probably because of the presence of the intact proximal segment of the middle cerebral artery, including the anterior insular arteries and the lenticulostriate arteries (Fig. 60b). In this baby girl the motor deficit was observed for the first time at the age of 2 years! In CASE 47, total occlusion of one middle cerebral artery resulted in the remarkable clinical finding of a complete symmetrical spastic tetraparesis. Presumably the contralateral hemisphere was also considerably damaged, although its lateral ventricle was only slightly enlarged (Fig. 61a).

In CASE 48 the 'hypoplasia' of one carotid artery (Fig. 62b) merits special mention. This finding was assumed to be secondary to a fetal or perinatal thrombosis of undetermined cause, and not a congenital variant. In this case, it must be assumed that an adequate collateral circulation had developed from the opposite side. Cases have been reported of carotid aplasia or hypoplasia resulting from defective embryonal development, which occurred both unilaterally (Töndury 1934, Lagarde et al. 1957, Priman and Christie 1959, Burmester and Stender 1961, Turnbull 1962, Tharp et al. 1965, Lhermitte et al. 1968) and bilaterally (Hills and Sament 1968). Such malformations are often accompanied by other defects, particularly saccular arterial aneurysms.

Fisher (1959) reported two remarkable cases of unilateral atrophy of the internal carotid arteries occurring after apparent thrombosis in early life. Both patients died of cerebral haemorrhage from dilated collateral vessels.

CASE 46

After normal pregnancy and birth, and after the major infantile milestones had been normally passed, it was noticed that this girl had a clumsiness of the left hand.

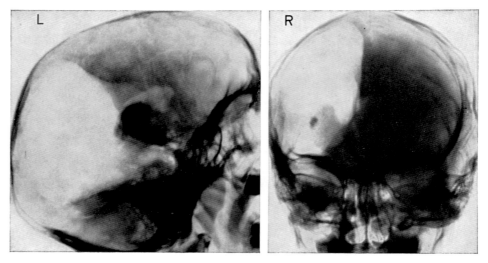

Fig. 60a. Extensive porencephaly in the territory of the middle cerebral artery distribution (Case 46).

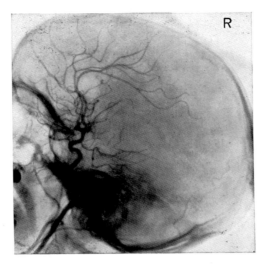

Fig. 60b. Fetal occlusion of the middle cerebral artery (Case 46).

At the age of 6½ years she began to experience attacks of a psychomotor nature (dreamy states).

At the age of 7 years and 10 months she was found to have a spastic left hemiparesis of medium severity involving particularly the arm, as well as a left homonymous hemianopia. The cause was shown to be a huge porencephalic cyst in the territory of supply of the right middle cerebral artery. Carotid angiography revealed the presence of an occlusion of the middle cerebral artery distal to the origin of the posterior insular vessels (Fig. 60b).

Follow-up examination at the age of 14½ years revealed a considerable disturbance of deep sensibility, and a slight disturbance of superficial sensibility, practically confined to the left arm (the leg was intact).

The clinical history made it likely that the time of onset of the middle cerebral artery occlusion was during fetal life. An attack as severe as this one after birth would almost certainly have produced a severe acute clinical picture.

The intellectual deficit in the patient was comparatively small. Prophylactic drug treatment was almost completely effective in suppressing symptomatic epilepsy.

CASE 47

This child was born a microcephalic and underweight, after a completely normal pregnancy and delivery at term. Clinical examination at the age of 3½ months revealed a severe degree of symmetrical cerebral palsy.

The surprising discovery of a huge porencephalic cyst of the right cerebral hemisphere (Fig. 61a) correlated with the angiographic demonstration of an occlusion

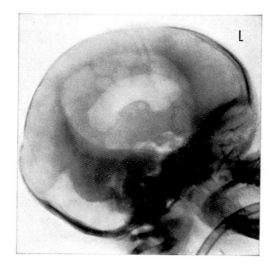

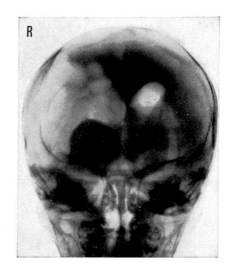

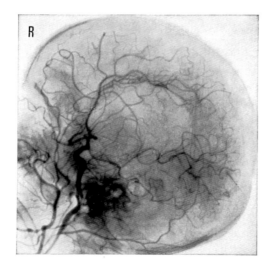

Fig. 61a (*above*). Extensive porencephaly in the territory of the middle cerebral artery distribution (Case 47).

Fig. 61b (*left*). Fetal occlusion of the middle cerebral artery (Case 47).

of the middle cerebal artery (Fig. 61b). This occlusion had undoubtedly occurred during fetal life, probably following a thrombosis which cut off the blood supply to the affected parts of the hemisphere.

Enlargement of the left lateral ventricle, and slight enlargement of the fourth ventricle in the presence of a very large cerebello-medullary cistern, combined with the bilateral abnormality of the EEG, indicated the widespread nature of the intra-uterine damage. A noteworthy feature was the symmetrical clinical nature of the cerebral palsy, with the absence of growth disturbances of the contralateral extremities, in the presence of a massive unilateral porencephaly of vascular origin.

106

CASE 48

The right hemiparesis which was first noticed in the fourth month of life was caused by an occlusion of the left common carotid artery (Fig. 62b). The ipsilateral cerebral hemisphere showed a massive degree of atrophy (Fig. 62a). The pathogenesis is a matter of speculation: a thrombotic occlusion during fetal life is thought to be the most likely explanation. The case history supports this view, since the hemiparesis was noted by the parents to have developed over a period of time. If the thrombotic occlusion had been a postnatal event, e.g. occurring during an influenzal infection at the age of 4 months, a dramatic acute disease picture, including an obvious hemiplegia, would have been present. The differential diagnosis should also include congenital aplasia of the carotid artery, although the author believes the latter to be extremely unlikely in view of the gross cerebral hemispherical atrophy; one of the features of such an aplasia would be a well-developed collateral circulation through arteries on the circle of Willis—a feature not demonstrated in the angiogram (Fig. 62b).

For more detailed reports of CASES *46-48 see pages 257-259.*

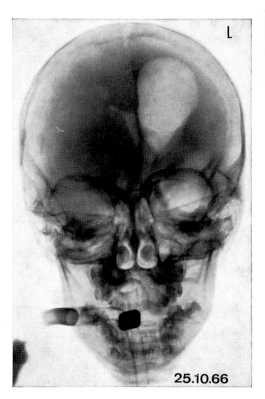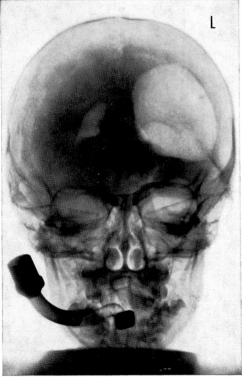

Fig. 62a. Massive atrophy of the left hemisphere, with displacement of the ventricular system to the left side and enormous enlargement of the ipsilateral ventricle (Case 48).

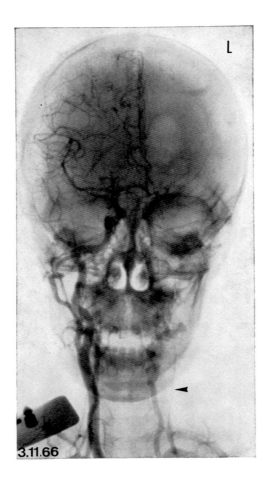

Fig. 62*b*. Fetal occlusion of the carotid artery in the neck. Arch angiogram. The left common carotid is unusually thin in its origin from the aorta, and shows progressive narrowing of its lumen (arrow) and complete interruption of the contrast column in the region of the bifurcation. No filling of the left internal carotid artery or its branches. Normal filling of the right carotid and both vertebral arteries (Case 48).

CHAPTER 15

Vasospasm

In scarcely any field of cerebral pathophysiology do the views of physiologically-oriented clinicians and others differ so fundamentally as over the phenomenon of vasospasm. The question is whether ischaemic cerebral insults may occur as a result of cerebral vasoconstriction.

Schneider (1961), Bernsmeier (1963) and others reject the theory of neurovasomotor spasm producing ischaemic deficits. They argue that the tone of the cerebral vessels is autonomic in type and is not mediated by the sympathetic nervous system. The cerebral arteries have few autonomic nerve fibres, and, except for the vessels of the circle of Willis, there are only elastic-type arteries in the brain. Therefore vasoactive drugs have little or no effect on the cerebral circulation, and the threshold levels for satisfactory stimulation are higher than those in other vascular territories. Metabolic factors (oxygen deprivation in the tissues, an increase in the carbon dioxide tension of the arterial blood) have by far the greatest effect on the cerebral circulation.

The authors mentioned above, as well as a number of other workers including Pickering (1951) and Denny-Brown (1951), regard the commonest cause of so-called 'vasospastic cerebral insult' to be disturbances of the extracerebral circulation (*e.g.* acute haemodynamic insufficiency), in lesions involving the cerebral circulation such as arteriosclerosis. In such cases cerebral ischaemia does not result from an active vasospastic process in a cerebral artery, but the cerebral perfusion becomes inadequate because of a disturbed systemic circulation.

On the other hand, there can be no doubt of the existence of local reversible constrictions of cerebral arteries in patients with intact cardiovascular systems. This type of vasospasm is most typically seen in cases of ruptured aneurysm (Pool 1958, Fletcher *et al.* 1959, Du Boulay 1963, Allègre *et al.* 1963, Krayenbühl and Yasargil 1965). Arterial spasm has also been observed in cases of head injury (Friedenfelt and Lundström 1963), raised intracranial pressure (Krayenbühl and Yasargil 1965), and migraine accompagnée (Dukes and Vieth 1964, see page 173). Lende (1960) and Raynor and Ross (1960) reported analogous findings following experimental mechanical stimulation. Buckle *et al.* (1964) published the case report of a 16-year-old girl who died following a vasospastic cerebral insult, presumably migrainous. Angiography revealed extreme narrowing of the internal carotid artery and its branches at the level of the cavernous sinus, while the proximal vessels were of normal calibre. At autopsy severe ischaemic parenchymal lesions were demonstrated in the vasospastic territory; however, the blood vessels themselves were intact.

The angiographic observation of spastic cerebral arteries has been the subject of unusually sharp criticism, which has been expressed in detail by Tönnis and Schiefer (1958). It is well known that spastic vascular changes very commonly accompany poor technique in cerebral angiography, whereas they rarely accompany a skilled technique. The author has observed—on the basis of more than 500 carotid angiograms performed under general anaesthesia in children—that vasospasm recurred in patients in whom the clinical picture suggested the presence of a vascular disturbance; on the other hand, it was extremely rare in patients with an intact vascular system (cerebral tumour, abscess, cerebral malformation). It is therefore concluded that an abnormal, functionally labile vascular situation leading to vasospasm is present in the former group. Three cases from the author's series will serve as illustrations. In CASE 49 a generalised status epilepticus with post-ictal hemiplegia occurred in association with a simple upper respiratory tract infection. The carotid angiogram, performed under general anaesthesia and without technical difficulty (one puncture only made at the first attempt), revealed gross spasm in the terminal segment of the internal carotid artery. Upon repeated contrast injections, and also at subsequent follow-up examination, a normal vascular pattern was shown (Figs. 63a and b). CASE 50, a child with hemiseizures occurring during an intestinal infection and post-ictal hemiplegia, exhibited unusually narrow cerebral vessels in the presence of a normal internal carotid artery (Fig. 65a).

In CASE 51, angiospastic occlusion of the anterior cerebral artery must be assumed. The first contrast injection revealed a completely normal vascular tree. During the second injection the point of the needle was inadvertently displaced towards the head, so that it came in contact with the carotid bulb. In the serial films obtained, the anterior cerebral artery failed to fill, while good filling of the internal carotid and middle cerebral arteries, including their peripheral branches, was obtained. At the same time, the vertebral and basilar arteries filled in a retrograde direction. The third injection, made after withdrawal of the needle into the common carotid, again showed normal opacification of the anterior cerebral artery (Fig. 66). The uniform and dense contrast opacification of the internal carotid artery rules out the phenomenon of laminar flow as a cause. Another possible explanation is a sudden fall in blood pressure following stimulation of the carotid bulb, causing collapse of the anterior cerebral artery. Against this theory is the good opacification of the middle cerebral branches into the peripheral fields, as well as the retrograde filling of the basilar artery as far as the junction of the vertebral arteries.

The author believes that vasospasm—at least in children—produces ischaemic deficits which are usually reversible. A causative factor (e.g. inflammation, abnormal metabolic products, trauma) is usually present to cause irritation of the cerebral vessels.

CASE 49

The patient, at the age of 15 months, experienced an attack of sunstroke shortly after an upper respiratory tract infection. Immediately afterwards she exhibited status epilepticus lasting several hours. A residual hemiplegia followed, at first flaccid but later spastic, but no significant intellectual deficit occurred. The cause of the status epilepticus was not clear: the negative clinical findings tended to rule out an acute infection.

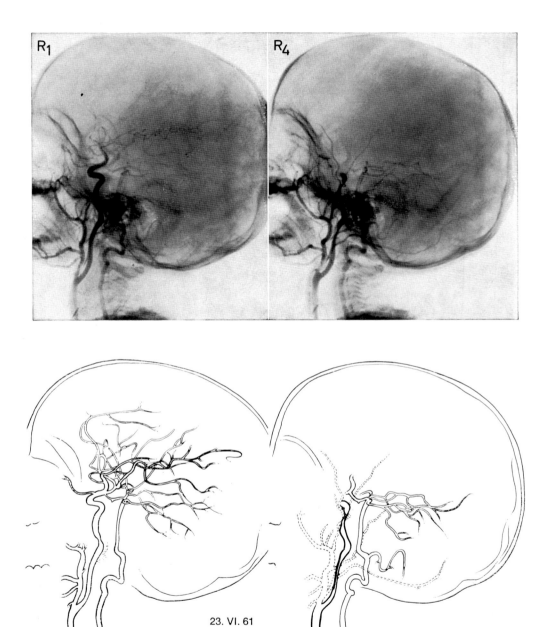

Fig. 63a. Vasospasm in the course of carotid angiography. *Left:* first contrast injection, early phase. *Right:* second contrast injection, early phase (see Fig. 63b) (Case 49).

111

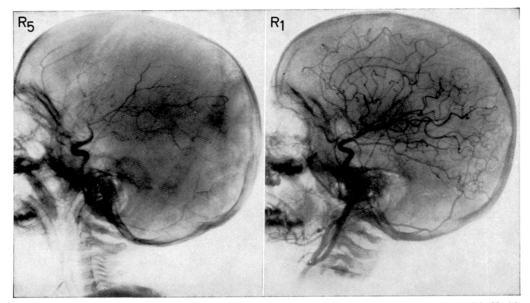

R₅   R₁

21. X. 62

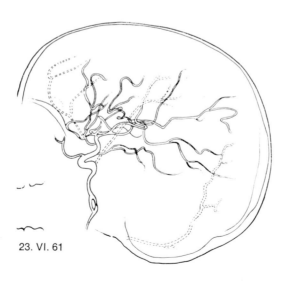

23. VI. 61

Fig. 63*b. Above left:* second contrast injection, late phase. *Above right:* follow-up angiogram 15 months later, showing normal appearances. *Left:* line drawing of above left. (see text, case 49).

112

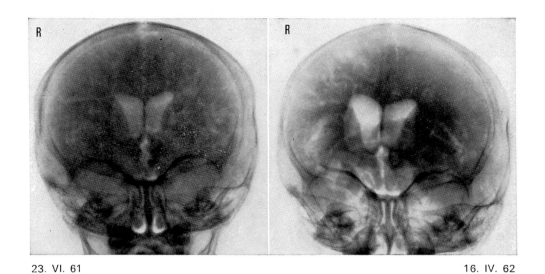

23. VI. 61   16. IV. 62

Fig. 64. *Above left:* normal pneumoencephalogram at the time of the vasospasm.
Above right: definite atrophy of the right hemisphere 10 months later.

Right: bilateral hemispherical atrophy 4 months later (Case 49).

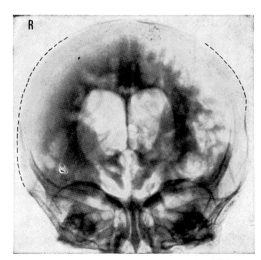

15. VIII. 62

According to the mother, who appeared to be a reliable witness, the epileptic seizures were all of a generalised nature, and no lateralising features, apart from conjugate deviation of the eyes to the left side, were present. Carotid angiography provided an explanation for the appearance of a permanent hemiparesis, namely severe spasm of the internal carotid artery and its branches (Figs. 63a and b).

Naturally, it is impossible to ignore the valid objection that the fluctuating vasospasm present with the three contrast injections in this patient might have been the result of the examination itself. While this is a possibility, it is thought to be unlikely, because no technical difficulty was experienced with the arterial puncture, and no contrast medium was injected intramurally or paravasally. The author believes that a circulatory deficit of the right hemisphere led to irreversible damage during the status epilepticus when the oxygen demand of the affected brain tissue was greatest. Two features support this view: firstly, the right hemisphere atrophy was not present during the acute phase but developed later, as demonstrated in the first pneumo-encephalogram; secondly, follow-up carotid angiography $1\frac{1}{2}$ years later revealed a completely normal vascular tree. No explanation can be advanced for the cause of the vasospasm.

The patient's subsequent course took a tragic turn. During an acute hyperpyrexial infection 9 months later, a second status epilepticus occurred, which severely affected the right side of the body. Gross atrophy of the left hemisphere followed. Unfortunately, a left carotid angiogram was not performed.

CASE 50

This girl from a severely handicapped family appeared to develop normally until the age of about 2 years. During an intestinal infection she experienced an attack of severe hemiconvulsions which resulted in a permanent hemiplegia. A hydrocephalus was demonstrated (Fig. 65b), which had probably been present long before the convulsive attack. Carotid angiography revealed diffuse narrowing of all the intracranial arteries in the presence of an internal carotid artery of normal calibre (Fig. 65a). Unfortunately, no angiogram of the opposite carotid artery was made.

CASE 51

This 10-month-old girl exhibited unusual angiographic findings. During investigation of a severe postictal hemiplegia following hemistatus epilepticus which occurred during an acute intestinal infection, a carotid angiogram was performed (three injections for an antero-posterior series and stereoscopic lateral series). The arterial puncture and injection, made under general anaesthesia administered by an anaesthetist, presented no technical difficulty. The first angiogram series showed normal appearances. Before the second injection, the needle was advanced further up the artery and its point directed into the mouth of the internal carotid artery. The injection was made without incident. Immediately preceding and following it, the heart rate was controlled by the anaesthetist who noted nothing unusual. However, the second angiogram series showed defective filling of the intracranial vessels: the anterior cerebral artery and its branches failed to opacify, and the middle cerebral group were considerably narrower in calibre and more weakly opacified than they were in the

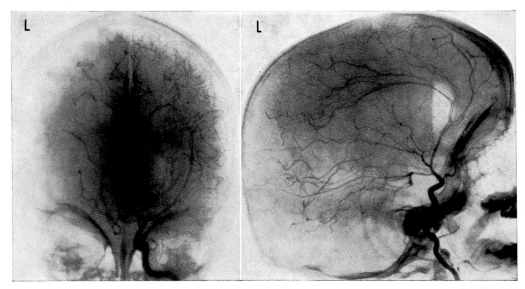

11. VII. 56

Fig. 65*a*. Carotid angiogram following hemistatus epilepticus. Abnormally thin cerebral arteries with an exceptionally well filled internal carotid artery (Case 50).

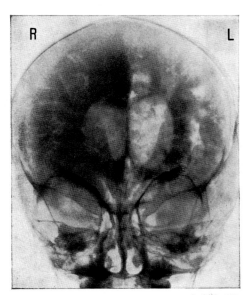

Fig. 65*b*. Progressive internal hydrocephalus (Case 50).

4. VII. 56

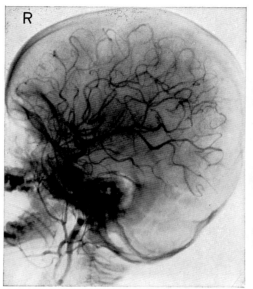

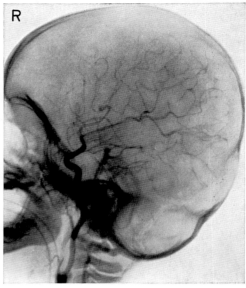

Fig. 66. Spastic occlusion of the anterior cerebral artery during carotid angiography. *Above left:* first contrast injection, blood vessels showing normal appearances. *Above right:* spastic occlusion of the anterior cerebral artery and spastic narrowing of the middle cerebral artery, in the presence of excellent filling of the internal carotid artery. Note retrograde filling of the vertebrobasilar tree.

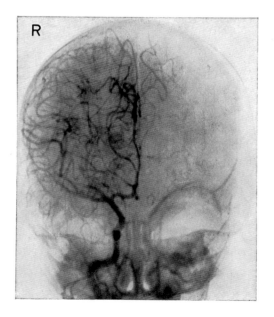

Left: third injection, vessels showing normal appearances (see text, Case 51).

first angiogram series; the internal carotid showed identical appearances following both injections. Retrograde filling of the vertebro-basilar tree was also noted following the second injection (Fig. 66).

This finding illustrates clearly the onset of arterial spasm. An artefact in the sense of a laminar flow phenomenon can be excluded by the uniform and normal opacification of the internal carotid artery. The possibility must be considered of damage to the arterial intima during the contrast injection, producing an acute hypotensive episode. There was no positive evidence of this (unfortunately no serial blood pressure recordings were made). Against this is the retrograde filling of the vertebro-basilar tree, including its peripheral branches, which would not be expected with a severe fall in blood pressure.

CASE 52

In this healthy 7-year-old boy, the pathogenesis of the acute right-sided complete motor hemiplegia, which did not involve the facial muscles or disturb speech, and lasted only a few hours, is a matter of speculation. It was presumed to be a vaso-spastic insult triggered off by a hot bath.

For more detailed reports of CASES *49-52 see pages 260-264.*

PART III

Venous Occlusions

CHAPTER 16

Venous Thrombosis

Intracranial venous thromboses are usually classified into those that are bland, *i.e.* without pyogenic micro-organisms, and those that are septic, *i.e.* infected. The bland form is caused either by changes in the blood components favouring thrombosis, or by damage to the vascular wall, *e.g.* in cases of cyanotic heart disease with polycythaemia and an increased blood viscosity (Byers and Hass 1933, Delille *et al.* 1936, Barnett and Hyland 1953, Weber 1957), in cases of severe dehydration, particularly in infants (Byers and Hass 1933, Toomey and Hutt 1949, Barnett and Hyland 1953), in diabetic coma (Ata 1965), in sickle cell anaemia as a result of the crystallising out of the abnormal haemoglobins in oxygen deficiency (Arena 1935, Greer and Schotland 1962), in therapeutically induced hypercoagulaemia in afibrinogenaemia (Huhn 1965), in thrombotic microangiopathies (O'Brien and Sibley 1958), and in post-traumatic thrombosis in non-penetrating head injuries (Carrie and Jaffé 1954, Pollack 1956, Askenasy *et al.* 1962, Huhn 1965).

In children, septic or infected thrombophlebitis is, in the author's experience, far more common than bland thrombosis. In the vast majority of cases it is caused by a focal infection in the region of the head. The most common cause is a purulent thrombosis of the transverse sinus in otitis media, with or without mastoiditis (Bernheim and Larbre 1956, Ford 1966); also common is involvement of the cavernous sinus due to its close proximity to the tonsils, pharynx and nasal and paranasal cavities. According to Toomey and Hutt (1949) the superior sagittal sinus is the least likely to be the site of an infected thrombosis, either in the course of a purulent meningitis or as a result of retrograde spread of a transverse sinus thrombosis. The anatomical relationships were described in detail by Weber (1957).

The clinical picture depends in the first instance on the site and the extent of the venous occlusion. Cerebral symptoms appear when the thrombosis involves the cerebral veins. In children the disease often runs a dramatic course, even in the presence of bland thrombosis (Carrie and Jaffé 1954). Various disease patterns have been described by Bernheim and Larbre (1956). In septic thrombophlebitis, which is the most common form in children, fever, headache, vomiting and clouding of consciousness are as a rule observed. Focal or generalised epileptic seizures are only rarely absent. The typical 'encephalitic' picture has been particularly emphasised by the French school (Girard and Devic 1954, Bernheim and Larbre 1956, and others).

The most constant abnormal finding in the CSF is an elevated protein level, but this may be absent. The cell count is usually normal or only slightly raised. An admixture of blood or xanthochromia is typical, indicating the presence of a haemorrhagic cerebral infarction; according to Weber (1957) this finding also may not be present.

The author has gained the impression that cases of septic thrombophlebitis have been less frequent since the era of antibiotics, and also perhaps less severe.

This trend was clearly shown in the paper of Toomey and Hutt (1949).

Only those cases of intracranial thrombosis in children accompanied by acute hemiplegia are discussed here. Mitchell (1952) described 10 cases in a paper that has been widely quoted. Supported by the findings of Symonds (1937, 1940) he attributed an acute hemiplegia in a local infection to cerebral venous thrombosis, and believed that many cases of acute hemiplegia in apparently healthy children could be attributed to this mechanism. The diagnosis of cerebral venous thrombosis can be regarded as likely in only one of Mitchell's 10 cases, and then only on the grounds of a visible and palpable thrombosed mastoid emissary vein. In a second case a preretinal haemorrhage in the eye contralateral to the paralysis was advanced as evidence of an intracranial venous thrombosis. Such haemorrhages have been described, for example, in 'otitic hydrocephalus' (Symonds 1931, 1932), a disease entity resulting from intracranial venous thrombosis. Although less common, this phenomenon is also seen in occlusions of the carotid artery (Walsh 1957). In the remaining 8 cases, the diagnosis of cerebral venous thrombosis was made entirely on the basis of the clinical picture. However, as has been pointed out in the previous chapter, identical symptoms may be produced by arterial occlusions. The differential diagnosis can be made in life only by means of angiography, particularly in those cases without a focal infection running a septic course.

Mitchell (1952), in his paper, also discussed the question of a traumatic cause of cerebral venous thrombosis, and rejected it in 3 of his cases with histories of mild head injury. Carrie and Jaffé (1954), on the basis of 2 autopsy cases, provided evidence for the presence of intracranial venous thrombosis in closed head injuries in children.

In the literature, septic phlebothrombosis accompanied by acute hemiplegia in childhood has been described by Bernheim and Larbre (1956) and Carels and Henneaux (1959). All these cases were diagnosed without angiography, solely on the basis of the clinical findings. Dekaban and Norman (1958) described the case of a 2½-year-old boy with acute hemiplegia, who was shown at autopsy to have a septic thrombosis of the superior sagittal sinus which spread into the cortical veins of one hemisphere. Angiographically verified hemiplegic forms in children have been reported by Weber (1957), Krayenbühl (1959), and Greer and Berk (1963).

In the author's series there are 3 cases (53-55) of angiographically confirmed septic thrombophlebitis of the cerebral veins. In 2 children the venous occlusion developed in the course of an otitis media complicated by an upper respiratory tract infection (CASES 53 and 54). In the third patient (CASE 55) cyanotic heart disease (Fallott's tetralogy) played the major rôle. While one child recovered completely, the other two died and the diagnosis was confirmed at autopsy.

CASE 54 is of unusual interest in that the patient survived for 5 months. Bailey (1959) reported similar cases in which death occurred very late in the course of the illness. The clinical courses of CASES 53-55 are presented graphically in the Table on page 199.

CASE 53

This boy, at the age of 13½ years, suffered an acute febrile throat infection from which he did not completely recover. He continued to experience headaches, lassitude and loss of appetite, and vomited repeatedly. Three weeks after the onset of the infection he became worse, with signs of a septicaemia (febrile, raised ESR, leucocytosis) with somnolence, confusion and sudden deterioration in vision, followed by Jacksonian seizures and motor hemiparesis. Carotid angiography revealed a localised cerebral venous thrombosis in the left parieto-occipital region (Fig. 67). The EEG initially revealed the presence of two epileptogenic foci in the opposite hemisphere, from which it was concluded that a multifocal cerebral infection was present. Treatment with antibiotics, anticoagulants and anticonvulsants resulted in the boy's complete recovery within a few weeks. Follow-up examinations over 9 years have confirmed the complete restitution to normal.

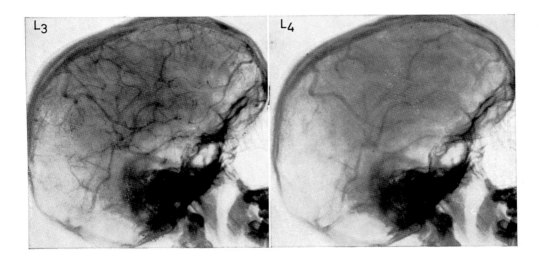

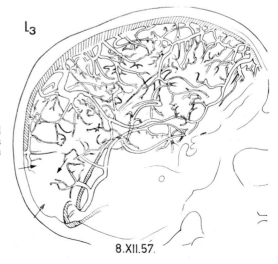

Fig. 67. Thrombophlebitis of the occipital lobe. Circumscribed area of non-filling in the venous phase of the serial angiogram (arrows in the line drawing) (Case 53).

A noteworthy feature was the result of CSF examination at the height of the illness: the only abnormalities were an elevated protein level and massive changes in the colloidal reactions, pleocytosis and xanthochromia being completely absent.

CASE 54

This boy fell ill at the age of 7 years and 3 months during an influenzal infection apparently complicated by otitis media; the picture was one of continuous status epilepticus (uncontrollable with anticonvulsants) with hemiseizures and hemiparesis, in a patient with generalised signs of severe inflammation. The level of consciousness remained clear, even when the clonic seizures spread to the opposite side.

The presence of a brain abscess was ruled out by ventriculography, so that only a cerebral thrombophlebitis or encephalitis were considered in the differential diagnosis. Retrospectively, the presence of xanthochromia and frank red cells in the CSF, as well as the virtually uncontrollable focal status epilepticus, favoured a cerebral thrombophlebitis far more strongly than an encephalitis. Carotid angiography, which, unfortunately, was only performed 7 weeks after the acute onset of the illness, revealed an almost complete blockage of cerebral drainage in the presence of a widespread thrombosis (Fig. 68), the large draining venous sinuses being particularly

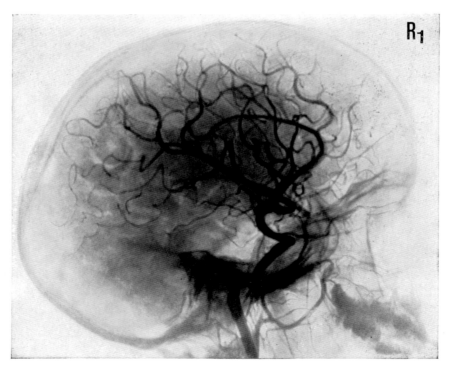

Fig. 68 (*above and facing page*). Extensive thrombophlebitis of the dural sinus and intracranial veins. Stasis of contrast medium in serial angiogram. In the capillary phase (R2) and even in the venous phase (R3) the arteries remained contrast filled (Case 54).

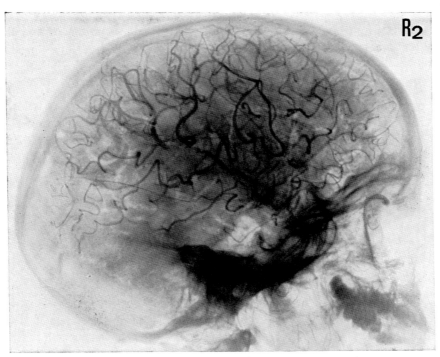

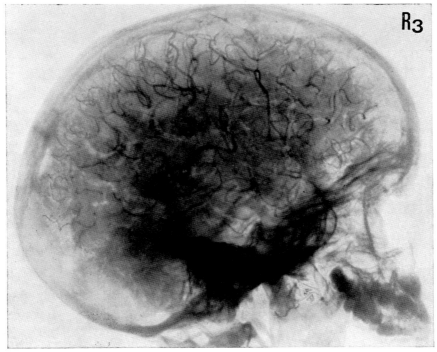

affected. The cause of the intracranial thrombophlebitis was most probably a purulent otitis media. No anticoagulant treatment was given, on the assumption that the case was one of encephalitis. Unfortunately, the angiographic findings were misinterpreted. The child, after 4½ months of progressive thrombosis, died in a state of severe marasmus.

CASE 55

This baby girl had developed normally, despite the presence of a congenital heart lesion (tetralogy of Fallot), and recovered remarkably well from pneumonia at the age of 2½ months. At 11 months she contracted an apparently harmless pyodermia which in no way influenced her general condition. It seems reasonably certain that this skin infection was the source of haematogenous metastasis into the

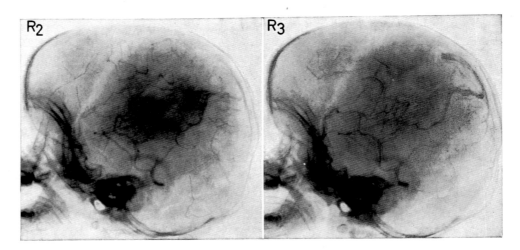

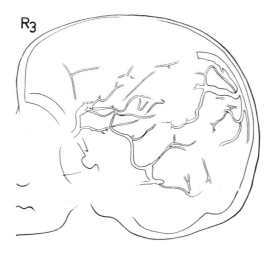

Fig. 69. Cerebral thrombophlebitis in Fallot's tetralogy. Incomplete filling of cerebral veins in the venous phases (R2 and R3) of the serial angiogram (Case 55).

cerebral veins through the congenital by-pass of the lung filter. A generalised epileptic seizure heralded a fatal course in an apparently healthy child. The clinical picture consisted of status epilepticus, severe signs of generalised inflammatory disease and considerable cardiac decompensation which was dominated by generalised cyanosis. At times the seizures were only right-sided, with a spastic hemiparesis during the seizure-free intervals; together with the presence *ab initio* of a conjugate deviation to the right side, this picture indicated a predominant lesion of the left cerebral hemisphere. Later, the clinical picture altered, and a spasticity of the left side of the body developed. At this point the EEG showed mainly a non-specific disturbance on the right side. Right carotid angiography (Fig. 69) demonstrated a thrombosis of ascending cortical veins and of the superior sagittal sinus. A strong pointer to cerebral thrombosis was the presence of xanthochromic CSF, which also contained erythrocytes and a slightly increased number of mononuclear lymphocytes.

The primary differential-diagnostic consideration was cerebral abscess. Retrospectively, the alteration in the neurological deficit in respect of the cerebral hemispheres, as well as the above-mentioned findings in the CSF, favoured the presence of a cerebral thrombophlebitis, and, thus, treatment with anticoagulants.

For more detailed reports of CASES *53-55 see pages 264-267.*

PART IV

Cerebral Diseases

CHAPTER 17

Postictal Hemiplegia

Epileptic attacks of the grand mal type, particularly status epilepticus, may produce severe and irreversible brain damage, quite apart from the precipitating cause of the attack. Fundamental morbid-anatomical studies were made by Spielmeyer (1927) and Scholz (1951). Both authors postulated vasospasm as the cause of elective ischaemic cerebral lesions. Earle *et al.* (1953) advanced a new hypothesis, namely that hippocampal sclerosis is the consequence of perinatal brain damage (temporal lobe herniation and anoxia) and therefore the cause, not the effect, of temporal lobe epilepsy. Meyer *et al.* (1955) assumed that the same pathological mechanism is present in status epilepticus or other postnatal cerebral affections. Lindenberg (1955) likewise regarded postictal cerebral lesions as secondary to compression of the arteries at the base of the brain. Gastaut *et al.* (1957) combined this concept with Scholz's (1951) interpretation to define the 'HHE syndrome' (hemiconvulsion-hemiplegia-epilepsy). They pointed out the various grades of irreversible brain damage which may follow compression of the cerebral arteries at various levels by cerebral oedema, which, in turn, may be secondary to a primary inflammatory, vascular or traumatic lesion. Norman (1962) rejected this interpretation, that diffuse cortical atrophy in post-epileptic hemiplegia can be explained by compression of a specific cerebral artery. Cavanagh (1962) attributed the neuronal necrosis to the cerebral oedema.

Adrian and Moruzzi (1939) and Jung (1953) observed electrophysiologically an excessive discharge frequency compared with the normal, and drew attention to an enormously increased metabolic turnover in the ganglion cells participating in the epileptic discharge. The period of electrical silence corresponded to the existence of a state of neuronal exhaustion. According to Scholz (1951), seizures following one after the other in rapid succession provoke the most severe brain damage through the lack of an adequate recovery interval.

In some cases the pathological mechanism of the postictal neurological deficit is not clear. Nowadays most workers subscribe to the view that extensive circulatory disturbances play the most important part. Schneider (1967) interpreted the findings of Scholz (1951) as a shock-like disturbance of the cerebral microcirculation, in which platelet and red cell clumping, as well as changes in their shape, lead to an increased flow resistance and hypoxia. A vicious circle is therefore produced through a general reduction in respiratory and circulatory efficiency, disturbances of the microcirculation and disturbances of the blood-brain barrier leading to the production of cerebral oedema.

Scholz's view that the degree and development of psycho-organic defects bear a relationship to the number and severity of the epileptic attacks, was questioned by Bamberger and Matthes (1959). These authors emphasized the importance of the primary disease causing the epilepsy, while acknowledging status epilepticus as the cause of irreversible brain damage.

Gastaut *et al.* (1957) grouped cases of hemiplegia in childhood following convulsions due to various causes (excluding cases of pre-existing brain damage) as the 'HHE syndrome' (hemiconvulsions-hemiplegia-epilepsy syndrome). These authors found that, in their series of 150 patients, over 80 per cent of cases of chronic epilepsy occurred after a free interval of less than one year and 50 per cent of cases of psychomotor epilepsy after more than 3 years. In the author's smaller series of cases fulfilling the criteria of the 'HHE syndrome', on the other hand, a much smaller percentage of cases of chronic epilepsy was observed — only 3 examples (CASES 57, 65 and 106), as opposed to 10 without early epilepsy (CASES 59, 85, 86, 93, 95, 97, 100, 101, 105 and 107) (see Table of Cases, pages 200-203). (This discrepancy may perhaps be attributed in the author's cases to prolonged prophylactic anticonvulsant treatment.)

The cases grouped in the Table of Cases under the title 'Para- and post-infectious hemiplegia' were classified according to the clinical findings. Excluded from this group were cases of clinically certain or probable encephalitis. The author is aware that this classification is arbitrary and based on criteria that are open to criticism. However, it was possible to identify the area of transition between benign postictal hemiparesis ('Todd's paralysis') and irreversible neurological deficits of varying degrees of severity. Permanent localised deficits following focal seizures were described by Penfield and Jasper (1954). Fowler (1957) published 5 cases, 4 of which were submitted to autopsy, which showed severe anoxemic cerebral necrosis after 'febrile convulsions'. The author regards these cases as a direct complication of epileptic attacks.

Postictal unilateral cerebral oedema was observed in 4 patients in this series (CASES 56-59), and these are described in detail. In one (CASE 56, Figs. 70*a*, and *b*) it disappeared surprisingly quickly—within 24 hours—despite the continual presence of hemiparesis and dementia from the time of the hemistatus epilepticus (duration of case history of 11 years).

CASE 58 is regarded as an example of irreversible ictogenic cerebral damage. The patient, a girl with a classical positive family history of febrile convulsions in infancy, initially experienced three generalised attacks during a febrile infection, and recovered promptly on each occasion. The fourth attack, which again occurred during a banal febrile 'influenzal infection', progressed to status epilepticus, with seizures confined to one half of the body and lasting for 12 hours. Serial pneumoencephalography (Fig. 71) revealed the presence of a persistent unilateral cerebral oedema for over two weeks, despite a normal CSF. Within two months atrophy of the affected hemisphere was observed. Hyperosmotic treatment started on the fifth day (repeated intravenous drip infusions of 40 per cent urea) proved to be of no value, perhaps because it was started too late.

No convincing correlation between the duration of the attacks on the one hand, and the duration and the severity of the postictal neurological deficit on the other hand, could be demonstrated in this series. Invariably, patients with severe and permanent deficits had suffered from status epilepticus with recurrent seizures lasting several hours, but two patients (CASES 86 and 111) who had experienced persistent

132

hemiconvulsions over several hours made a complete clinical recovery within a few days, while another (CASE 85), in whom the convulsions had lasted for a considerably shorter period, took 2 weeks.

In the vast majority of children with postictal hemiparesis, a history of febrile infection was present. In this series, only 3 out of 25 such patients (CASES 109-111; see Table of Cases, page 200), presented no evidence, either in the history or the clinical examination, of a primary or accompanying illness. All 3 recovered completely, despite the fact that one child (CASE 111) experienced a hemistatus epilepticus lasting for many hours. Individual constitutional factors undoubtedly play a part.

CASE 56

The patient was born before term (birth weight 970 g) and showed a retarded psychomotor development. He was prone to upper respiratory tract infections and had suffered many 'febrile convulsions' by the age of 13 months when he was submitted to detailed clinical examination. Pneumoencephalography revealed a symmetrically enlarged ventricular system (Fig. 70b), but EEG showed no abnormal findings.

At the age of $2\frac{1}{2}$ years, during a hyperpyrexial influenzal illness, he experienced 10 hours of hemistatus epilepticus which resulted in a severe and permanent hemiparesis. On the twelfth day of this illness, massive unilateral cerebral oedema was demonstrated by pneumoencephalography (Fig. 70a). The differential diagnosis included subdural haematoma, and on the following day a carotid angiogram was performed. To the author's surprise, the ventricular displacement had now completely disappeared (Fig. 70b). It is possible that the high concentration of contrast medium used (10 ml of 50 per cent Diodone for the lateral series, a few minutes before the second injection for the antero-posterior series) played some part in the reduction of the swelling.

Two and a half years later, the patient was admitted for the third time during an episode of fever. Despite physiotherapy, the severe spastic hemiparesis remained virtually unaltered. Psychological testing showed the patient to be an imbecile.

This case is an impressive example of irreversible severe brain damage following status epilepticus. An associated encephalitic process can by no means be ruled out. On the basis of the early history, however, the case appears to be one of exclusively unilateral ictogenic cerebral damage in a child with previous slight and diffuse cerebral damage.

CASE 57

The child, at the age of 2 years and 10 months, experienced a hemistatus epilepticus of many hours duration in the course of a febrile upper respiratory tract infection. She was left with a residual flaccid subtotal hemiplegia, which regressed completely within weeks. Pneumoencephalography revealed transitory unilateral cerebral oedema of moderate severity. The EEG showed persistent focal epileptic activity over the affected hemisphere.

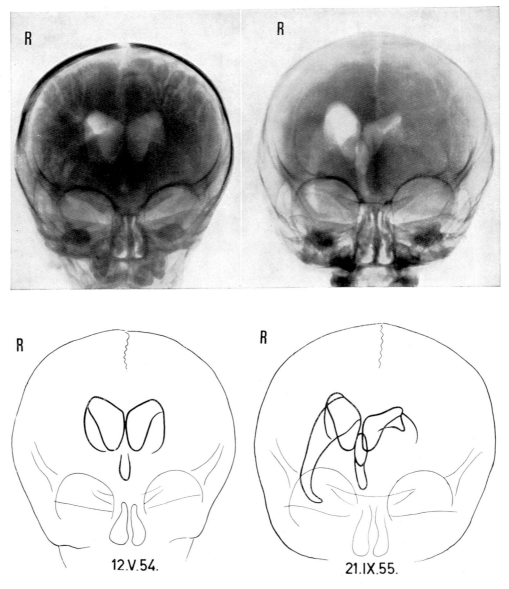

Fig. 70*a*. Unilateral cerebral oedema after hemistatus epilepticus. *Left:* symmetrical internal hydro-cephalus (see text, Case 56). *Right:* massive left-sided cerebral oedema, with displacement of the ventricular system to the right side (compare Fig. 70*b*).

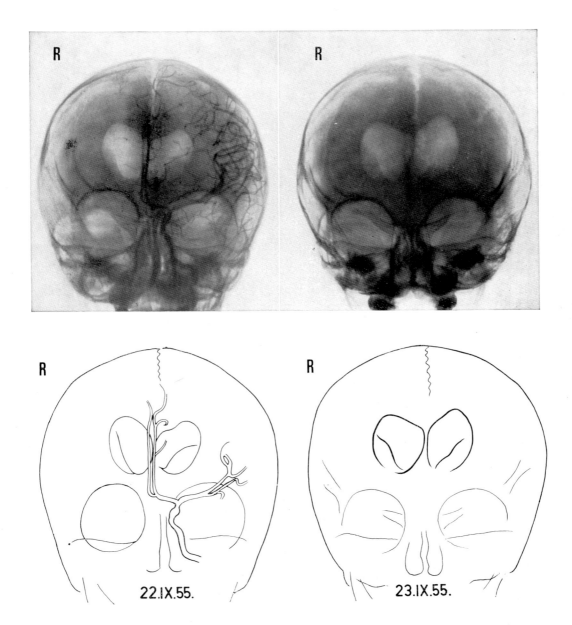

Fig. 70*b*. *Left:* carotid angiogram made 24 hours after pneumoencephalography in the oedema stage (see Fig. 70*a*). Cerebral oedema largely subsided. *Right:* follow-up pneumoencephalogram made 24 hours later. Symmetrical hydrocephalus. Cerebral oedema completely disappeared (Case 56).

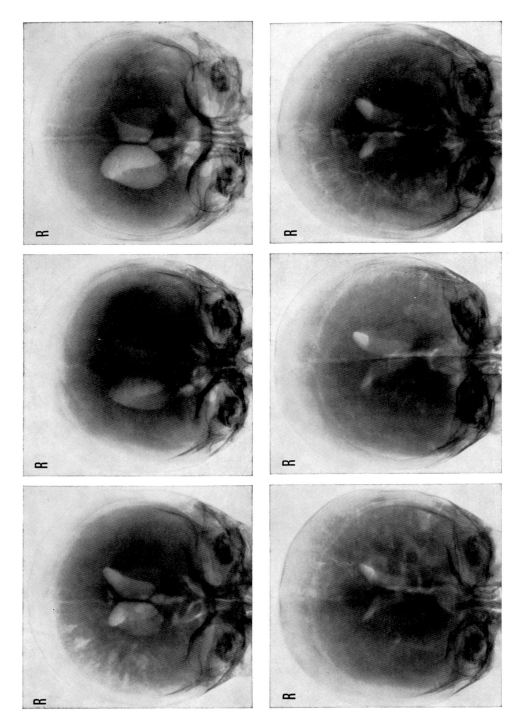

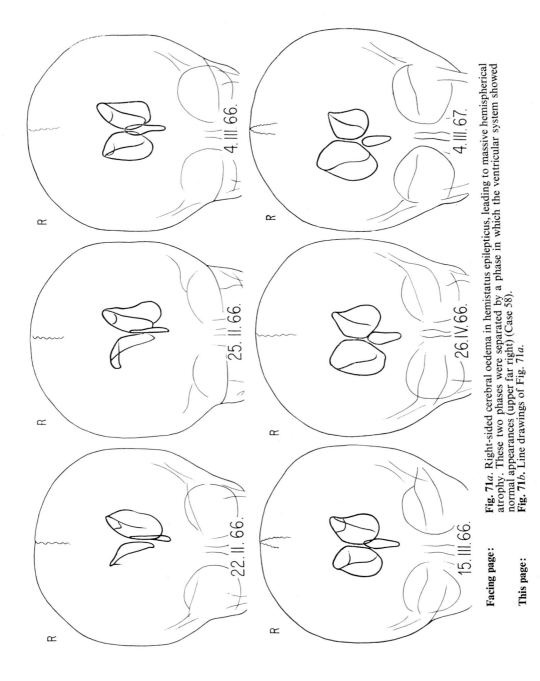

R   4. III. 66.

R   25. II. 66.

R   22. II. 66.

R   4. III. 67.

R   26. IV. 66.

R   15. III. 66.

Facing page: **Fig. 71a.** Right-sided cerebral oedema in hemistatus epilepticus, leading to massive hemispherical atrophy. These two phases were separated by a phase in which the ventricular system showed normal appearances (upper far right) (Case 58).

This page: **Fig. 71b.** Line drawings of Fig. 71a.

CASE 58

This patient had a multiple family history of febrile convulsions. At the ages of 4½, 9 and 12 months, during hyperpyrexial influenzal attacks, he experienced generalised seizures which once lasted for 4 hours. Each time the child recovered promptly and completely.

At the age of 14 months the patient experienced, on the second day of a febrile illness, a status epilepticus that lasted for more than 12 hours and recurred on the following day; the seizures were confined strictly to the left side of the body. Recovery of consciousness revealed a complete flaccid left hemiplegia, which over the course of weeks became spastic.

Serial pneumoencephalograms revealed the presence of a massive unilateral oedema during the acute phase of the illness, which gradually disappeared in 3-4 weeks. After 10 weeks, a fairly marked atrophy of the affected hemisphere was demonstrated (Fig. 71).

This case is an impressive example of irreversible cerebral damage which, according to the author's view, resulted from hemistatus epilepticus. It is, of course, impossible to exclude the possibility of a focal 'encephalitis'. The author assumes that the neurological deficit could have been prevented by prompt and appropriate management of the seizures. Understandably, the case history suggested an optimistic prognosis of the status epilepticus. Clearly, long-lasting convulsions must always be taken seriously.

CASE 59

The patient, a little girl, experienced at the age of 14 months a status epilepticus, comprising predominantly left-sided hemiseizures, during an acute febrile attack of tonsillopharyngitis. The seizures were followed initially by a flaccid left hemiplegia, which gave way to a permanent and severe spastic hemiparesis affecting mainly the

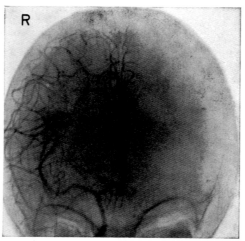

Fig. 72a. Carotid angiogram during the phase of unilateral oedema. Displacement of the anterior cerebral artery to the left side, but blood vessels in other respects normal (Case 59).

15. IV. 65

138

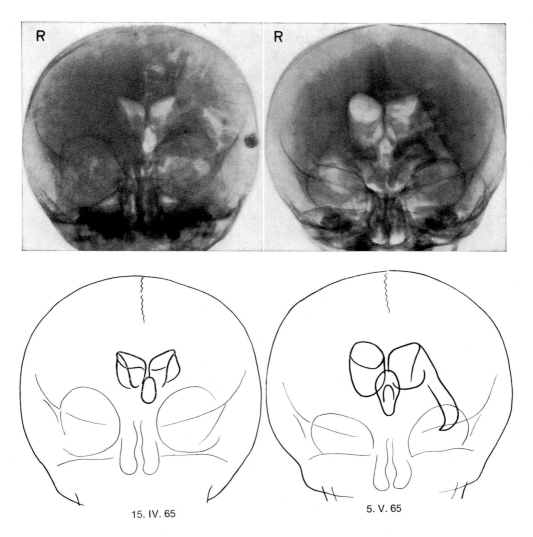

Fig. 72b. Unilateral cerebral oedema following hemistatus epilepticus (left) and secondary hemispherical atrophy (Case 59).

hand. Echoencephalography on the 3rd day of the illness revealed a significant displacement of the mid-line structures to the left side. Pneumoencephalography and carotid angiography on the 11th day still showed the presence of unilateral cerebral oedema (Figs. 72a and b). Serial EEG showed the persistence of a massive depression over the corresponding hemisphere. Hemispherical atrophy developed within a month, as was demonstrated by serial pneumoencephalography (Fig. 72b).

It is presumed that the status epilepticus, of which the hemiseizures had lasted for several hours, played a major rôle in the development of the irreversible brain damage. It was not possible, on the basis of the clinical findings, to decide to what extent the transient unilateral cerebral oedema could be attributed to convulsive damage, or whether an encephalitic component or another type of lesion (*e.g.* ischaemia following a primary circulatory disorder) could have been responsible for it.

For more detailed reports of CASES *56-59 see pages 268-271.*

CHAPTER 18

Pre-ictal Hemiplegia

Two patients in the author's series (CASES 60 and 61) illustrated the unusual phenomenon of the epileptic attack being preceded by a flaccid hemiplegia. In CASE 60 the course of events was fully documented from start to finish. The author can advance no explanation of the pathogenic mechanisms. Penfield and Jasper (1954) described this form as inhibitory or akinetic epilepsy. According to these authors, epileptic discharges, even when they occur in the motor cortex, may lead to inactivity or weakness instead of activity, peripherally. It can also be assumed that this motor inactivity arises from specific inhibitory centres, *e.g.* the caudate nucleus. In CASE 60 the cause was far more likely to have been an acute circulatory disturbance, *e.g.* in the sense of migraine accompagnée (see page 171). The onset, with a feeling of queasiness and unilateral paraesthesiae, is in keeping with this assumption. However, during the entire period of observation of 3 years in this patient, no migrainous disturbances have manifested themselves, nor are there any known cases of migraine in the family, so the author's assumption is probably incorrect. Clinically the case was definitely one of epilepsy, although repeated EEG examinations failed to reveal any specific epilepsy potentials.

CASE 60

This patient, a boy, when aged 8 years and in perfect health, experienced a left hemisensory disturbance, followed immediately by a complete flaccid left hemiplegia without loss of consciousness. After this attack, which lasted one hour, the patient lost consciousness and exhibited clonic convulsions of the left upper extremity. While he regained consciousness completely within 2 hours, the hemiplegia took 9 hours to disappear.

Repeated brief focal clonic attacks occurred during the succeeding days, usually without loss of consciousness or paralysis. Clinical examination remained negative throughout. No more attacks occurred and the patient was still free from attacks 3 years later under regular phenobarbitone medication. Follow-up examinations revealed a normal neurological status.

CASE 61

This child with perinatal brain damage presented at the age of 8 months with generalised epileptic attacks. Following admission to hospital for clinical evaluation at the age of 12 months, a pre-ictal attack of complete hemiplegia lasting several minutes was observed, without loss of consciousness. The succeeding attack followed the typical Jacksonian pattern, commencing on the side opposite to the paralysis and involving only the paralysed extremity and the face during the stage of generalisation. An EEG made 4 days later revealed an increase of slow waves over the posterior part of the right hemisphere. However, recovery from this attack led to complete disappearance of the paralysis.

The question arises of whether this attack of pre-ictal hemiplegia occurred after a hemiconvulsion that had gone unnoticed. The author believes this to be extremely unlikely, since the child was under the care of an attentive nursing sister in a small 5-bed ward, and a convulsion would hardly have been missed.

For more detailed reports of CASES *60 and 61 see pages 272-273.*

CHAPTER 19

Encephalitis: Toxic-infectious and Neuroallergic Encephalopathy

Strict clinical criteria were used to group cases of hemiplegia into the encephalitis category, *i.e.* toxic infectious or neuroallergic encephalopathy. This arbitrary designation was used firstly to separate cases of para- or post-infectious postictal hemiplegia, in which the accompanying illness is regarded as possessing only a triggering effect without actually involving the brain substance, from cases of encephalitis in which definite participation of the brain in the disease process is assumed. Examples are cases with cerebral complications following smallpox vaccination, measles, chickenpox and whooping cough. Four cases of encephalitis in the more widely-accepted sense are also described. CASES 62-67 are reported in detail, while CASES 98-108 are projected graphically in the Table of Cases (pages 202-203).

The question of why the cerebral involvement is unilateral, or, to be more accurate, shows a unilateral preponderance, can only be answered by speculation. Autopsy examination in children with this type of encephalitis invariably provides evidence of a marked swelling of the brain, usually with hyperaemia. It is presumed that, in the hemiplegic form, a more extensive unilateral cerebral oedema leads to catastrophe. The decisive factor is, perhaps, damage to the cerebral circulation, with which cerebral oedema is always linked in the form of a vicious circle. The damage is particularly aggravated if the increased metabolic requirements of the affected neurones are unsatisfied because of the presence of epileptic seizures.

CASE 63, a patient with post-vaccinal encephalitis, may be cited as an example. In a series of pneumoencephalograms (Fig. 73) it was possible to demonstrate massive unilateral cerebral oedema, which disappeared only after 2 weeks, and the development in the course of the succeeding few months of a severe hemispherical atrophy. Hyperosmotic treatment (30 per cent urea solution by intravenous drip infusion) for 9 days had no effect, perhaps because it was commenced too late—24 hours after the onset of the hemistatus epilepticus. The course and findings were roughly similar to those in CASE 58, in the group of para-infectious postictal hemiplegia (see page 138).

French workers (Bernheim *et al.* 1954, Girard and Devic 1954, and others) have expressly referred to the clinical picture of encephalitis in children with cerebral venous thrombosis. In this series of cases of acute hemisyndromes in children, only 3 cases of venous thrombosis were found (see page 121). In the 3 children with encephalitis who were examined *post mortem*, the findings in this respect were negative in two (CASES 62 and 108), whilst in the third (CASE 67) the cerebral venous thrombosis was almost certainly a secondary feature. None of the patients examined angiographically in the acute phase (CASES 102, 104, 106, 108, also CASES 56, 58, 59, 85, 89, see Table of Cases, pages 200-203) showed any suspicious changes in the

143

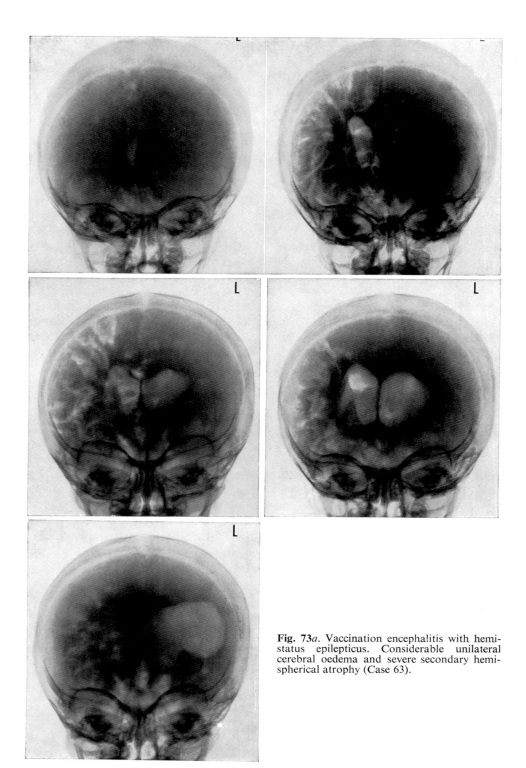

Fig. 73a. Vaccination encephalitis with hemi-status epilepticus. Considerable unilateral cerebral oedema and severe secondary hemispherical atrophy (Case 63).

144

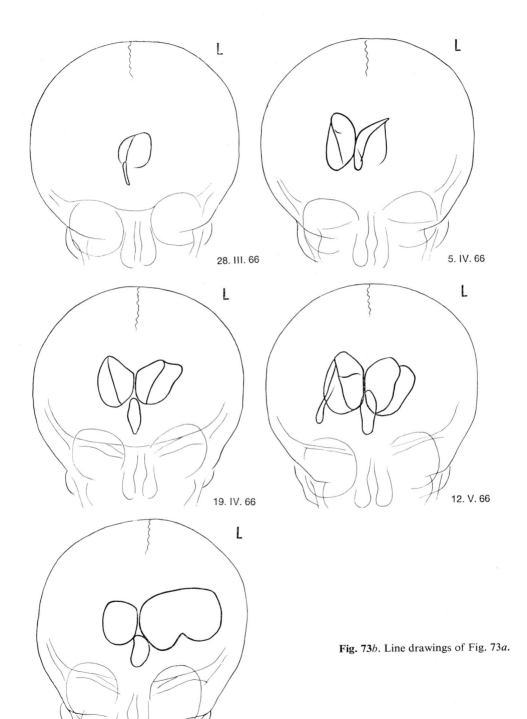

28. III. 66

5. IV. 66

19. IV. 66

12. V. 66

19. VII. 66

Fig. 73*b*. Line drawings of Fig. 73*a*.

145

venogram. It should, of course, be pointed out that occlusions of the smaller cerebral veins would probably not be visible in the serial angiogram.

Of the patients in this series with pure encephalitis, two are of particular interest. In CASE 66, which is described in detail, an acquired focal toxoplasmosis encephalitis was probably present, since a significant rise and fall of the titres was demonstrated in the Sabin-Feldmann test. This boy made a complete recovery. Only a few similar cases are described in the literature (Sabin 1941, Hedenström *et al.* 1958, Lelong *et al.* 1960).

The other case (67), a patient with acute necrotising leucoencephalitis, was dramatic and fatal. Hurst (1941) described this rare form of encephalitis, commencing in completely healthy subjects and running a fulminating course, which possesses specific histological features; these are almost exclusive involvement of the white matter, severe damage to the walls of blood vessels, perivascular haemorrhages and necrosis around larger veins as well as around precapillaries, focal demyelinisation, intense polymorphonuclear exudation and oedema. The autopsy findings in the author's case (Fig. 78) corresponded to this picture. Specifically, the necrosis was confined to the white matter of the left hemisphere: the areas of softening in the remaining parts of the brain and spinal cord were regarded as secondary changes that occurred terminally in the course of the week for which the patient was kept alive artificially on a respirator.

CASE 107, a patient with a predominantly unilateral leptospiral encephalitis, has been reported in detail by Gsell and Prader (1953) and CASE 99, a patient with predominantly unilateral measles encephalitis, by Fanconi (1955).

As indicated graphically in the Table of Cases (pages 202-203), patients with the hemiplegic form of encephalitis carry an unfavourable prognosis. Three children died, 8 were left with a very severe residual spastic hemiparesis, 2 showed some regression of the motor deficit, 1 developed late epilepsy of a psychomotor type, and only 3 children showed complete clinical recovery. One patient with a cerebral abscess (CASE 68) is discussed in the next chapter.

CASE 62

At the age of 2 years and 4 months, this little girl became acutely ill with a high fever and a hemistatus epilepticus. Death from circulatory failure followed a persistent state of coma. Autopsy indicated the presence of a virus encephalitis. The unilateral distribution of the symptoms could not be explained at autopsy.

CASE 63

The patient, a baby girl aged 14 months, experienced a bout of fever 4-7 days after an initial smallpox vaccination. On the 16th day a second bout of fever occurred, followed by a hemistatus epilepticus lasting many hours and then by a flaccid hemiplegia which later became severely spastic. A transient spasticity of the extremities was present on the opposite side. Pneumoencephalography revealed massive unilateral cerebral oedema during the first fortnight. In the course of less than 4 months progressive atrophy of the affected hemisphere developed, particularly of the anterior parts (Fig. 73). The EEG revealed persistence of an almost complete depression in this hemisphere (Figs. 74a, b and c).

The clinical diagnosis was encephalitis, predominantly unilateral, due to an influenzal infection complicating a smallpox vaccination.

It must be assumed that the hemistatus epilepticus contributed significantly to the development of severe and irreversible brain damage. A primary vascular cause appeared unlikely. Carotid angiography, performed on the 12th day of the illness, revealed normal intracranial blood vessels.

CASE 64

During an infection (for which neither a bacteriological nor a virological agent could be isolated), accompanied by two peaks of high temperature and transient diarrhoea, this 11-month-old baby girl experienced first generalised seizures and then, after an interval of 2 days, recurrent clonic seizures of the left side of the body followed by hemiplegia. An incomplete recovery from the latter occurred, leaving the child with a moderate spastic incomplete hemiplegia. It is to be assumed that the persistently low IQ of 75 (Brunet-Lézine) was a result of the severe brain damage.

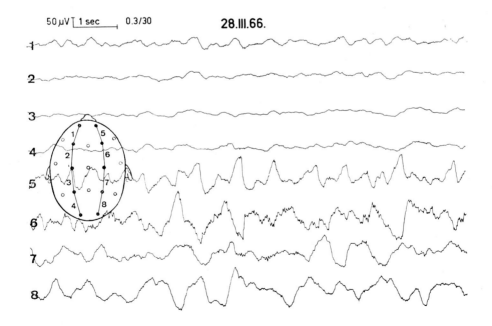

Fig. 74a. EEG made during the phase of left-sided cerebral oedema. Depression of cerebral activity over the left side and severe non-specific disturbance of the right hemisphere (Case 63).

14.IV.66.

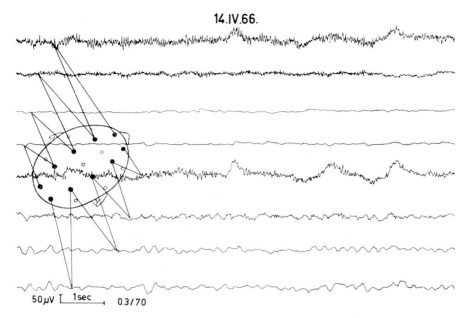

50 µV ⌊ 1sec ⌟ 0.3/70

Fig. 74b. EEG made after subsidence of left-sided cerebral oedema. Persistent depression over the left hemisphere; widespread recovery over the right hemisphere. Muscle infarcts over frontal leads (Case 63).

50 µV ⌊ 1 sec ⌟ 0.1/30 **19.VII.66.**

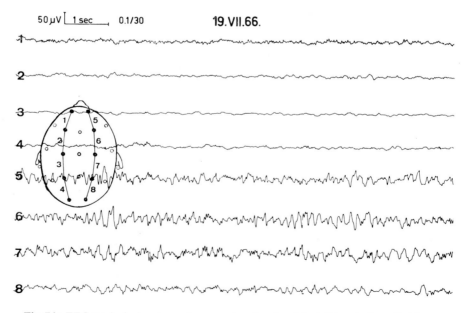

Fig. 74c. EEG made during stage of progressive atrophy of the left hemisphere. Persistent depression of cerebral activity over the left hemisphere. Rapid dysrhythmia over the right hemisphere; in other respects activity normal for patient's age (Case 63).

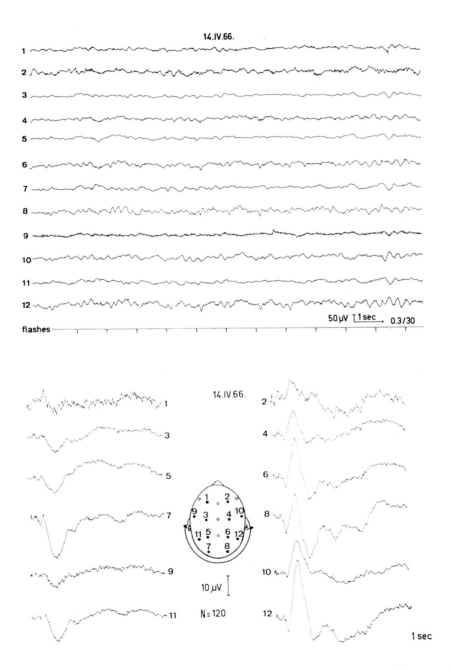

Fig. 75. Evoked responses during photic stimulation in simultaneous electroencephalograms. Left hemisphere: depression of the background rhythm and absence of evoked responses (the deviations with reversed polarity originate from the reference electrode). Right hemisphere: normal background activity with well shown normal visual evoked responses (by kind permission of Dr G. Dumermuth) (Case 63).

149

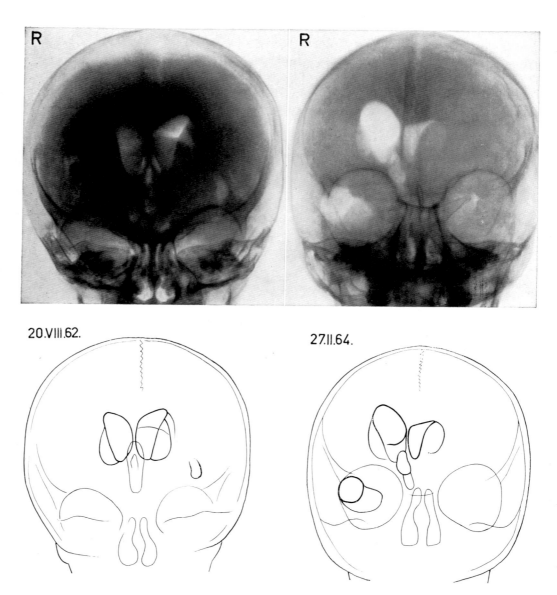

Fig. 76a. Hemispherical atrophy following encephalitis with hemiconvulsions. *Left:* mild symmetrical enlargement of the ventricular system 3 months after the onset of the illness. *Right:* massive unilateral cerebral atrophy $1\frac{1}{2}$ years later (Case 64).

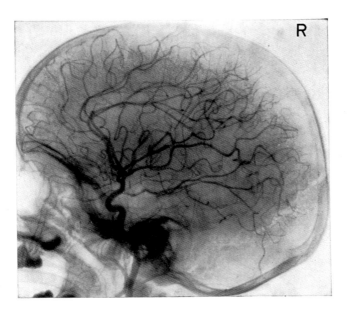

27. II. 64

Fig. 76*b*. Normal carotid angiogram in the presence of massive hemispherical atrophy (Case 64).

The pneumoencephalogram made 3 weeks after the onset of the illness showed a virtually normal ventricular system, yet 15 months later massive atrophy of the right hemisphere was present (Fig. 76*a*), in the presence of normal angiographic appearances (Fig. 76*b*). The problem of demonstrating the cause of the unilateral cerebral atrophy remains unsolved. A toxic-infectious encephalopathy can be assumed to be the most likely cause, but the unilateral involvement is unusual. The normal appearances of the blood vessels supplying the affected hemisphere 15 months after the acute episode do not exclude a vascular cause, *e.g.* an angiospastic insult or a large-vessel thrombosis with recanalisation. It is also possible that irreversible damage was produced by the repeated epileptic attacks.

CASE 65
    The patient, a girl, was submitted to smallpox vaccination at the age of 1 year and 6 months, and 10 days after the inoculation developed a hyperpyrexial, virtually unilateral encephalitis with hemiconvulsions and unconsciousness lasting for 3 days. A severe residual left-sided hemiplegia remained. Six and a half years later Jacksonian and psychomotor-type attacks commenced, which were resistant to treatment and became increasingly frequent, and a considerable intellectual deterioration and personality disturbance now appeared. Eight and a half years after the encephalitis, the patient was submitted to hemispherectomy; the hemisphere was found to be severely atrophic. The operation made no difference to the spastic hemiplegia, but the severe personality disturbances largely disappeared and the patient's IQ rose

151

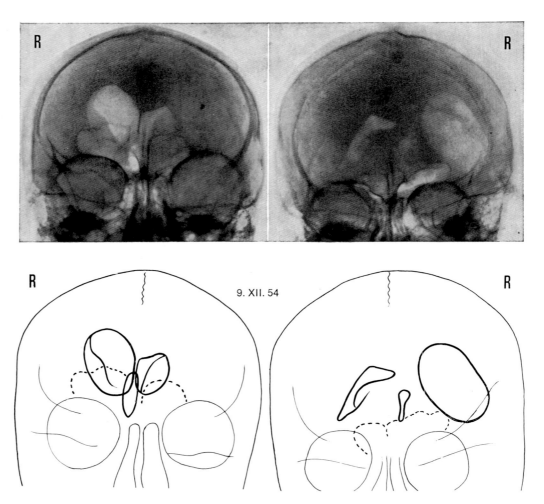

Fig. 77. Severe unilateral hemispherical atrophy 8 years after vaccination encephalitis with hemistatus epilepticus (Case 65).

from 34 to 50. With regular anticonvulsant treatment, the child remained free from attacks for the following 10 years. She now manages to do some housework and can read, write and knit, but she still cannot do sums (Fig. 77).

CASE 66

The patient, a healthy 12-year-old boy, experienced an acute attack of left-sided headache, slight fever, vomiting and a speech disturbance. On clinical examination a severe parietal-lobe (Gerstmann's) syndrome (acalculia, agraphia and a disturbance of body image) was found, in addition to aphasia and a homonymous hemianopia (the latter perhaps due to 'inattention'). EEG provided confirmation of the clinical picture in demonstrating a focal area of depressed cerebral activity in the left parietal region. The acute phase of the illness lasted less than a week.

It is believed that this case represents one of acute toxoplasmosis encephalitis. The titre of toxoplasmosis antibodies in the blood rose from 1:1024 to 1:6400 and fell, two years later, to 1:10—a significant finding. Convalescence extended over more than 2 months, dominated by a slight organic psychosyndrome in the form of a generalised slowing and forgetfulness. Follow-up examination 2 years later revealed no residual effects.

CASE 67

The patient, a 13-year-old boy, presented with a fulminating illness 10 days after an ordinary upper respiratory tract infection. Within hours, a hemisensory syndrome progressed into a complete flaccid hemiplegia. Purulent CSF was obtained, but no micro-organisms could be cultured from it. A perforating brain abscess was suspected, so carotid angiography was undertaken: no space-occupying process was demonstrated, but the cerebral circulation was markedly slowed. After this investigation the patient deteriorated, and was kept alive for several days by artificial respiration.

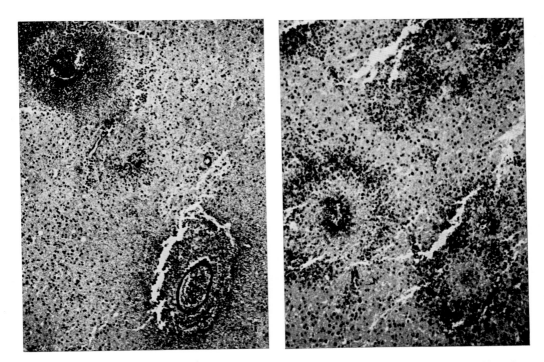

Fig. 78. Necrotising leucoencephalitis (Hurst). *Left:* very vascular cell infiltration (above left) and ring-shaped haemorrhages (below right) into the cerebral hemisphere. Magnification 100x. *Right:* dense cellular infiltration, haemorrhages and necrosis into the white matter of the cerebral hemisphere. Magnification 130x. (Pathological Institute, University of Zurich) (Case 67).

Autopsy revealed the picture of Hurst's necrotising leucoencephalitis. Secondary changes were present (cerebral and spinal cord softening, marantic thrombosis), attributable to the 8-day period that the patient was kept alive before cardiac arrest (Fig. 78).

For more detailed reports of CASES *62-67 see pages 274-280.*

CHAPTER 20

Cerebral Abscess

Adjacent focal infections are the commonest causes of cerebral abscess, as is the case with cerebral thrombophlebitis. According to Ford (1966), otitis media, particularly the chronic form, is most frequently responsible. Of the 20 children with cerebral abscess seen in the past 20 years at the Children's Hospital, Zurich, otitis media was the most probable cause in 4, purulent meningitis in 3, tonsillectomy in 2 and injury to the facial skeleton, ethmoidal sinusitis, lacrimal-duct infection, nasal furuncle and pneumonia in 1 each. Cyanotic congenital heart lesions play a significant rôle in the pathogenesis of cerebral abscess (Gluck *et al.* 1952, Keith *et al.* 1958, McGreal 1962), a fact underlined by the presence of 5 such cases in the present series. Pyogenic micro-organisms (according to Keith mostly haemolytic streptococci), from peripheral parts of the body, by-pass the lung filter through the venous-arterial communication in the heart and seed out metastatically in the brain. Remarkably, the child with cyanotic heart disease rarely suffers this complication before the age of 2 years (Keith *et al.* 1958), while cerebral abscesses arising from other causes show no age predisposition (the youngest patient in the author's series was 6 weeks old). Staphylococci represent the most frequent micro-organism responsible, although mixed infections with anaerobic organisms are also seen, and sterile abscesses are not rare.

The clinical course is usually acute or sub-acute. After a latent interval of days or weeks following an infectious process, various symptoms appear, the commonest of which are anorexia, headache, disturbances of consciousness and signs of raised intracranial pressure. Initially a fever may be absent (in 5 of the author's 20 cases), as may a leucocytosis in the blood (3 of the 20 cases); however, the ESR is elevated almost without exception. Meningism may only appear after several days. The CSF in the vast majority of cases shows a pleocytosis and an increased protein content, although lumbar puncture may be made hazardous by the risk of tonsillar herniation in the presence of raised intracranial pressure. After the abscess has formed, appropriate neurological signs appear, depending on its site. However, they may be absent if a silent area of the brain (*e.g.* frontal or temporal lobes) is involved. In such cases, one relies upon EEG and/or sonoencephalography to lateralise the lesion. Occasionally, focal or even generalised epileptic attacks may be early manifestations of cerebral abscess. The combination of cyanotic heart disease and neurological deficit should always prompt the suspicion of cerebral abscess.

Only rarely does a cerebral abscess present the clinical picture of an acute hemisyndrome. Raimondi *et al.* (1965) recorded 2 such cases in their series of 19 patients with cyanotic heart disease.

One patient in the author's series (CASE 68) presented with an acute expressive aphasia, 6 days after a minor injury to the maxillary region of the face, which was subsequently shown to be the presenting symptom of a cerebral abscess. A remarkable feature was the initial well-being of the patient, as well as the absence at first of fever and inflammatory blood changes. This case is described in detail below.

The prognosis depends in great measure on early diagnosis and treatment. According to the experience of the Department of Neurosurgery, University of Zurich, the best results are obtained with early radical removal of the abscess, under antibiotic cover with chloramphenicol or some other broad spectrum antibiotic. Of the 20 cases reported here, 5 died, all in the 1946-56 period, while the subsequent 12 cases survived. Four have so far developed late epilepsy.

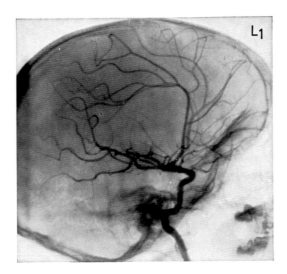

Fig. 79. Cerebral abscess in the opercular region. *Above left:* depression of middle cerebral artery, stretching of anterior cerebral artery. *Above right:* avascular region in the capillary phase. *Left:* displacement of the anterior cerebral artery across the mid-line (Case 68).

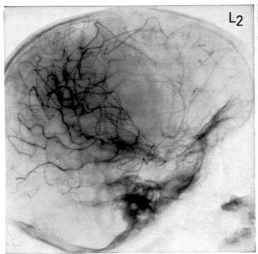

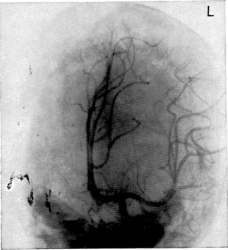

The patient, a 4-year-old boy, presented with an expressive aphasia and moderate headache 6 days after a minor injury to the mouth. In the succeeding few days weakness and twitching of the right angle of the mouth appeared, followed by drowsiness and a mild weakness of the right arm. One week after the onset of the illness an encapsulated abscess was removed from the left operculum (Fig. 79). The boy made a perfect recovery without residual effects, other than a minimal facial palsy. He remained free of attacks with prophylactic anticonvulsant treatment (length of history $6\frac{1}{2}$ years).

For a more detailed report of CASE *68 see page 281.*

CHAPTER 21

Intracranial Tumours

Horster and Walter (1961), in a study of 4,000 brain tumour cases, found 30 adults who presented with an apoplectiform onset due to haemorrhage into the neoplasm. These cases included benign as well as malignant tumours.

In children, acute hemisyndromes are observed only with the greatest rarity as part of the early picture of brain tumours. Of 160 cases seen at the Children's Hospital, Zurich during the past 20 years, only a single case could be found, which is described in detail below (CASE 70). In this 9-year-old boy with a slow-growing glioma of the white matter of the cerebral hemisphere, there were no signs of haemorrhage, and a postictal functional epileptic disturbance could also be ruled out as a cause of the recurrent hemiparesis. The most likely explanation was thought to be a disturbance of perfusion, possibly as a result of perifocal oedema.

In 7 children with supratentorial tumours in the above series, the onset of the illness was heralded by focal epileptic attacks without definite subsequent paralysis. Four children with infratentorial tumours presented with focal seizures as the first striking sign of the illness, in one case as a result of haemorrhage from an angio-reticuloma.

A 7½-year-old girl (CASE 69), in apparent good health, suddenly experienced a massive apoplectiform cerebral haemorrhage which was later shown to have occurred from an ependymoma. This case illustrates the importance of a careful histological examination of the 'haematoma membrane'.

CASE 69

The patient, a healthy girl aged 7½ years, presented with right frontal headache and vomiting. During the course of one night she developed a left hemiparesis and became drowsy. Carotid angiography revealed a large space-occupying process which immediate operation revealed to be a haematoma the size of a hen's egg in the right temporal lobe. After evacuation, the patient made a remarkably rapid recovery and was left only with a discrete residual facial palsy. Six months later she developed, in the course of one week, progressive signs of raised intracranial pressure, without neurological deficit. Operation revealed a large ependymoma of the right frontal and temporal lobes. Despite microscopic total excision and radiotherapy, the patient died 8 months later (Fig. 80). After the first operation, the cause of the haematoma was attributed to an arteriovenous malformation that had ruptured, and clearly was incorrect.

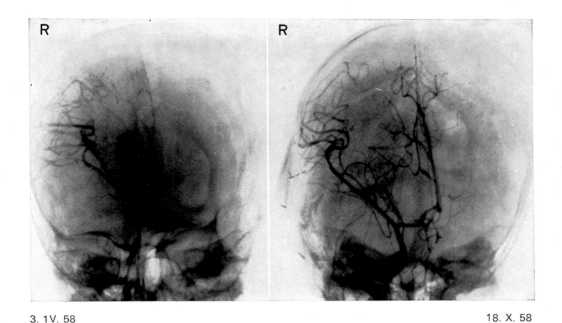

3. 1V. 58   18. X. 58

Fig. 80. Haemorrhage from a tumour in the right temporal lobe. *Left:* massive elevation of the middle cerebral vessels and displacement of the anterior cerebral artery across the mid-line prior to evacuation of the haematoma. *Right:* similar angiographic findings 6 months later, now due to a large ependymoma of the right temporal lobe (Case 69).

CASE 70

The patient, a 9-year-old boy, suffered for several mornings from right-sided headache, vomiting and a transient feeling of heaviness of the left foot. During the day he was free from complaints. One week later he developed a sudden incomplete left hemiplegia with paraesthesiae of the left arm and nausea, but without loss of consciousness; the attack lasted 10 minutes. During the following 5 weeks he had 5 more such attacks, although none were as severe as the first one. Clinical examination revealed no definite weakness and EEG showed only a discrete, doubtful disturbance in the right post-central region. However, pneumoencephalography proved a mass in the parasagittal white matter (Fig. 81), and a cystic astrocytoma was radically removed. The boy made an excellent recovery. Six years later only slight residual weakness is present in the left extremities. No intellectual defects and no epilepsy have been observed (duration of case history, 6 years).

For more detailed reports of CASES *69 and 70 see page 282.*

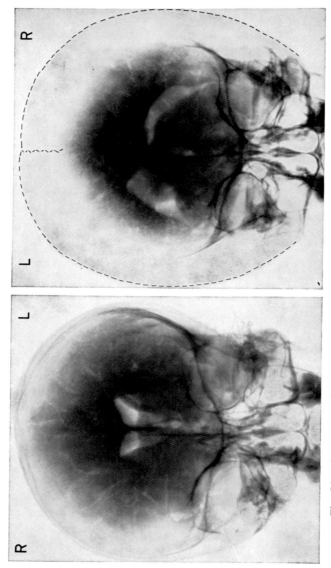

Fig. 81a. Astrocytoma in the white matter of the right parietal lobe. *Left:* antero-posterior pneumoencephalogram, showing slight depression of the roof of the cella media on the right side. *Right:* postero-anterior pneumoencephalogram, showing definite displacement of the right lateral ventricle (Case 70).

160

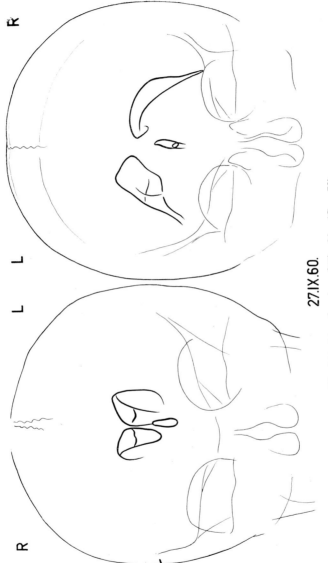

27.IX.60.

Fig. 81b. Line drawing of Fig. 81a. (Case 70).

161

CHAPTER 22

Multiple Sclerosis

Sandifer (1962), in discussing non-vascular causes of acute hemiplegia in childhood, referred to the encephalitides of neuroallergic origin, and postulated their transition into multiple sclerosis. Uchimura and Shiraki (1957) and Palffy and Mérei (1961) demonstrated convincingly the passage of cases of serologically proven encephalomyelitis into the disease picture of multiple sclerosis. The concept of a neuroallergic pathogenesis has become increasingly acceptable, since none of the earlier aetiological theories (syphilis, viruses, etc.) has ever been substantiated. Baasch (1966), in an interesting paper, has implicated the heavy metals, particularly mercury (*e.g.* in dental fillings), as the allergen responsible for the disease.

Multiple sclerosis is a disease of young adults and only rarely affects children (Low and Carter 1956, Gall *et al.* 1958, Isler 1961). One patient from the author's case material who presented with an acute hemiplegia in the initial phase of the illness (CASE 71) is described in detail below.

The diagnosis of multiple sclerosis is usually a retrospective one, made on the basis of a disease pattern consisting of characteristic bouts of multifocal symptomatology and remissions. Signs of inflammation (fever, leucocytosis, shift to the left of the haemogram, and increased sedimentation rate) form no part of the disease picture. No reliable laboratory methods of making the diagnosis have yet been devised: the CSF usually shows typical changes, but none of these is pathognomonic; plasmocytes are of some diagnostic value. It should be pointed out that occasionally in the first attack the multifocal nature of the neurological deficits may prompt suspicion of the diagnosis, particularly when further focal deficits occur and others regress.

CASE 71

At the age of $6\frac{1}{2}$ years, this girl experienced an acute episode of left-sided motor and sensory paralysis. The disturbance in the leg was milder and less prolonged than that in the arm. A transient partial left third nerve palsy was also present, indicating the multifocal nature of the disease process. A slightly raised protein content was found in the CSF, in the presence of a normal cell count; the colloidal gold curve was shifted slightly to the left side. The diagnosis at that time was a neuritis of unknown aetiology. After complete remission, when the patient was 17 years old, a second attack occurred, which took the form only of paraesthesiae (case-record information). It is of interest that she passed the menarche at the age of 15 years free of symptoms. Third and fourth acute attacks occurred 5 and 6 years later, dominated by subjective sensory deficits in the lower extremities. Trembling of the hands and ataxia of gait indicated cerebellar involvement. Although both these remissions were subjective, clinical examination 6 weeks after the fourth remission revealed evidence of involvement of the optic nerves, the pyramidal tract, the cerebellum and modalities of sensation.

Retrospectively, the acute illness experienced by the patient at the age of $6\frac{1}{2}$ years must be regarded as the first attack of multiple sclerosis. A remarkable feature is the 17-year remission.

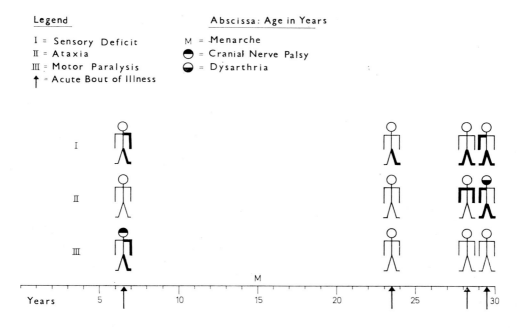

For a more detailed report of CASE *71 see page 283.*

CHAPTER 23

Subdural Haematoma

Subdural haematomas in childhood follow a definite age pattern. They appear almost exclusively in infants and young children up to the second or third years of life. Usually they result from a mild head injury which disrupts the delicate subdural bridging veins. In the Children's Hospital, Zurich, about 6 new cases on average are seen each year. In only about half of these is there a reliable history of trauma. Most show no radiographic evidence of fracture. When cases are referred early, bulging fontanelles or an abnormally large circumference of the skull are typical findings, as well as tonic and clonic convulsions (generalised or unilateral), vomiting, disturbances of consciousness and anaemia; however, none of these features need be present. A highly significant feature is the presence of fundal haemorrhages. A combination of the three symptoms mentioned above - increased intracranial pressure (*e.g.* bulging fontanelle, fundal haemorrhages, vomiting), convulsions (focal or generalised) and anaemia - virtually proves the presence of a subdural haematoma. Later on, the anaemia regresses and the symptom picture is that of a generalised increase in intracranial pressure. Many cases are referred with the diagnosis of 'progressive hydrocephalus'.

An acute hemiparetic course in children with subdural haematomas is unusual. In the only case in the author's series, whose course is described in detail below (CASE 72), no information about either the preceding convulsions or the episodes of mild trauma was available at the time of emergency admission. The clinical picture at that time consisted of an acute hemiparesis accomanied by a clouding of consciousness.

In the author's experience, the subdural haematoma can be of any size, and in the vast majority of patients it is found to be bilateral. Diagnosis is simple, by means of subdural puncture (in infants through one side of the anterior fontanelle, in older children through the coronal suture which is usually diastased). If the case is referred sufficiently early, it is possible to evacuate the haematoma by repeated punctures. However, once a haematoma membrane has formed (commencing after about 8-10 days), neurosurgical intervention is almost unavoidable.

CASE 72

In this 13-month-old baby girl, the hemiparesis resulted from an acute subdural haematoma which was probably traumatic in origin. Because of the defective case history, it is not possible to evaluate the rôle of epileptic seizures in the hemiplegia. After repeated evacuation of the subdural haematoma, the hemiplegia showed a partial regression within a month.

For a more detailed report of CASE *72 see page 284.*

PART VI

Migraine Accompagnée

CHAPTER 24

Migraine Accompagnée

No satisfactory definition of migraine has yet been found. The author subscribes to that of Vahlquist (1955) and Bille (1962) which includes the following generally accepted symptoms: paroxysmal attacks of headache with symptom-free intervals, associated with at least two of the following criteria:

> Unilateral distribution of the headache (63 per cent)*
> Nausea (80 per cent)*
> Prodromal visual disturbances (50 per cent)*
> Family history (78 per cent)*

By the term *migraine accompagnée* or *associée* (Charcot 1892) is understood attacks of migraine that are associated with neurological deficits, such as hemiparesis, hemianopia, aphasia, and ocular muscle palsies.

By the term *migraine equivalents* is understood the various paroxysmal disturbances, seen in patients with migraine, which appear without headache, *e.g.* disturbances of vision, attacks of vomiting, abdominal pain, and paroxysmal tachycardia.

The incidence of migraine in children was first determined by the systematic studies of Vahlquist (1955) and Bille (1962). These workers found that the frequency in unselected pupils in Uppsala schools was 2·5 per cent in 7 to 9-year-olds, 4·6 per cent in 10 to 12-year-olds and 7·4 per cent in 16 to 19-year-olds. Selby and Lance (1960), in a series of about 500 cases, found that the onset in 21 per cent was before 10 years of age, and Balyeat and Rinkel (1931), in a series of 200 cases, put this figure at 30 per cent. Vahlquist and Hackzell (1949) described 31 cases commencing between the first and the fourth years of life.

The pathogenic mechanism of migraine is still not fully understood, but clearly a functional vascular disturbance plays the major part. According to Wolff (1948, 1955), Friedman and Merritt (1959), Ostfeld (1960) and others, the typical migraine attack exhibits the following phases:

(1). Prodromal phase, characterised by vasoconstriction of the blood vessels supplying the brain and the retina. Mental changes, visual disturbances and sensory and motor disturbances can be attributed to the resulting disturbance in circulation.

(2). The phase of headache, with arterial dilatation, particularly of the branches the of external carotid artery. The throbbing nature of the headache is attributed to over-distension of the atonic vessel during the pulse wave. It is possible that autogenous chemical substances that reduce the pain threshold also play a part. The vascular dilatation extends to the small vessels, and leads to secondary perivascular oedema because of a disturbance of membrane permeability.

---

* Percentages according to Bille (1962), on the basis of 347 cases.

(3). Late headache phase. The dilated vessel wall becomes oedematous and rigid. When this occurs, the headache loses its throbbing nature and becomes more of a continuous dull pain. Focal tissue damage may occur as a result of the disturbance of membrane permeability and the action of autogenous chemical substances (polypeptides).

Heyck (1956) offered a completely different pathomechanical explanation of migraine. He suggested that abnormal arteriovenous shunts appear which result in tissue ischaemia, and this in turn reduces the pain threshold. Heyck attributed the pulsating nature of the pain to an increase in blood perfusion resulting from hypoxia of sensitive arteries.

Friedman and Merritt (1959) considered that both pathogenic mechanisms (vessel atonia and abnormal arteriovenous shunts) could be responsible for precipitating an attack of migraine.

Ophthalmoplegic migraine occupies an exceptional position in relation to migraine accompagnée. While it is rare, it usually commences in childhood (ver Brugghen 1955, Bickerstaff 1964). It is characterised by the feature that, as the migraine headache fades away, an ocular motor palsy (more rarely also a cochlear and abducent paralysis) develops, which persists for days and may occasionally be permanent. The cause is presumed to be compression of the oculomotor nerve between the dilated posterior cerebral and superior cerebellar arteries.

Hemiplegic migraine is a specific form of migraine accompagnée. Two varieties may be distinguished:
(1). Hemiplegic migraine with transitory neurological deficits during the prodromal phase. The actual attack of migraine varies greatly in its nature. Sporadic and familial cases have been described (Whitty 1953, Rosenbaum 1960, Bradshaw and Parsons 1965).
(2). Familial hemiplegic migraine, exhibiting a motor hemiplegia lasting for hours or days in association with the fading migraine headache. This variety, which exhibits a very marked familial pattern, tends to produce an identical syndrome in a sib and always affects the same side of the body (Dynes 1939, Symonds 1950, Whitty 1953, Blau and Whitty 1955).

Bradshaw and Parsons (1965) widened considerably the definition of 'hemiplegic migraine', so that it included, as well as motor deficits, purely sensory disturbances of all grades of severity. This definition allows the vast number of cases to be included which exhibit paraesthesiae in the prodromal phase. Bille (1962) found in 73 cases of severe migraine affecting children that 70 per cent exhibited visual disturbances, and 20 per cent paraesthesiae in the prodromal phase.

Basilar artery migraine (Bickerstaff 1961a and b) is another specific form of migraine accompagnée. In the majority of cases it appears in girls at the time of puberty and is usually associated with ordinary attacks of migraine. The symptoms arise as a result of circulatory disturbances in the territory of the basilar artery, viz. the region of the brain-stem, cerebellum and occipital lobes. The neurological symptoms appear in varying combinations during the prodromal phase, in the form of visual disturbances, vertigo, ataxia of gait, dysarthria and various degrees of disturbance of consciousness. They may last for minutes or for any time less than an hour. Lees and Watkins (1963) endorsed Bickerstaff's interpretation and discussed the pathogenic mechanism as a trigger factor of epileptic attacks. The author believes that CASE 82, which is described in detail below, belongs to this variety.

Although migraine accompagnée most frequently affects young adults, it may commence in childhood. Ophthalmoplegic migraine, in particular, frequently begins before the 12th year of life (Friedman *et al*. 1962, Bickerstaff 1964, Ford 1966). Many authors have described the hemiplegic form of migraine in children (Osler 1909, Clarke 1910, Dynes 1939, Symonds 1950, Whitty 1953, Blau and Whitty 1955, Heyck 1956, Ross 1958, Connor 1962, Ford 1966). Bickerstaff (1961*a* and *b*) described transient brain-stem disturbances in basilar artery migraine occurring in older children.

Of great importance is the pathogenic mechanism responsible for the neurological deficit. There is unanimity over the concept that a disturbance of vascular function is involved. Most authors assume it to be arterial vasospasm with secondary tissue ischaemia. In cases showing prolonged neurological deficits, some authors postulate a circumscribed cerebral oedema, provoked by brief tissue ischaemia resulting from vasospasm (Whitty 1953, Blau and Whitty 1955, Rosenbaum 1960, Bradshaw and Parsons 1965), while Symonds (1950) suggested a thrombosis of aterioles following vasospasm. Connor (1962) discussed focal tissue necrosis resulting from prolonged vasospasm or vascular occlusion or haemorrhage. Heyck (1956) attributed tissue ischaemia to abnormal arteriovenous shunts. Direct observations of vasospasm in the retinal vessels have been reported by Graveson (1949), Friedman (1951) and Connor (1962). Montgomery and King (1962) advanced their view that vasodilatation leading to secondary transient cerebral oedema causes similar deficits.

The clinical application of arteriography has produced further support for the vascular nature of the neurological deficit. Many normal angiograms in cases of migraine accompagnée contrast with individual cases in which interesting pathological features have been demonstrated. Dukes and Vieth (1964) were able to make serial angiograms in a 44-year-old man before, during and after a typical migraine attack, and demonstrated a progressive narrowing of the lumen in the internal carotid territory. After fading of the prodromal symptoms (scotomata), the lumen of the artery again returned to its normal width, and this was followed shortly afterwards by a transient hemiplegia! Walsh and O'Doherty (1960) were able to demonstrate in 2 cases of ophthalmoplegic migraine a narrowing of the distal part of the internal carotid artery on the side of the paralysis, while the opposite artery showed normal appearances. These authors quoted a similar finding reported by Alpers and Yaskin (1951) and ver Brugghen (1955). They concluded that a transient oedematous swelling of the arterial wall produces compression and/or ischaemia of the nerves supplying the external ocular muscles through the vasa vasorum in the cavernous sinus. Bickerstaff (1964) reported a similar finding in an 11-year-old boy in whom the internal carotid narrowing had disappeared and returned to normal dimensions in the control angiogram made after regression of the oculomotor palsy. Friedman and co-workers (1962) examined 6 patients during an attack of ophthalmoplegic migraine, and found that all 6 showed normal angiographic appearances. In one case which was submitted to vertebral angiography as well, a segmental narrowing of the basilar artery was demonstrated between its superior cerebellar and posterior cerebral branches. Brain

(1954) described patients with permanent hemianopia following attacks of migraine, in whom occlusion of one posterior cerebral artery was demonstrated angiographically. He attributed the arterial occlusion to thrombosis resulting from arterial spasm. Connor (1962) examined a 26-year-old man during an attack which resulted subsequently in a permanent hemianopia and hemiparesis, and demonstrated defective filling of the corresponding posterior cerebral artery. Examination 7 months later showed normal opacification of the previously occluded artery, while pneumo-encephalography revealed enlargement of the homolateral ventricle.

Cerebral swelling occurring during attacks of migraine accompagnée has been the subject only of isolated observations. Walsh and O'Doherty (1960) quoted Naffziger (personal communication), who observed the displacement of the calcified pineal gland during an attack, and its subsequent return to a normal mid-line position when the attack had ceased. These authors also quoted Goltman (1936) who observed swelling of the brain directly, through a defect in the cranium in the course of an attack.

Guest and Woolf (1964) described a significant and impressive finding at autopsy in a 28-year-old man who had died during an attack (hemiparesis and disturbance of consciousness). They found areas of focal ischaemic necrosis, mainly in the anterior cerebral territory, and ischaemic brain stem changes in the presence of a completely intact cardiovascular system, including the cerebral vessels. The authors concluded that the pathogenic mechanism had been vasospasm of one or more cerebral arteries.

Buckle et al. (1964) published an equally impressive fatal case. The patient, a 16-year-old girl, had died during an attack. Carotid angiography revealed severe narrowing of the terminal part of the internal carotid artery and the larger cerebral vessels, while the cervical carotid was of normal calibre. There was no morbid anatomical evidence of any intrinsic disease of the blood vessels while severe ischaemic tissue changes with gross cerebral oedema were present throughout the territory of supply of the internal carotid artery; the tissues in the vertebro-basilar territory showed normal appearances. The authors ascribed the fatal course to vascular spasm.

The majority of so-called normal angiograms in cases of migraine accompagnée are not carried out in the critical phase, but during an interval between attacks or at the conclusion of one. For this reason, the case of Dukes and Vieth (1964) is invaluable: the segmental arterial narrowing was present only in the prodromal phase and disappeared promptly at the beginning of the headache phase. It is noteworthy that a transient hemiplegia appeared shortly after the attack faded; no further angiographic study was made.

From the paper of Friedman et al. (1962) it appears that the vascular disturbance may be sought in the wrong territory; these workers found in a patient with ophthalmoplegic migraine that the carotid angiogram was normal, while the vertebral angiogram revealed abnormal findings.

The findings may be normal even when the appropriate artery is examined angiographically at the appropriate time, since the vascular disturbance may involve smaller arteries than it is possible to opacify with the contrast medium. A normal angiographic result by no means excludes a disturbance of local perfusion, as Ekberg et al. (1965) have demonstrated by regional blood flow measurements.

Ten cases (73-82) of migraine accompagnée with acute hemisyndromes in the author's series will be described in detail. Carotid angiography was carried out in 4 children, although only in 2 (CASES 77 and 81) during the presence of residual neurological deficits—and then only when the latter were regressing. No definite abnormality was demonstrated. On the other hand, the EEG showed massive unilateral non-specific changes, sometimes strikingly focal, in all the children examined during an attack (CASES 73-75, 77, 79-82); these changes were slow to regress and exceeded the period of clinical recovery. These findings are interpreted as the result of ischaemia.

The pathogenic mechanism of migraine accompagnée still awaits complete clarification. On the basis of all the evidence so far accumulated, an ischaemic mechanism can no longer be questioned.

CASE 73

The patient's mother suffered from migraine and Raynaud's disease. The boy suffered, from the age of 5 years, from attacks of headache, usually accompanied by vomiting, which became more frequent after he entered school at 7 years. The attacks of headache were first accompanied by a hemisensory syndrome (contralateral paraesthesiae, with pain in the face, tongue and arm) at the age of 11 years. Some weeks later another attack of a migraine was complicated by visual disturbances. The headache was again followed by paraesthesiae and, after 1 hour, by an expressive dysphasia. A hemihypaesthesia and hemianalgesia (the leg was uninvolved), as well as pupillary dilatation and fundal venous engorgement in the contralateral eye, could also be observed. The EEG reflected the local disturbance in the form of a depression of cerebral activity, which disappeared after the clinical signs had regressed. A similar attack occurred 3 months later (Figs. 82a and b).

A noteworthy feature was an episode lasting several weeks, 1½ years later, which was heralded by attacks of severe abdominal pain accompanied by retching.

In this patient a diagnosis of migraine accompagnée was made. The episode of abdominal pain was regarded as a migraine equivalent.

CASE 74

This 13-year-old boy suffered from frequent and unusually stereotyped attacks of migraine accompagnée, which presented as a hemisyndrome confined to the left parietal region. The course of the attacks could be precisely described. Physical examinations performed in the intervals between attacks revealed a normal neurological system. However, EEG revealed a mild focal disturbance of function which correlated well with the clinical picture. The patient was examined by a doctor in the course of an attack, and the latter confirmed the clinical features of the deficit.

CASE 75

The patient experienced his first attack of migraine at the age of 14 years. Initial unilateral headache, unaccompanied by other complaints, was followed by an intermittent hemisyndrome without headache. Prominent features were brief disturbances

20.II.53.

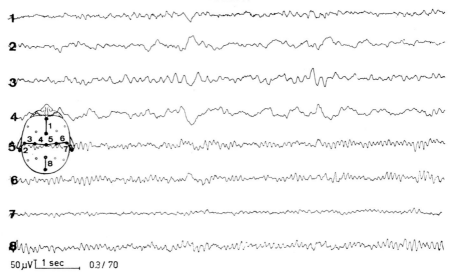

50 μV ⎍ 1 sec ⎍ 0.3 / 70

Fig. 82a. EEG recorded during an attack of migraine accompagnée. Delta focus and slow background activity over the left central area (Case 73).

24.II.53.

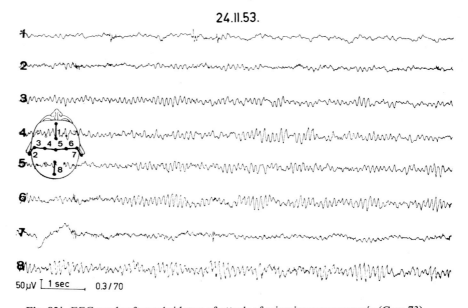

50 μV ⎍ 1 sec ⎍ 0.3 / 70

Fig. 82b. EEG made after subsidence of attack of migraine accompagnée (Case 73).

176

of sensory and motor function, which, on the basis of the clinical features and the EEG findings, indicated a disturbance of function in the posterior and anterior central gyri. In this patient, the hemisyndrome appeared as a migraine equivalent.

CASE 76

The patient, a young girl, had no family history of migraine. She experienced her first attack at the age of 15 years: a rapidly spreading motor paralysis commencing in the right hand and accompanied by dysarthria. This hemisyndrome, which occurred without warning or other manifestations, lasted only 10 minutes. Two months later a similar disturbance occurred, on this occasion accompanied by sudden nausea and headache. Clinical examination gave negative results.

During the next year two further attacks occurred, consisting of headache, nausea and paraesthesiae in the right arm; on neither occasion was there a motor deficit.

This case was diagnosed as one of migraine accompagnée.

CASE 77

The patient, a girl, when aged 8 years, experienced an attack of migrainous headache which was heralded by prodromal symptoms in the form of transient paresthesiae and weakness of the left hand. An exacerbation led after a few hours to severe bilateral frontal headache which persisted for 2 days, despite two bouts of vomiting, and which was accompanied by an incomplete left hemiparesis. No convulsions or loss of consciousness occurred.

The neurological findings were reflected in the EEG as a marked depression in the right hemisphere, with a maximum in the precentral region (Figs. 83a and b). Carotid angiography suggested the presence of oedema in the right insular region and arterial spasm in individual branches of the sylvian vessels.

The acute episode was regarded as migraine accompagnée, because of the following features: history of classical migraine in the patient's father, prodromes in the form of paresthesiae, the presence of vomiting, complete disappearance of all symptoms, a rapidly increasing headache. On the other hand, the long interval free from attacks (up to the time of writing, over one year) is unusual.

This fact raises the question of whether the author's interpretation of this case as one of migraine accompagnée was inaccurate. The carotid angiogram revealed the presence of oedema, albeit discrete. Also, some of the sylvian vessels appeared to be in spasm. According to Wolff et al. (1948), vasoconstriction may occur at various levels of the arterial tree during the second phase of the migraine attack (headache phase with dilatation of the intracranial arteries). The oedema can be explained as a reaction to ischaemic parenchymal damage; however, it is possible that tissue damage may have been caused by Wolff's 'headache substance' (neuroquinine), or a combination of both mechanisms.

Some other cause for the patient's disease picture (e.g. epilepsy, encephalitis, or poisoning) appears unlikely on the basis of the clinical history and physical examination. In any event, the picture can best be explained as a transient vascular disturbance in a case of migraine accompagnée.

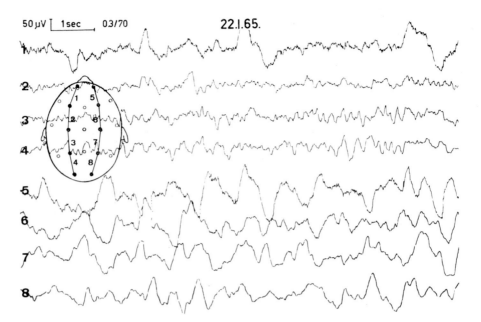

Fig. 83a. EEG made during an attack of migraine accompagnée. Massive disturbance with depression of the background activity over the right hemisphere (Case 77).

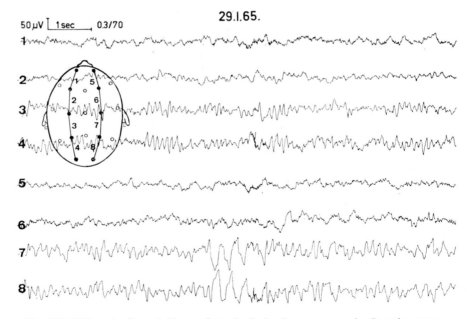

Fig. 83b. EEG made after subsidence of attack of migraine accompagnée. Great improvement in cerebral activity. Intermittent disturbance over the posterior part of the right hemisphere (Case 77).

CASE 78

The patient, a 12-year-old boy from a family with a history of migraine on the maternal side, experienced his first attack of migraine during sleep. An unusual feature was the fact that before regression of the attack a second phase occurred, which consisted of exacerbation of the unilateral headache, and was accompanied by hemiparaesthesiae and difficulty with articulated speech.

At irregular intervals of a few months, the patient experienced further migraine attacks, all of which commenced regularly with fortification spectra. Thorough clinical examination in the interval between attacks revealed no abnormal findings, and ancillary tests (EEG, skull radiography, and CSF examination) all gave negative results.

A severe attack of migraine accompagnée occurred 3½ years after the onset of the migraine, consisting of a hemiparesis and dysphasia lasting 2 hours, followed by typical unilateral headache.

The patient has been free from symptoms since his last attack 18 months ago.

CASE 79

The patient, a girl, experienced her first severe attack of migraine at the age of 13½ years. This attack produced morning headaches in the left temporal region for 2 weeks. The migraine accompagnée symptoms presented an unusually fluctuating picture in this case. Even during the phase of onset, the hemianopic disturbance indicated an upset of cerebral cortical function. Next, a motor and sensory hemiplegia

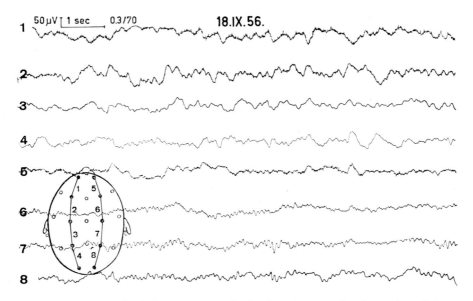

Fig. 84a. EEG made during an attack of migraine accompagnée. Depression of the background activity over the left hemisphere (Case 79).

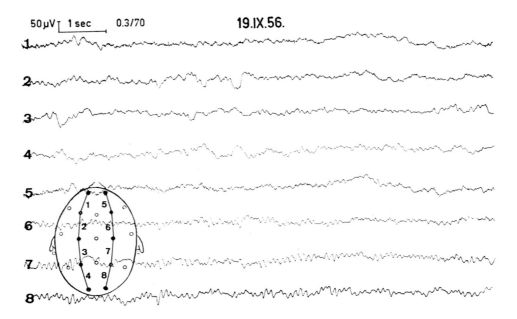

Fig. 84b. EEG made during subsidence of an attack. Improvement in the left-sided disturbances of cerebral activity (Case 79).

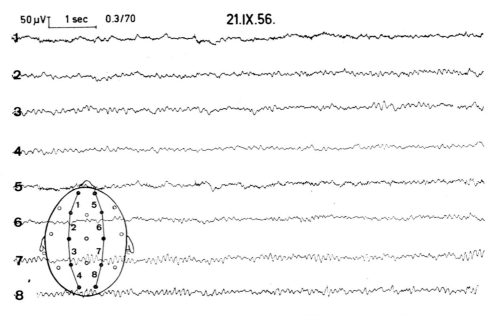

Fig. 84c. EEG made after subsidence of the attack. Mild disturbances still present (increased theta waves) over the left hemisphere (Case 79).

suddenly occurred, which regressed and then reappeared in a less intense form. At the height of the neurological deficit, the girl was severely confused and amnesic. EEG revealed a massive disturbance of cerebral activity in the form of a depression (Fig. 84a). The syndrome disappeared completely within 36 hours, and the EEG revealed a corresponding return to virtual normality (Figs. 84a and b). However, the intermittent generalised slow-wave complexes present in the recording indicated that the brain-stem, as well as the cortex, had suffered functional damage.

A neutrophilic leucocytosis and a raised ESR prompted the suspicion of an infection as the provoking cause; however, none could be detected clinically. The CSF revealed an abnormal colloidal gold reaction and a protein content at the upper limits of normal, and no plausible explanation could be offered for these findings. Apart from the absence of a family history of migraine, an unusual feature was the rarity of the subsequent attacks.

CASE 80

The patient, a perfectly healthy girl, at the age of 13½ years experienced an attack of left-sided migraine accompagnée associated with a disturbance of speech and writing ability. From the clinical deficit, a functional disturbance in the region of the angular gyrus was assumed, which was reflected in the EEG as a depression of cerebral activity. The EEG disturbance lasted several days longer than the clinical deficit (Figs. 85a and b).

Subsequently, sporadic, typical migraine attacks occurred, which were successfully treated with Cafergot.

CASE 81

The patient, a boy from a family with a history of migraine, experienced an unusually severe and prolonged attack of migraine accompagnée at the age of 14½ years in a situation of mental stress. The headache followed clinical deficits which pointed to involvement of the angular gyrus and the left occipital lobe, viz. sensory aphasia, apraxia, alexia, agraphia, acalculia and hemianopia. No abnormality was demonstrated either by carotid angiography or upon clinical examination of the cardiovascular system, but the severe functional disturbance was reflected in the EEG finding of a depression of cerebral activity. The focal disturbance shown upon EEG remained present for several weeks after clinical recovery was complete (Figs. 86a, b and c).

The acute hemisyndrome at the age of 5 years (speech disturbance, central facial plays and distal weakness of the right arm) with simultaneous redness of the face, which appeared acutely and showed prompt spontaneous regression, was retrospectively viewed as an attack of migraine accompagnée. The mild head injury several hours before the attack was dismissed as a possible cause for it, partly because of the absence of any signs of concussion, and partly because of the presence of emotional factors triggering the attack.

Further typical migrainous attacks occurred at irregular intervals (fortification spectra, unilateral headache), some accompanied by speech disturbances and paraesthesiae.

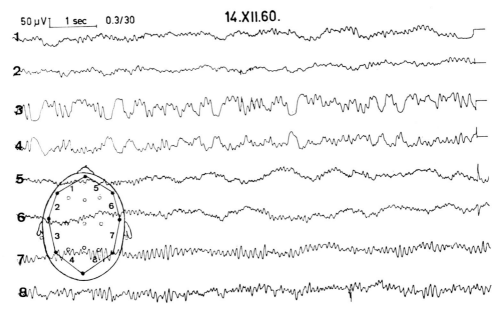

Fig. 85a. EEG made immediately after subsidence of an attack of migraine accompagnée. Delta focus in the left temporo-occipital region (Case 80).

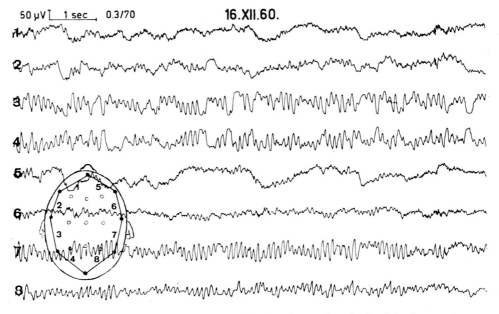

Fig. 85b. EEG made 2 days later. Only a slight disturbance of cerebral activity (increased delta waves) remaining in the left temporo-occipital region (Case 80).

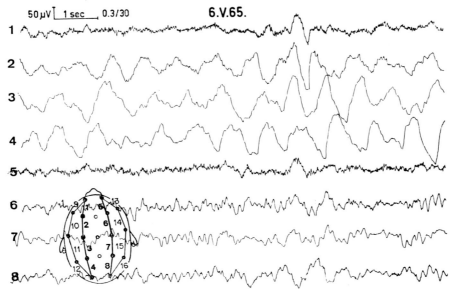

Fig. 86a. EEG made during migraine accompagnée status. Massive disturbance and depression of background activity over the left hemisphere. Mild right-sided disturbance (increased delta waves) (Case 81).

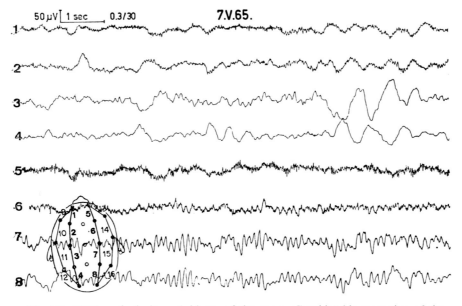

Fig. 86b. EEG made during subsidence of the status. Considerable regression of the functional disturbances over the left hemisphere. Normal right cerebral activity (Case 81).

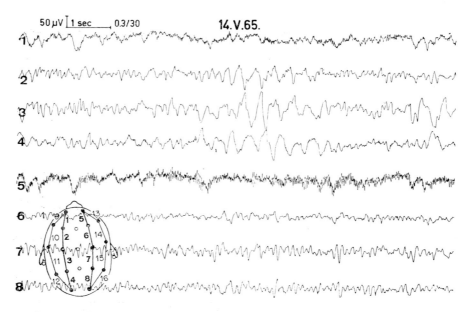

50 µV | 1 sec , 0.3/30   14.V.65.

Fig. 86c. EEG made one week after subsidence of the status. Intermittent disturbance of cerebral activity over the left hemisphere. The slow rhythms indicate a disturbance of subcortical function (Case 81).

CASE 82

The patient, a 7-year-old girl, showed acute transient disturbance of perfusion in the vertebro-basilar territory, with ataxia, visual disturbances and clouding of consciousness. EEG revealed a marked slowing of cerebral activity over both occipital regions, which was interpreted on the one hand as evidence of brain-stem involvement and on the other as impairment of blood flow in the posterior cerebral arteries.

This patient was regarded as a case of basilar migraine. The strong family history of migraine supports the diagnosis.

For more detailed reports of CASES *73-82 see pages 285-294.*

Conclusions

Conclusions

Acute hemiplegia in childhood is by no means a rare condition. However, the apparent uniformity of the clinical picture is not consistent with the wide variety of aetiologies.

Aetiologically, two main groups may be distinguished: vascular and non-vascular diseases. Only in the vascular group do a considerable number of cases present with a characteristic clinical picture: *i.e.* attacks of sudden hemiplegia occurring without convulsions.

There are no reliable clinical symptoms which permit differentiation between cerebral arterial occlusion and cerebral haemorrhage. One symptom which was found in most of our cases with spontaneous cerebral haemorrhage was leaking in the subarachnoid space which produced neck rigidity. However, as this prominent sign of subarachnoid haemorrhage is absent during coma, diagnosis ultimately depends on lumbar puncture. Spontaneous cerebral haemorrhages are mostly caused by vascular malformations (*e.g.* arteriovenous aneurysms, microangiomas, saccular aneurysms); other, rare causes are hypertension (CASE 28 with coarctation) and tumours (CASE 69).

As a rule, apoplectiform hemiplegia, occurring without loss of consciousness, without convulsions and without neck rigidity, points to arterial occlusion, but does not exclude intracerebral haemorrhage (*e.g.* CASE 10, with arteriovenous aneurysm). On the other hand, cerebral arterial thrombosis, as well as embolism, may also lead to immediate coma.

Many different vascular diseases may cause arterial occlusion, as described in Chapters 6-15. Cerebral angiography is particularly useful in the diagnosis of specific diseases.

Thrombotic arterial occlusions may regress spontaneously within a few days, as was observed in CASE 35. Dalal *et al.* (1965, 1966) have reported the spontaneous disappearance of emboli, either within hours or within days. These observations indicate clearly that the pathogenesis may only be revealed by early angiography. On the other hand, repeat angiography at a later stage in the course of the illness may also be of great importance, as is evident from CASE 21. This young girl developed a mycotic aneurysm as a result of a local inflammation of the arterial wall, and it was thus possible, retrospectively, to explain the pathogenesis of the acute hemiplegia. Reference has already been made to similar findings reported by Bickerstaff (1964) (see page 42).

The venous phase of the angiogram merits special attention. As illustrated by CASE 14, significant pathological lesions may go unrecognised in routinely performed angiography. Under certain conditions, *e.g.* in cases of venous malformations and suspected cases of cerebral venous thrombosis, several late exposures may be essential for the diagnosis.

The objection that carotid angiography represents a risk that may well aggravate the patient's condition should not be dismissed lightly. However, in the hands of an experienced operator, and with the use of general anaesthesia administered by a competent anaesthetist, angiography can be approached without serious misgivings, even in children with acute and severe hemisyndromes. The results are by no means only of academic interest, but may have therapeutic consequences, *e.g.* in opening the way for evacuation of a cerebral haematoma, for operation on an arteriovenous malformation, and for anticoagulant treatment in cerebral thrombophlebitis.

Although sudden hemiplegia occurring without epileptic seizures in the acute stage can be ascribed with a fair degree of certainty to a vascular insult, the aetiology of acute hemiplegia accompanied by convulsions is far less uniform. As a general rule, any cerebral disturbance is apt to produce seizures, and children are more prone to convulsions than adults.

By far the commonest and most peculiar form of hemiplegia in children is characterised by an abrupt onset of hemiconvulsions associated with an ordinary infection (usually of the upper respiratory tract), and an absence of any clinical evidence of encephalitis. This picture is found almost exclusively in children under the age of 4 years, or, in effect, in the same group of children that is prone to benign febrile convulsions. The aetiology of febrile convulsions is still unknown. Millichap (1968) has sharply opposed the widely advocated view that they are related to an inherited predisposition. He considers immaturity of the brain and structural cerebral pathology to be aetiologically significant factors, along with various miscellaneous mechanisms such as electrolyte imbalance, lack of immunoglobulins and hypersensitive reactions to bacteria, toxins and drugs. The author suspects pre-existing but, for the most part, clinically silent cerebral damage to be one of the principal causes of 'febrile hemiconvulsions'.

As shown on page 131, long-lasting tonic-clonic convulsions may produce ictogenic brain lesions, independently of the causative disease. In this respect, cerebral oedema may play a decisive rôle, as was demonstrated in CASE 62 by follow-up pneumoencephalography.

In this series, the absence of cerebral seizures in the acute stage was most striking in patients who suffered spontaneous and para- and post-infectious arterial occlusions of sudden onset. It would seem that ischaemia of a cerebral hemisphere may be so abrupt that the latter loses its ability to produce hypersynchronous discharges—a function which persists, however, during gradually increasing hypoxia. Illustrative examples are CASE 21 (with local inflammatory involvement of the carotis), CASE 29 (with traumatic carotid thrombosis) and CASE 42 (showing initial intermittent attacks, with thrombosis of the middle cerebral artery).

A particular diagnostic problem is presented by patients in whom hemiconvulsions commence homolaterally to the brain lesion (*e.g.* CASE 1, with a ruptured arteriovenous aneurysm, and CASE 29, with traumatic carotid thrombosis), or in whom EEG demonstrates epileptic discharges in the hemisphere contralateral to the brain lesion (*e.g.* CASE 5, with a ruptured arteriovenous aneurysm). This misleading side localisation may be explained by structural (haemorrhagic) and/or functional (ischaemic) obstruction of the affected hemisphere, which prevents that hemisphere from taking part in a proper generalised seizure.

Convulsions may be disastrous in cases with inadequate cerebral circulation, as is illustrated by CASE 21. The author believes that severe residual unilateral cerebral atrophy in this patient was caused more by the convulsive damage than by the defective circulation. Bearing in mind the damage which convulsions can cause, it should again be emphasised how frequently epileptic attacks occur in association with disturbances of the venous circulation (*e.g.* thrombophlebitis, venous malformations), when tissue hypoxia is also present or can be confidently postulated.

Unfortunately, following an acute hemiplegia, the majority of children are left with severe neurological sequelae, not only in respect of motor and sensory function, but also of an intellectual and emotional nature. Brandt (1962), in order to explain the mental damage that is frequently present, presumed that, in children with acute hemiplegia, bilateral cerebral damage occurs. The majority of such patients either experience severe seizures during the acute phase of the illness or develop late epilepsy, so the involvement of both hemispheres could result from convulsive activity. However, in CASES 34 and 40 of this series (both with spontaneous cerebral artery occlusions), epileptic complications did not accompany the apoplectiform insult, nor did they occur during the years which followed; there were similar findings in CASE 22 (with post-inflammatory carotid thrombosis). Nevertheless, all three children exhibited a definite organic psychosyndrome following unilateral damage.

Apart from hemiplegic encephalitis, acute occlusion of cerebral arteries has the worst prognosis, as irreversible cell damage occurs within minutes of total interruption of the cerebral blood supply. As has been shown by several examples (see Chap. 13), if the brain is to recover following an arterial occlusion, a satisfactory collateral circulation must develop rapidly. Little is known of the reasons why, in many cases, the collateral circulation fails to open up promptly. Inadequately developed collateral channels may offer a partial explanation.

Patency of the lenticulostriate arteries is a critical factor in patients who recover from hemiplegia. If these arteries are deprived of their blood supply, the cerebral damage is irreversible. CASE 43 illustrates this point. CASE 37 demonstrates clearly that even a total occlusion of the middle cerebral artery may be accompanied by minimal neurological deficit. In this patient, the thrombosis took some time to become complete, a factor which probably facilitated the development of a satisfactory collateral circulation.

An essential pre-requisite for the functional integrity of the collateral circulation is the maintenance of a well-functioning general systemic circulation; this has been stressed by Denny-Brown (1951), Meyer and Denny-Brown (1957), Bernsmeier (1963) and others. It is known that, in the presence of an intact vascular system, the cerebral circulation is autonomically regulated, so that its perfusion pressure and oxidative metabolism are held at an extraordinarily constant level, to a large extent independent of the systemic blood pressure. This regulation of the cerebral circulation is affected by alterations in the calibre of the blood vessels, and by the extent of oxygen depletion in the blood. The carbon dioxide content of the blood and the degree of oxygen deprivation of the brain tissues are among the most important factors involved in the regulation of the cerebral circulation. Under normal conditions, however, a transient general circulatory insufficiency may be enough to provoke irreversible brain damage in a critically irrigated region (Meyer and Denny-Brown 1957, Cavanagh 1962).

Therapy

The importance of maintaining a continuously sufficient systemic circulation and adequate ventilation needs no comment, and treatment will not be discussed here.

The immediate objective should be suppression of a status epilepticus. In this respect, diazepam (Valium 'Roche', 5-10 mg per m^2 body surface, i.v.) proved its value in most cases. If this drug should fail, fast-acting intravenous barbiturates are usually effective (*e.g.* amobarbital sodium 'Lilly' 100-200 mg/m^2, slowly, i.v., or Somnifene 'Roche'—which is identical to Hypnophen 'Gattiker'—200-400 mg/m^2, slowly, i.v., or Evipan sodium, 100-150 mg/m^2, slowly, i.v.). In the rare cases in which convulsions persist, anaesthesia is necessary. In small children, rectal chloral hydrate (2-3 g/m^2 body surface) is invaluable.

Anticonvulsant treatment for approximately one week is appropriate in all children with hemiplegia accompanied by convulsions. If seizures occur, or epileptic discharges become apparent on EEG, either during convalescence or later, long-term anticonvulsant treatment should be commenced (*e.g.* with phenobarbitone and/or Dilantin).

Treatment with anticoagulants is thought to be indicated in all cases with cerebral thrombophlebitis or venous thrombosis. The author starts therapy with rapidly effective heparin (15,000 U/m^2/24 hours, i.v.; adjustment of the dose is made by frequent determinations of the anti-thrombin time). Starting one to two days later, Marcumar 'Roche' (approximately 3 mg/m^2 body surface/24 hours, orally; adjustment of dose depending on Quick test) is used for at least one month. A period of hospitalisation is necessary for adjustment of the dosage of an anticoagulant.

No significant results can be given concerning the use of anticoagulant treatment in cases with cerebral arterial occlusion.

In cases with hyperpyrexia (*e.g.* encephalitis, thrombophlebitis), the author uses 'cocktail-treatment', aimed at lowering the patient's temperature to a level compatible with an adequate systemic circulation and ventilation. (Composition of 'cocktail': pethidine 50 mg = 1 ml, Largactil 50 mg = 2 ml, NaCl 0.9 per cent = 7 ml. Dose: 0.1 ml/kg body weight, every 3-4 hours). If this treatment is not effective within 12 hours, cooling of the body may be achieved by the use of a fan, alcohol spray, and ice bags.

Antibiotic treatment of cases with bacterial infection will not be discussed here.

The problem of how to treat brain oedema remains unsolved. The usefulness of hypertonic solutions is debatable. In all cases with prolonged convulsions, brain oedema is more than likely to be present. In such cases, the author uses sorbitol 40 per cent ($2\frac{1}{2}$ ml/kg body weight, in a single dose, by i.v. drip infusion). In his opinion, early treatment (*i.e.* within hours of the start of convulsions) is essential. In cases of advanced oedema this treatment is no longer of value (*e.g.* CASES 58 and 63). Oedema may also be treated with the saluretic furosemide (Lasix 'Hoechst', 0.5-1.0 mg/kg body weight pro dosi orally, or i.m. or i.v.). It should be pointed out that such a treatment can only be administered in patients with compensated systemic circulation. Cortico-steroids are also widely used in the treatment of brain oedema.

There is, so far, no convincing evidence of the efficacy of drugs in the treatment of a pathological circulation (*i.e.* in opening up collateral channels in cases with cerebral arterial occlusion or in cases with suspected brain oedema due to prolonged convulsions). Papaverine, advocated as one of the most potent drugs in this respect, exerted no significant effect in many of the cases in this study, even when given in large doses (up to 200 mg/m^2 body surface/24 hours).

Vascular surgery (*e.g.* thrombectomy) is briefly discussed in Chapter 13 (see page 80).

This study has revealed an unexpected multiplicity of causes of acute hemi-syndromes in children. Cerebral angiography has provided the aetiological explanation in many cases of so-called 'hemiplegia of obscure origin'. However, it has been found that in certain cases one should hesitate before drawing any conclusions from the angiographic appearances, for negative findings by no means rule out the possibility of a vascular aetiology. Successful demonstration of the presence of a vascular lesion may depend not only upon an adequate angiographic technique but also upon the instant during the course of the illness at which the angiogram is made. A sentence from the first aphorism of Hippocrates—'the right time is only a moment'—possesses a dual validity in this instance: in the treatment as well as in the elucidation of the cause of the illness.

Table of
Case Histories

KEY

◁	Primary illness
◀	Hemisyndrome
▨	Hemiconvulsions
▤	Generalised seizures
URTI	Upper respiratory tract infection
I	Influenzal illness
GI	Gastro-intestinal infection
Vacc.	Vaccination
T	Head injury
S	Subarachnoid haemorrhage

#	Epileptic attacks
→	Attacks
?	Onset not precisely known
E	Vomiting
C	Carotid angiogram
P	Pneumoencephalogram
V	Vertebral angiogram
Ⓚ	Duration of history
OP	Operation
+	Death

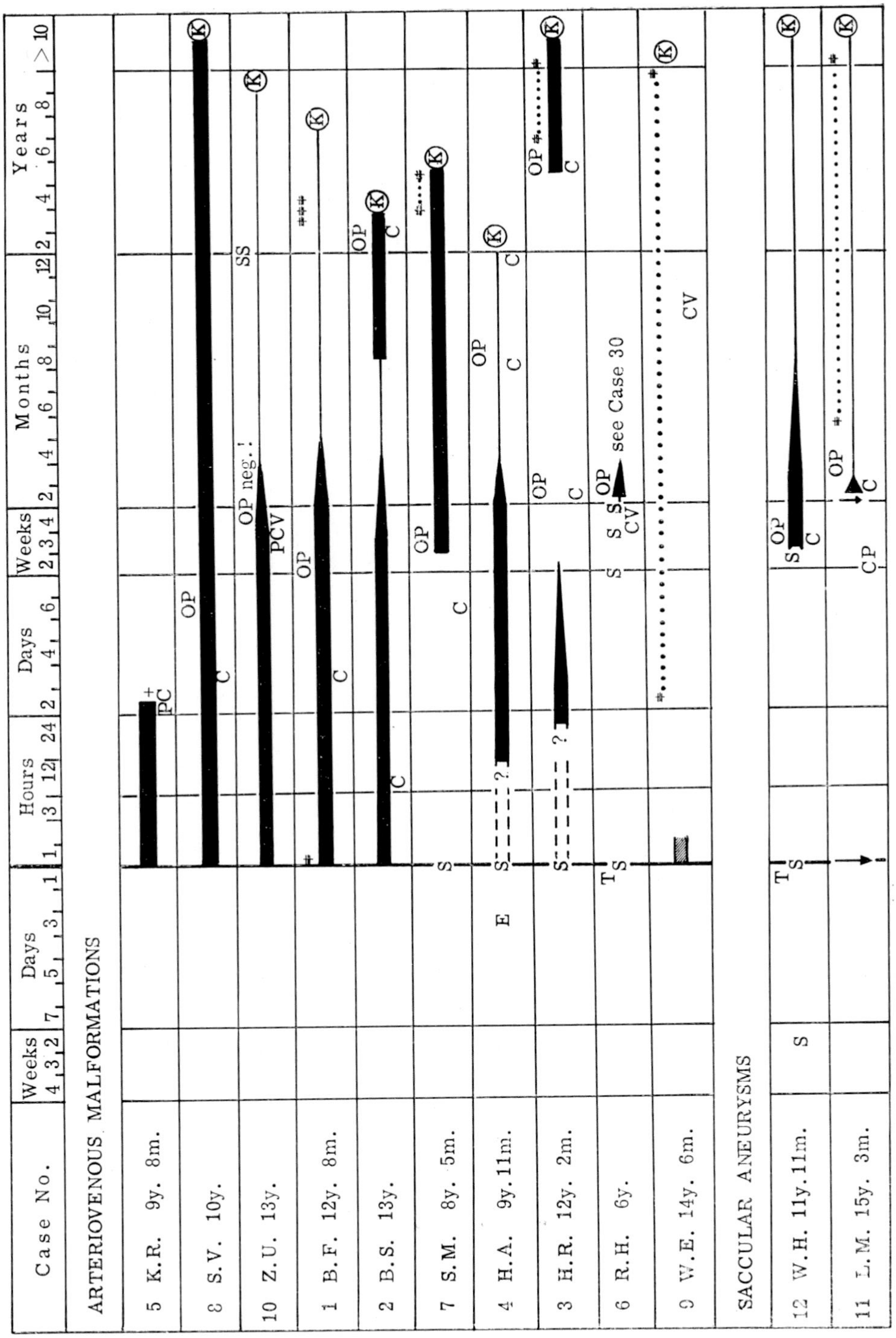
Case No.
Weeks 4 3 2
Days 7 5 3 1
Hours 1 3 12 24
Days 2 4 6
Weeks 2 3 4
Months 2 4 6 8 10 12
Years 2 4 6 8 > 10
ARTERIOVENOUS MALFORMATIONS
5 K.R. 9y. 8m.
8 S.V. 10y.
10 Z.U. 13y.
1 B.F. 12y. 8m.
2 B.S. 13y.
7 S.M. 8y. 5m.
4 H.A. 9y. 11m.
3 H.R. 12y. 2m.
6 R.H. 6y.
9 W.E. 14y. 6m.
SACCULAR ANEURYSMS
12 W.H. 11y. 11m.
11 L.M. 15y. 3m.
PC
OP
OP neg. !
PCV
SS
see Case 30
CV
CP

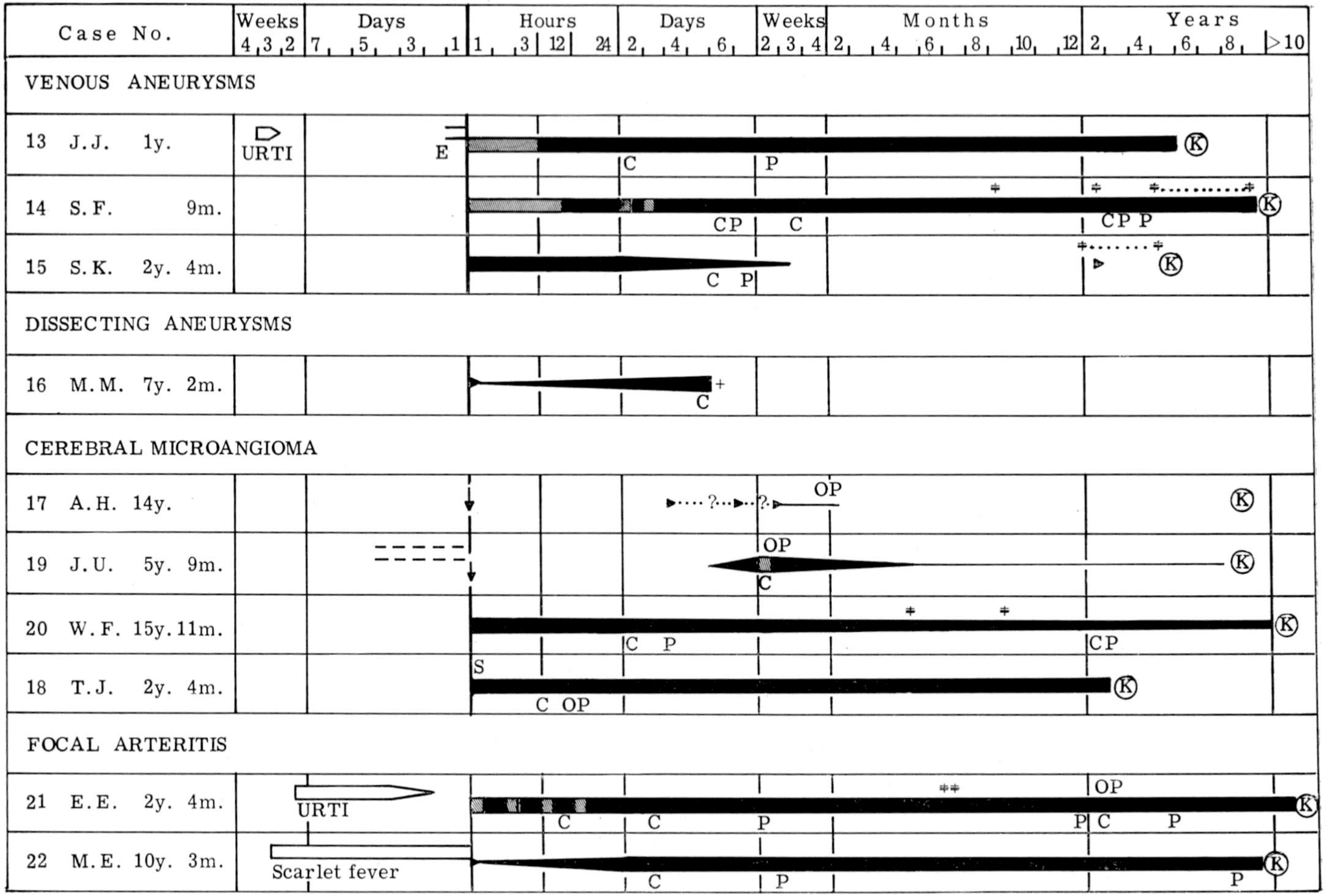
Case No.
Weeks 4 3 2
Days 7 5 3 1
Hours 1 3 12 24
Days 2 4 6
Weeks 2 3 4
Months 2 4 6 8 10 12
Years 2 4 6 8 >10
VENOUS ANEURYSMS
13 J.J. 1y.
URTI
E
C P
K
14 S.F. 9m.
CP C
CP P
K
15 S.K. 2y. 4m.
C P
K
DISSECTING ANEURYSMS
16 M.M. 7y. 2m.
C
+
CEREBRAL MICROANGIOMA
17 A.H. 14y.
? ?
OP
K
19 J.U. 5y. 9m.
OP
C
K
20 W.F. 15y. 11m.
C P
CP
K
18 T.J. 2y. 4m.
S
C OP
K
FOCAL ARTERITIS
21 E.E. 2y. 4m.
URTI
C C P
OP
P C P
K
22 M.E. 10y. 3m.
Scarlet fever
C P
P
K

Years | Months | Weeks | Days | Hours | Days | Weeks

Case No.

FIBROMUSCULAR HYPERPLASIA

23 R.G. 2y. 9m.

MULTIPLE OCCLUSIONS WITH UNUSUAL NET-LIKE COLLATERALS ('Moyamoya Disease')

24 F.D. 8m.

25 H.B. 6y. 8m. — — — URTI

HYPERTENSION

27 A.R. 8y.10m. E E Renal hypertension

28 G.M. 13y. Aortic stenosis

TRAUMATIC CEREBRAL ARTERIAL OCCLUSION

29 P.F. 3y. T

30 R.H. 6y. 4m. T 3.5m. previously

EMBOLISM

31 A.E. 9y. 4m.

32 R.A. 2y.10m. Carditis

For KEY to Table see page 194

SPONTANEOUS CEREBRAL ARTERIAL OCCLUSION

Case No.	Weeks 4,3,2	Days 7,5,3,1	Hours 1,3,12	24,2,4,6 Days	Weeks 2,3,4	Months 6,8,10,12 Years 2,4,6,8 >10
39 S.K. 16y.11m.					C	‡‡ Ⓚ
40 U.H. 9y.	T		OP	C		Ⓚ
38 S.F. 14y. 7m.			C	C	C	‡‡ CP Ⓚ
35 H.B. 11y. 5m.			C		C Ⓚ	
37 N.R. 5y.				C	C	C Ⓚ
34 B.H. 2y. 1m.	E			C	C	Ⓚ
33 A.I. 12y.	‖‖▲			V	VC ▲	Ⓚ
36 H.M. 13y.10m.				C	C	Ⓚ

198

PARA- AND POST-INFECTIOUS CEREBRAL ARTERIAL OCCLUSION

Case No.	Weeks 4,3,2	Days 7,5,3,1	Hours 24 2,1	Days 2,4,6	Weeks 2,3,4	Months 6,8,10 12	Years 2,4,6,8 >10

41 G.E. 2y. 4m. — URTI — ? C — P — ♯ Ⓚ C

43 H.M. 1y. 2m. — ? C — Ⓚ C.P.

44 I.L. 1y. 5m. — Pneumonia — PC — C — ♯ Ⓚ C

45 M.M. 5y. 3m. Tonsillect., measles — C P — C — CP — Ⓚ

42 G.M. 1y. 2m. II URTI — P C — C — Ⓚ

HEMIPLEGIA WITHOUT CONVULSIONS

52 S.H. 7y. 3m. — Ⓚ

112 R.H. 7y. 2m. — C — P — Ⓚ

113 F.M. 5y. 4m. Otitis media — P — Ⓚ

INFECTIOUS THROMBOPHLEBITIS

53 B.G. 13y. 7m. E — URTI — C P — ♯ + Ⓚ

54 S.K. 7y. 3m. GI Otitis — P — C +

55 G.M. 11m. Congen. heart disease — URTI — CP +

199

Case No.

Weeks 4, 3, 2 | Days 7, 5, 3, 1 | Hours 3, 12 | 24, 2 | Days 4, 6 | Weeks 2, 3, 4 | Months 8, 10, 12 | Years 2, 4, 6, 8 | >10

POSTICTAL HEMIPLEGIA WITHOUT INFECTION

109 H.T. 5y. 4m. — ? — PC — C — Ⓚ

110 G.W. 3y, 7m. — ? — C — P — Ⓚ

111 A.C. 2y. 11m. — Ⓚ

POSTICTAL HEMIPLEGIA, PARA- AND POST-INFECTIOUS

56 H.F. 2y. 5m. — GI ? — PCP — Ⓚ

59 W.S. 1y. 2m. — URTI — ? — PCP — Ⓚ

58 P.R. 1y. 2m. — GI — CP P — PPCPPP — Ⓚ

57 G.C. 2y. 11m. — URTI — P P — Ⓚ

114 Z.B. 2y. 1m. — URTI — P — Ⓚ

115 V.A. 1y. 1m. — URTI — Ⓚ

116 W.V. 1y. 8m. — URTI — P — Ⓚ

83 Z.C. 1y. — URTI — Ⓚ

84 G.Y. 2y. 11m. — URTI — PC

200

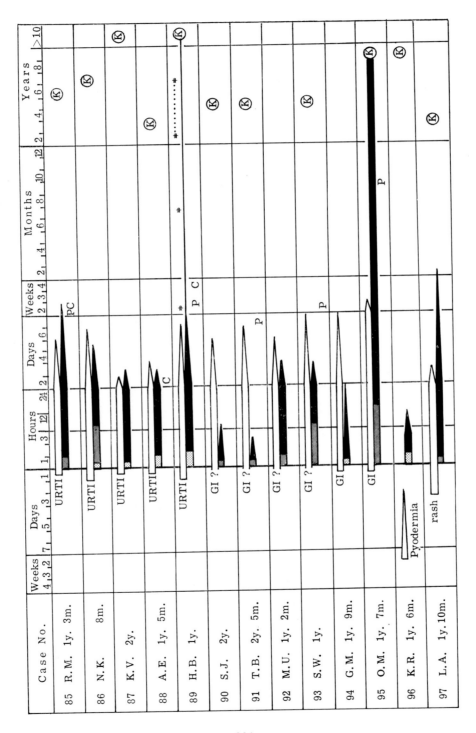

HEMIPLEGIA IN ENCEPHALITIS

Case No.								
	Weeks	Days	Hours	Days	Weeks	Months	Years	
62 A.B. 2y. 4m.	'Virus encephalitis'							
64 B.R. 10m.	I							
65 G.M. 1y. 6m.	Vacc•							
63 B.B. 1y. 2m.	Vacc•							
66 S.V. 11y.10m.	Toxoplasmosis encephalitis							
67 F.E. 13y. 4m.	URTI Necrotising leucoencephalitis							
68 R.C. 3y.10m.	T Cerebral abscess							
98 K.S. 1y. 2m.	Measles							
99 I.F. 7y. 4m.	Measles							
100 I.R. 1y. 3m.	Chicken-pox							
101 D.B. 1y. 3m.	Vacc•							
102 J.G. 3y.10m.	GI Vacc.							

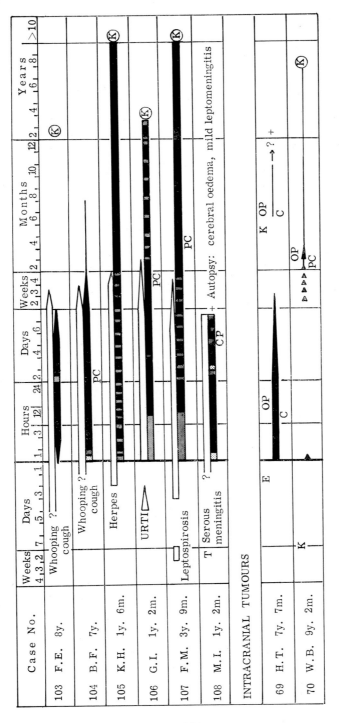

For KEY to Table see page 194

203

MIGRAINE ACCOMPAGNEE

204

Detailed Case
Reports

Detailed Case Reports

CASE 1

B.F., born 3 November 1947 (372/60, 515/60).*

FAMILY HISTORY. Nil relevant.

PREVIOUS HISTORY. Pregnancy normal. Birth at 8 months gestation. Birth weight 2500g; healthy baby. Development normal. Appendicectomy in 1953. Bruising of right forehead in Autumn of 1959, without signs of brain damage.

PRESENT ILLNESS. On 10 July 1960, the patient, then a healthy boy aged 12 years 8 months, went outside after his midday meal to work on his bicycle. A few minutes later he returned inside, complained of severe headache and nausea, and said 'blood has suddenly flowed into my head'. He vomited and collapsed unconscious. Immediately, coarse convulsive movements commenced in the right arm and leg, recurring every 5-10 minutes; the left extremities remained flaccid and immobile.

Admission to Children's Hospital, Zurich (10-15 July 1960).

FINDINGS ON ADMISSION. Admitted 1½ hours after the attack, the child was deeply unconscious and did not react to painful stimuli. Clonic seizures involving the right side of the body occurred every few minutes, the left extremities remaining flaccid and immobile. Knee and ankle jerks were normal on both sides of the body; bilateral Babinski responses were present. The right abdominal reflex only was present. The pupils were equal, reacting promptly to light. The eyes diverged slightly and were directed upwards. The nasal margin of the optic discs appeared somewhat blurred, but the blood-vessels were normal and no haemorrhages were present. Neck muscles were flaccid and there was no meningism. Auscultation of the skull proved negative. Blood pressure 125/85 mm. Pulse 64/min, regular.

Lumbar Puncture. Pressure 40 cm H_2O, CSF grossly and uniformly blood-stained. Total

*Admission numbers allocated by the Children's Hospital, Zurich. Cases without numbers are from the Department of Neurosurgery, University Hospital, Zurich.

protein 2790 mg/per cent, glucose 67 mg/per cent, chloride 447 mg/per cent. Blood: Hb 72 per cent; reticulocytes 21 per cent; leucocytes 6400, juvenile forms 9 per cent, mature forms 59 per cent; eosinophils 3.9 per cent; monocytes 6 per cent; lymphocytes 22.5 per cent; platelets normal. ESR 6/18 mm. Axillary temperature 37.8°C.

EEG (11 July 1960). Constant focus of delta activity in the right central/postcentral region, with very severe and diffusely disturbed cerebral activity. No epilepsy potentials were observed.

Right Carotid Angiogram (12 July 1960). A mass of blood vessels 1 x 0.5 cm in size was demonstrated precentrally at the level of and lateral to the callosomarginal artery. Excellent opacification was present in the arterial phase of the serial angiogram. A solitary large vein drained the contrast blood into the superior sagittal sinus. No definite displacement of cerebral vessels was shown (Figs. 1 and 2).

Left Carotid Angiogram (12 July 1960). With compression of the contralateral carotid artery, the right anterior cerebral artery was seen to be supplying the arteriovenous aneurysm by cross-flow through the anterior communicating artery. The left cerebral vessels appeared normal.

COURSE. The level of consciousness improved to the extent that the child could be spoken to 7 hours after the attack. He complained of severe pains in the neck and right forehead, and vomited repeatedly. A flaccid left hemiplegia and facial palsy were present. With the return of consciousness, severe neck stiffness appeared, the patient adopting an opisthotonic position. On 11 July 1960, the patient remained dazed, spatially disorientated and answered questions with slow slurred speech. A flaccid paralysis was present in the left arm and a spastic paralysis in the left leg. The deep reflexes were increased on the left side and the Babinski response remained positive. The meningism did not diminish and the boy complained of a continuous severe headache. Towards evening of the same day, a state of psychic excitement supervened. The patient was incontinent of urine and faeces.

207

Transfer to Department of Neurosurgery, University Hospital, Zurich (15 July 1960).

FINDINGS ON ADMISSION. Physical findings were virtually unchanged. The left arm showed withdrawal from painful stimuli. The modality of pain was preserved over the paralysed left half of the body. The left corneal reflex was diminished.

OPERATION (18 July 1960). Right fronto-parietal craniotomy. An abnormal subpial vascular mass was found 4 cm lateral to the mid-line in the precentral region, upon which numerous tortuous vessels converged from the medial and lateral sides. A single large vein passed mediallv from the mass towards the superior sagittal sinus. The cortex in this region showed a blackish discolouration, with an 8 x 6 x 6 cm haematoma protruding into the brain substance and rupturing the lateral ventricle beneath. The vascular formation was removed and the haematoma evacuated.

Histological Examination (Department of Pathology, University of Zurich). Extirpated vascular mass found to be angioma arteriovenosum aneurysmaticum.

COURSE. The child regained complete consciousness on the evening following the operation. Three weeks later the first slight voluntary movements returned in the paralysed extremities. With constant physiotherapy (27 July-10 September 1960) the hemiparesis showed an amazing regression, only slight distal spasticity and facial palsy involving the mouth remaining. The boy started regular school lessons again in the Autumn of 1960, but his results were not as good as they had been before the attack. Repeated EEG examinations (6 January 1961, 24 May 1961) revealed the presence of an epileptogenic focus in the right parietal region, but an otherwise normal background activity.

PROGRESS (to August 1966). Between March 1964 and November 1965 the patient experienced several epileptic attacks, despite anticonvulsant treatment. One such attack resulted in a twilight state which lasted several hours, in which the patient rode about aimlessly on a bus and was unable to recall anything of the incident. Other attacks were accompanied by clonic unilateral convulsions and brief losses of consciousness. The attacks disappeared with adjustment of the antiepileptic treatment. In 1963, the patient began

an apprenticeship as a machine fitter, which he has pursued to the present time with satisfactory results. The only residual deficit of the hemiplegia is a mild spastic paresis of the left upper limb, and some disturbance of function of the left hand. His gait is normal. The patient is known for his 'fussiness'.

CASE 2

B.S., born 4 September 1951 (2695/64, 4931/65, 7973/66).

FAMILY HISTORY. Nil relevant.

PREVIOUS HISTORY. Pregnancy normal. Caesarean section at term, due to abnormal position. Possible fetal asphyxia, but prompt recovery. Birth weight 3300g. Psychomotor development normal. Tonsillectomy following repeated attacks of acute tonsillitis up to the age of 2 years. Subsequently, no relevant illnesses or attacks. A bright pupil at school.

PRESENT ILLNESS. On 11 September 1964, while at morning toilet, the girl suddenly experienced an attack of right-sided hemiplegia with aphasia, without warning symptoms. She developed extreme pallor, vomited repeatedly and appeared not to recognise her mother.

Admission to Children's Hospital, Zurich (11 September-22 December 1964).

FINDINGS ON ADMISSION. Admitted 7 hours after the attack, the patient was somnolent, with complete right-sided hemiplegia (including the face) and motor aphasia. There was a diminution of tendon jerks in the right extremities (left side normal); a right Babinski reflex was present; right abdominal reflexes were absent. The child exhibited a bilateral Parinaud-type of paralysis of upward gaze, delayed pupillary reaction to light, and irregular fine spontaneous nystagmus to both sides. Marked meningism was present, accompanied by an apparently marked reduction of superficial and deep sensitivity over the entire right side of the body. She was afebrile, and her cardiovascular system was normal. Pulse about 100/min. Blood: Hb 13g per cent; leucocytes 12,800, juvenile forms 36.5 per cent, mature forms 57.5 per cent.

Lumbar Puncture. The fluid was uniformly blood-stained, and moderately xanthochromic after centrifugation. Pressure was normal.

Left Carotid Angiogram. (11 September 1964). An enormous arteriovenous aneurysm was demonstrated in the depths of the hemisphere, supplied by the middle cerebral artery and draining into the vein of Galen and the straight sinus (Figs. 1 and 3).

COURSE. On 12 September 1964, the patient fully recovered consciousness. Sub-total motor aphasia and complete anaesthesia and analgesia remained, with insensitivity to heat and reduced vibration and movement modalities over the entire right side of the body. The Parinaud Syndrome was no longer visible on 15 September, and there was some return of voluntary movement in the proximal muscles of the leg. Improvement was surprisingly good with intensive physiotherapy. Upon discharge before Christmas 1964, only a limited spastic paraplegia of the distal muscle groups was still present. Fine hand movements remained defective, the gait was only slightly disturbed by a mild degree of circumduction, and the facial palsy had disappeared completely. The right-sided diminution in superficial and deep sensory modalities persisted. A definite organic psychosyndrome was present, with a marked disturbance of recent memory. IQ (Stanford-Lückert) on 3 December 1964: 76.

Lumbar Puncture (3 December 1964). CSF clear. Protein 58 mg per cent; monocytes $5\frac{1}{3}$; erythrocytes $3\frac{1}{3}$.

EEG (4 December 1964). A non-specific low-grade disturbance was demonstrated over the postero-lateral parts of the left hemisphere, with isolated suspicious epilepsy potentials in these areas. Photostimulation produced more generalised disturbances with convulsive potentials.

The patient's condition remained stationary until the end of May 1965. On 29 May 1965, during the night, the patient suddenly cried out in her sleep. Her parents found her unconscious, vomiting, and incontinent of urine.

Re-admission to the Children's Hospital, Zurich.

FINDINGS ON ADMISSION. Admitted shortly after the attack, the patient was unconscious with complete spastic right-sided hemiplegia. Her arm was in flexion and her leg in extension. There was inconstant conjugate deviation of both eyes to the right and upwards, and the pupils were bilaterally constricted, with delayed reaction to light. Severe trismus was present. The girl showed no reaction to pinprick over the whole right side of the body, but prompt reaction on the left side. She was afebrile, but showed marked meningism and was incontinent of urine. Blood pressure 110/80 mm; pulse 100/min.

Lumbar Puncture. CSF grossly and uniformly blood-stained.

COURSE. By the following day the spasticity had disappeared, and a completely flaccid hemiplegia, with total motor aphasia, remained. The patient was apathetic and somnolent. An irregular oscillatory nystagmus was present, and she was unable to maintain focus for long. Tendon jerks in the right extremities were absent, and a right Babinski response was elicited. Jerks on the left side were greatly increased; left-sided voluntary movement was intact. The child was incontinent of urine and yawned persistently.

Recovery on this occasion took much longer and was less complete. A severe spastic hemiplegia persisted, as well as a right-sided homonymous hemianopia, partial motor aphasia, severe right-sided disturbances of sensory modalities, and a marked organic psychosyndrome.

EEG (12 November 1965). Moderately severe diffuse disturbances were demonstrated, with complete depression of the background rhythm over the left hemisphere. There was a very active epileptogenic focus over the left parietal region. Photostimulation produced generalised bursts of convulsion potentials.

OPERATION (19 January 1966). An operation was performed at the Department of Neurosurgery, University Hospital, Zurich, for ligation of the lenticulostriate, anterior cerebral and posterior communicating arteries on the left side.

Follow-up Left Carotid Angiography revealed that the malformation continued to fill, although it was less marked.

The patient suffered no ill effects from the operation.

EEG (15 February 1966). Only minor changes were shown compared with the findings of 12 November 1965. The epileptogenic focus was still present in the left anterior temporal region. However, photostimulation now produced no bursts of activity. The right hemisphere appeared to be scarcely involved.

PROGRESS. Up to July 1966 no change had occurred in the child's condition. She could get about on crutches.

CASE 3

H.R., born 7 March 1941.

FAMILY HISTORY. Nil relevant.

PREVIOUS HISTORY. Measles in 1949; scarlet fever in 1950.

PRESENT ILLNESS. On 13 May 1949, this 12-year-old boy suddenly, and without warning, experienced severe pain in the neck which radiated to the head. He recollected walking into his room and vomiting. He was found 1-2 hours later.

Admission to the Department of Medicine, Cantonal Hospital, Aarau (13 May-17 June 1953).

FINDINGS ON ADMISSION. The child was very drowsy, answering only 'yes' and 'no'. He had no neck stiffness and was afebrile. CSF was normal with a pressure of 23 cm. Leucocytes 8800 with 90 per cent neutrophils. ESR 21-50 mm. Blood pressure 135/85 mm; pulse 100/min. The cardiovascular system was found to be normal.

On 14 May the boy's temperature was 38°C, and he showed definite neck stiffness with flaccid paresis of the left arm. On 15 May he temporarily lapsed into a coma.

Lumbar Puncture revealed negative pressure, and cisternal puncture showed uniformly blood-stained CSF. Over the next few days speech returned to normal, but the patient remained dysarthric, and the paresis began to improve. About one week after the attack, he showed a temporary marked right central facial paralysis.

Lumbar Puncture (26 May 1953) revealed xanthochromic fluid.

Admission to the Department of Neurosurgery, University Hospital, Zurich (17 June-16 July 1953).

FINDINGS ON ADMISSION. The child's neurological state was unchanged and his CSF was normal.

EEG. Left frontal delta focus.

Left Carotid Angiogram. An arteriovenous aneurysm was demonstrated in the left frontal region.

OPERATION (29 June 1953). The arteriovenous malformation which lay between the anterior and middle cerebral arteries below the second and third frontal gyrus was sub-totally resected. A walnut-sized subcortical haematoma was evacuated.

COURSE. The patient was discharged on 16 July 1953, without neurological deficit. He remained free from complaints until mid-November 1957, when he suffered a febrile influenza-like illness from which he recovered within one week. On the morning of 8 December 1957 he awakened with a flaccid paralysis of the right arm, a skew mouth, and intense headache.

Second Admission to the Department of Neurosurgery, University Hospital, Zurich (11 December 1957-11 January 1958).

The child showed no mental disturbance, but severe spastic paresis of the right arm and a right central facial paralysis were present.

Bilateral Carotid Angiography and Vertebral Angiography. An extensive arteriovenous aneurysm was demonstrated in the left fronto-precentral region, supplied chiefly by the anterior cerebral artery. The malformation also received a supply from the opposite carotid through the anterior communicating artery, but not from the vertebro-basilar tree. There was extensive venous drainage through the precentral vein (vein of Trolard) and the internal cerebral vein (Figs. 1 and 4).

EEG. A left frontal delta focus was shown, with no epilepsy potentials. General physical examination revealed no abnormality. No scalp murmurs synchronous with the pulse could be elicited.

OPERATION (17 December 1957). A radical resection was made of the arteriovenous aneurysm which lay in the subcortical layer of the left precentral region and extended deep to the level of the ventricle. A large haemorrhagic cyst in the central part of the hemisphere was evacuated.

COURSE. Upon discharge on 11 January 1958 some mental slowing was present, while the spastic paresis of the arm remained unchanged. There was no sensory involvement.

PROGRESS. A gradual improvement occurred in the paralysis until the onset of epileptic attacks in July 1959. The boy found work as a joiner's assistant, and was able to use his right hand after a fashion. Despite prophylactic pheno-barbitone medication, he experienced an attack roughly every 3 months; sometimes these attacks were Jacksonian in type, at other times they took the form of generalised convulsions. He is now suffering from a marked psycho-organic syndrome with a memory defect as the presenting feature, and a partial motor aphasia is present in that he has difficulty in finding the correct word. The spastic paresis of the right arm has increased, and the hand is now functionally useless.

CASE 4

H.A., born 18 December 1945.

FAMILY HISTORY. Nil relevant.

PREVIOUS HISTORY. Measles at 6 years; pneumonia at 9 years; otherwise health had been good.

PRESENT ILLNESS. In November 1955, this 9-year-old boy complained of lack of concentration, repeated vomiting and disturbed sleep. During the night of 23 November 1955, he was taken ill with vomiting and faecal incontinence, marked irritability and drowsiness. The next morning, a right-sided hemiplegia and a speech disturbance became manifest; the child lapsed into unconsciousness and remained in this state for 10 days.

Angiography performed in a foreign hospital revealed a left arteriovenous aneurysm.

Admission to the Department of Neurosurgery, University Hospital, Zurich (3-27 July 1956).

The patient was suffering from marked right-sided distal hemiplegia. The leg was more severely affected than the arm, and the face was not significantly involved. There was a slight speech disturbance with stuttering. A general physical examination gave negative results. Blood pressure 100/75 mm.

Left Carotid Angiography and Vertebral Angiography. An extensive arteriovenous aneurysm was demonstrated which was supplied exclusively by the left posterior communicating artery (Figs. 1 and 5).

OPERATION (9 July 1956). Two arteries were ligated at the origin of the posterior communicating artery from the internal carotid artery. Post-operatively, there was no significant change in the neurological deficit.

PROGRESS.

Follow-up Angiogram (28 January 1957). The arteriovenous aneurysm was shown to be filling from the left anterior cerebral artery through the perforating arteries, and draining through enlarged venous channels into the inferior sagittal sinus.

Clinical examination revealed that the hemiparesis was stationary, the arm hypotonic,

and the leg spastic. No speech disturbance remained. There was a marked mental change, in that the boy encountered great difficulties at school and had to be taught privately at home.

CASE 5

K.R., born 3 February 1947 (783/56, autopsy 1630/56).

FAMILY HISTORY. Nil relevant.

PREVIOUS HISTORY. Measles and whooping cough as a child. Smallpox vaccination in 1955.

PRESENT ILLNESS. On 24 October 1956, when the child was 9 years 8 months old and in good health, he experienced without warning at 6.30 a.m. a severe headache of sudden onset, followed by repeated vomiting. 15 minutes later he was found, limp and unrousable, in the toilet. Some hours later the family doctor referred the boy to hospital as an emergency, on the suspicion of food poisoning.

Admission to Hospital

FINDINGS. On admission at 2 p.m. the child was stuporose, with neck stiffness, right mydriasis with a reduced reaction to light, and muscular hypotonia with reduced knee jerks. Only the left ankle jerk was present; a left Babinski response was elicited.

Blood pressure 135/105 mm, later 160/90 mm; pulse 60/min, later 72/min. The child was afebrile. Blood: leucocytes 12,600/cu mm; glucose 190 mg per cent.

Lumbar Puncture. Pressure 30 cm H_2O; CSF clear; cells 6/3, Nonne and Pandy reactions negative.

The patient was transferred to the Children's Hospital, Zurich, and from there immediately to the Department of Neurosurgery, University of Zurich, because of the intracranial pressure signs and the flaccid hemiparesis.

Admission to the Department of Neurosurgery, University Hospital, Zurich.

FINDINGS ON ADMISSION. On admission at 10 p.m., the boy was very drowsy and somnolent, and answered questions with difficulty. He was suffering from flaccid incomplete left-sided hemiparesis with central facial palsy. All tendon reflexes were diminished without lateralising differences; a left Babinski response was elicited. There was a suggestion of blurring of the nasal margins of the optic discs. Visual fields could not be evaluated, due to drug dilatation of the pupils. No signs of meningism were observed.

EEG (25 October 1956, 8 a.m.). The recording was severely abnormal, with diffuse disturbances and depression of the background activity over the right hemisphere. A right postcentral delta focus was observed. There were extensive epileptogenic areas over the left hemisphere, with numerous spikes, often in series, followed by slow waves with delayed final deflection.

On the morning of 25 October 1956, a total flaccid paralysis of the left arm and an incomplete paralysis of the left leg were present. Tendon jerks were elicited with difficulty on the left side, but were normal on the right side. There was a marked left Babinski response. There was evidence of complete right third nerve palsy. The patient was irritable, and experienced attacks of headache which were tolerated less well over the left side of the head than the right. He was markedly drowsy, but answered questions correctly.

The surprising EEG changes prompted a change of plan, and a pneumoencephalogram was begun, instead of carotid angiography. During induction of the anaesthetic, a transient respiratory arrest occurred, which was promptly reversed. Some hours later, gas was injected following lumbar puncture without anaesthesia, but the ventricular system failed to fill.

Ventriculogram. This was carried out from a frontal burr-hole and revealed displacement of the ventricular system to the left side.

Right Carotid Angiogram. A $2\frac{1}{2}$ x 2 cm, large arteriovenous aneurysm was shown to be applied to the parietal convexity of the right hemisphere. It was supplied entirely by an abnormally large middle cerebral artery, and drained by large venous channels into the superior sagittal sinus. The malformation, which filled chiefly from the angular branch of the middle cerebral artery, showed irregular contours, which were interpreted to represent extravasation (Figs. 1 and 6). One hour after the carotid angiogram, while preparations were being made for emergency craniotomy, acute pulmonary oedema supervened, and the child died at 10 a.m. on 25 October 1956.

AUTOPSY FINDINGS. The autopsy was performed at the Institute of Pathology, University of Zurich. A large plum-sized arteriovenous aneurysm was found in the parieto-occipital

lobe of the right hemisphere, with extensive haemorrhage into the surrounding brain tissue. Other findings included cerebral oedema, (weight of brain 1280g), pulmonary oedema, acute dilatation of the heart with flaccid myocardium, and acute venous congestion of the internal organs.

CASE 6

R.H., born 28 August 1952 (5353/58, 5781/59, autopsy 151/59).

FAMILY HISTORY. Father with renal stones; otherwise, nil relevant.

PREVIOUS HISTORY. After a normal pregnancy, birth and development were normal. Mumps, chickenpox and German measles without complications. Occasionally suffered asthmatic bronchitis. In the winter of 1957/58 he suffered a right perforated otitis media.

PRESENT ILLNESS. On 28 August 1958, the patient, a 6-year-old boy, sustained a slight head injury without signs of concussion. Two hours later, he suddenly developed severe frontal headache, and vomited repeatedly. In the succeeding few days, he experienced repeated attacks of headache of sudden onset but of brief duration; there were no other symptoms. On 5 September 1958, he had a severe headache with vomiting, and became confused.

Admission to the Children's Hospital, Zurich. (6 September–9 October 1958).

FINDINGS ON ADMISSION. The patient was drowsy but orientated. He was suffering from severe meningism, and there was a suggestion of bilateral Babinski responses, but no other abnormality was noted. Blood pressure 115/60 mm; temperature 37.7°C. Blood: leucocytes 19,500, juvenile forms 14 per cent, mature forms 73 per cent. ESR 18/40 mm.

Lumbar Puncture. The fluid was lightly but uniformly blood-stained, and xanthochromic upon centrifugation. Recent as well as altered erythrocytes were present.

EEG. A moderate, generalised disturbance was demonstrated in the occipital region, with signs of brain-stem involvement (paroxysmal generalised slow wave groups).

Bilateral Carotid Angiogram (22 September 1958). Findings on the right side were normal, but visualisation was technically poor on the left side.

Follow-up left carotid angiogram was normal.

Vertebral Angiogram (2 October 1958). An arteriovenous aneurysm of the left posterior inferior cerebellar artery was demonstrated (Figs. 1 and 7).

COURSE. Initially, the patient's condition improved markedly. On 19 September he experienced a sudden attack of severe headache, with repeated vomiting and marked meningism. A further, more severe, attack occurred on 27 September 1958, and *lumbar puncture* now showed a uniformly blood-stained CSF, which was xanthrochromic upon centrifugation. On 5 October 1958, a further similar attack occurred which left the boy drowsy, and from which he no longer made as good a recovery as from the earlier attacks.

Admission to the Department of Neurosurgery, University Hospital, Zurich (9-25 October 1958).

FINDINGS ON ADMISSION. The boy was apathetic and drowsy, and was developing bilateral papilloedema. He was suffering from severe meningism, generalised muscular hypotonia, and an inconstant horizontal nystagmus to the right side.

OPERATION (16 October 1958). Removal was made of the arteriovenous aneurysm which was located in the region of the left posterior inferior cerebellar artery and of the lateral surface of the left cerebellar hemisphere as far as the cerebellopontine angle. No haemorrhage into the cerebellum could be demonstrated.

Histological Examination. (Institute of Pathology, University of Zurich) confirmed that an arteriovenous aneurysm had been removed.

COURSE. The boy's recovery was slow. His gait remained ataxic and he had weakness in the legs; a horizontal nystagmus was present on both sides, and he suffered occasional bouts of vomiting. He died on 25 January 1959.

AUTOPSY. There was softening of the brain into the dissecting aneurysm in the left internal carotid artery. The boy had died as a result of the aneurysm spreading to the middle cerebral artery and cutting off the main arterial supply to the insular and surrounding softened areas.

CASE 7

S.M.T., born 15 July 1953 (4386/61, 4765/62, 1189/64, 3395/65, 6816/66).

FAMILY HISTORY. Nil relevant.

PREVIOUS HISTORY. Pregnancy, birth and delivery normal. Mumps, measles and whooping cough as a small child. A very bright pupil.

PRESENT ILLNESS. During the night of 24 December 1961, the child called her parents, and complained of a feeling of dizziness and nausea. A few minutes later she became unconscious and stiff in all four extremities. Within 15 minutes she recovered, answered questions correctly, and complained of severe occipital headache. Shortly thereafter, she again lapsed into unconsciousness, this time for longer than one hour, with flaccid extremities. Subsequently, she regained consciousness but remained drowsy.

Admission to the Children's Hospital, Zurich (24 December 1961-3 January 1962).

FINDINGS ON ADMISSION. The patient was drowsy, but rousable. She was disorientated in time and place, and had severe neck stiffness, but no neurological deficit was found. The fundi and eye fields were normal, and she was afebrile. Blood: leucocytes 14,350, juvenile forms 29 per cent, mature forms 66 per cent.

Lumbar Puncture. The CSF was uniformly and grossly blood-stained, and was definitely xanthochromic after centrifugation.

EEG (26 December 1961). The recording showed bilateral disturbances of moderate severity, with slow rhythms, over the posterior parts of both hemispheres.

Bilateral Carotid Angiogram (29 December 1961). The left side was normal. An arteriovenous aneurysm about the size of a hazel nut was demonstrated in the region of the lateral wall of the lateral ventricle (cella media), draining into the thalamostriate and internal cerebral veins (Figs. 1 and 8). During the venous phase, the lateral ventricles were outlined with contrast medium.

Admission to the Department of Neurosurgery, University Hospital, Zurich.

OPERATION (5 January 1962). The lateral ventricle was exposed through the prefrontal part of the right hemisphere. The arteriovenous aneurysm was found to lie in the lateral wall, and in the precentral part of the internal capsule. The terminal vein was shown to be 2-3 cm in diameter; it was congested with blood, and was supplying a vascular mass of greatly dilated veins and numerous smaller arteries. Radical resection was possible despite considerable difficulties, including damage to the tissues of the internal capsule.

Post-operatively, a sub-total left-sided hemi-plegia, with analgesia, was present. Over the course of several weeks, a massive spastic hemiparesis developed, with a complete loss of function of the arm, and a disturbance of gait. The condition remained unchanged, despite intensive physiotherapy for many months, and a rehabilitation programme lasting one year.

EEG (March 1962). A generalised epileptic seizure occurred for the first time during photic stimulation. Repeat EEG in January 1963 revealed an epileptogenic focus in the right anterior temporal region. In April 1964, a very active epileptogenic focus was shown over the right precentral region, as well as generalised seizure complexes.

EEG (January 1965). This recording revealed deterioration, in that the epilepsy potentials emanating from the very active precentral focus had spread over the entire hemisphere. Numerous generalised seizure complexes were again present.

COURSE. Regular anticonvulsant treatment was commenced in March 1962, and it was initially possible to suppress clinical attacks. On 6 April 1965, the patient, for the first time, experienced a clonic left-sided convulsion lasting 5-6 minutes; she was unrousable and drowsy. Despite stepping up of the dose of anticonvulsant, further focal seizures occurred within the next month, some accompanied by loss of consciousness.

EEG (January 1966). Apart from the very active epileptogenic focus in the right pre-central region, a second less active focus was now demonstrated over the anterior part of the left hemisphere, accompanied by generalised rhythmic sharp and slow waves.

With the clinical onset of epileptic attacks, and the resultant increased dose of anti-convulsant medication, a marked slowing occurred in the patient's intellectual develop-ment. In February 1964 her IQ was 87. Since February 1969 she has made no mental progress at all. Menarche in July 1965 (at the age of 12 years) was followed by irregular menses at 1-2 monthly intervals.

CASE 8

S.V., born 17 April 1940 (1734/50, 3978/51).

FAMILY HISTORY. Nil relevant.

PREVIOUS HISTORY. Pregnancy, birth and development normal. Acute tonsillitis in 1949. Measles and whooping cough as a small child, without complications. A bright pupil.

PRESENT ILLNESS. No symptoms appeared until 19 April 1950. On this morning, the parents heard the child go to the toilet and fall. They found her lying motionless and unconscious on the floor.

Admission to the Children's Hospital, Zurich (19 April-21 December 1950).

FINDINGS ON ADMISSION. On admission, 3 hours after the attack, the patient was unconscious, and showed a flaccid right-sided hemiplegia not involving the face. The tendon jerks could be elicited on both sides, without any definite lateralising differences; there was a right Babinski response; the right abdominal reflex was absent. Pupillary responses were normal. Blood pressure 140/100 mm. Pulse 116/min. Blood: Hb 80 per cent; leucocytes 25,000, juvenile forms 8 per cent, mature forms 77 per cent. ESR 9/18 mm. The child was afebrile.

Lumbar Puncture. The fluid was grossly and uniformly blood-stained, and was lightly xanthochromic after centrifugation.

Left Carotid Angiogram. An extensive arterio-venous aneurysm was revealed (Figs. 1 and 9).

COURSE. On 20 April 1950, the patient was rousable; however, she showed marked neck rigidity, a complete hemiplegia, and diminution of the tendon jerks in the paralysed leg, but normal responses in the upper extremities.

Admission to the Department of Neurosurgery, University Hospital, Zurich

OPERATION (25 April 1950). Ligation of the left internal carotid artery.

In the course of the succeeding few weeks, a progressive improvement in the level of con-sciousness occurred. At the same time, a severe motor and partial sensory aphasia, as well as a central facial palsy, became apparent.

Within weeks, the patient developed a near-complete spastic hemiplegia, maximal in the arm, but also marked in the leg. Speech remained severely defective for months, although the sensory aphasia disappeared within about 6 months. At the end of the period of intensive physiotherapeutic rehabili-tation in mid-July 1951, the arm remained functionally useless, but the child managed to run about with a limp. The motor aphasia remained noticeable during conversation, but the sensory aphasia could no longer be detected.

214

While pain sensitivity was retained over the paralysed half of the body, a marked disturbance of tactile sensitivity was present. Movement sensitivity was abolished over the paralysed extremity.

COURSE (until July 1966). In 1955 the child was admitted to a special school for cerebral palsied children. She was unable to complete any occupational training, and now works as an assistant in an electrical workshop. She can use the paralysed limb only by supporting it, the fingers remaining immobile. Her gait is grossly abnormal. A striking underdevelopment of the paralysed extremities is present. The facial palsy can no longer be recognised. The difficulty in finding words during conversation persists, and is aggravated by emotion and tiredness. A marked disturbance of tactile sensitivity and hyperalgesia are present over the right side of the body. Movement sensitivity has been lost in the hand and foot. No epileptic attacks have yet occurred. (Length of Case History: $15\frac{1}{2}$ years.)

CASE 9

W.E., born 11 August 1941.

FAMILY HISTORY. Mother suffers from migraine, and one of her brothers from febrile convulsions.

PREVIOUS HISTORY. Several episodes of antepartum haemorrhage, up to the sixth month. Birth 2 weeks before term, but delivery normal. Birth weight 3150g; healthy child. Development normal. Pneumonia at 2 months. Frequent attacks of diarrhoea up to the age of 2 years, and attacks of fever up to about 5 years. In addition, *cardiac enlargement* was detected upon routine clinical examination, but no explanation was given for it.

PRESENT ILLNESS. In February 1956, the patient, then a $14\frac{1}{2}$-year-old girl, experienced an epileptic attack, with loss of consciousness and clonic seizures (localisation?). Since that time, attacks have been frequent, sometimes one or more daily, sometimes with a free interval of up to $1\frac{1}{2}$ months. So far, however, only 3 attacks have occurred with loss of consciousness, once with transient weakness of the right arm. The nature of these attacks is consistent: the onset is stereotyped, with a numb feeling which appears first on the right side of the face, and then immediately afterwards in the right arm; this is followed by palpitations and clonic seizures of the right hand and the right side of the face. A feeling of cramp then develops in the right leg. During this phase, the patient often experiences illusions ('like a film'), or notices a difficulty in finding the correct word. The attacks last 1-15 minutes.

Admission to the Department of Neurosurgery, University Hospital, Zurich (16-20 December 1957).

FINDINGS ON ADMISSION. The patient's neurological state was normal. There was a soft murmur synchronous with the pulse over the left parieto-temporal region. Her heart was clinically normal (no chest radiograph or electrocardiogram was made). Blood pressure 110/65 mm.

EEG. A mild non-specific disturbance, with numerous polymorphic delta waves, was demonstrated in the temporo-occipital part of the right hemisphere(!).

Bilateral Carotid and Vertebral Angiography. A huge arteriovenous aneurysm was shown in the left insular region. The principal source of supply was the left middle cerebral artery, but additional feeding arteries came from the left anterior cerebral artery, from the opposite carotid, through the anterior communicating artery and the vertebral and posterior choroidal arteries. The main drainage was into the right cavernous sinus (Figs. 1 and 10).

COURSE. With regular anticonvulsant treatment, the patient has experienced only brief and infrequent disturbances, with paraesthesiae in the right side of the face and right hand, but no more actual epileptic attacks have occurred. She was married at the beginning of 1965, and her first child is expected in the Autumn of 1966. Sensory disturbances have been somewhat more frequent during pregnancy, occurring once or twice a month. She has no other complaints, save for infrequent headaches (which commence only with a change in the weather). She is free from physical disturbances, and does all her own housework.

CASE 10

Z.U., born 24 October 1945.

FAMILY HISTORY. One brother died in infancy of a heart complaint.

PREVIOUS HISTORY. Birth and development normal. Mumps and whooping cough as a small child. Influenza in 1957.

215

PRESENT ILLNESS. Until the age of 13 years, the boy was completely healthy. On the morning of 11 November 1958, he was found sitting on the edge of his bed in a confused state, having been incontinent of urine. Almost immediately, he sank to the floor, became unrousable, and showed a right-sided paralysis.

Admission to the Department of Medicine, Cantonal Hospital, Schaffhausen (11-24 November 1958).

FINDINGS ON ADMISSION. The patient had complete flaccid paralysis of the right arm, severe paralysis of the right leg, and right facial palsy with sparing of the forehead. His tongue was deviated to the right side. Hyper-reflexia, and a right Babinski response were seen, and the right abdominal reflexes were diminished. There was an inequality of the pupils, with the right pupil reacting better to light. A convergent squint had developed, with right sixth nerve palsy. The boy was conscious; his speech was dysarthric, but he had no aphasia. The fundi were normal. There were no signs of meningism, headache or vomiting. Blood: Hb 83 per cent; leucocytes 5200, with normal differential count. ESR 4/9 mm. Blood pressure 120/90 mm. Pulse 84/min. The patient was afebrile.

Lumbar Puncture. Pressure 14 cm. Fluid clear. Protein 33 mg per cent. Cells 3/3. Colloidal gold 334433221111.

On 13 November 1958, there was a slight improvement in the paralysis of the leg; on 17 November, the first flicker of voluntary movement in the forearm flexors appeared; on 24 November, he regained slight voluntary movement of the hand flexors, and was able to stand on his right leg.

Admission to the Department of Neurosurgery, University Hospital, Zurich (24 November-23 December 1958).

FINDINGS ON ADMISSION. The patient had severe flaccid right-sided hemiplegia, which was more severe in the arm than the leg, and a central facial palsy. Hyper-reflexia and a right Babinski response were observed, accompanied by hypalgesia and hypaesthesia of the right side of the body. The boy's speech was dysarthric, though he was not aphasic; he had a slight difficulty with mental arithmetic. He was fully conscious.

EEG (25 November 1958). A circumscribed intermittent theta focus was demonstrated in the lateral part of the central part of the left hemisphere.

Pneumoencephalogram. The ventricular system was normal in size, shape and position.

The *CSF* was normal in all respects.

Left Carotid Angiogram (1 December 1958). A $2\frac{1}{2}$ x 2 cm arteriovenous aneurysm was shown in the paramedian part of the left hemisphere, in the region of the basal ganglia, supplied by branches of the middle cerebral artery and also the posterior communicating artery. The principal drainage was through an enlarged vein of Galen. No vessel displacement was shown (Figs. 1 and 11).

Right Carotid Angiogram (3 December 1958). The vessels were normal, and there was no filling of the arteriovenous aneurysm.

Vertebral Angiogram (3 December 1958). The vessels appeared normal, and there was no definite filling of the arteriovenous aneurysm.

OPERATION (8 December 1958). Left parieto-occipital craniotomy. During exploration of the midbrain, the greatly dilated vein of Galen could be demonstrated. The malformation itself was not visible, being buried in the basal nucleus. There was no evidence of previous haemorrhage.

COURSE. The hemiparesis slowly and gradually improved with prolonged physiotherapy. In February 1959 the boy went back to school, did well, and was promoted to the next class in the Spring of 1960. He took part keenly in sporting activities. Follow-up examination at the beginning of October 1960 revealed only the presence of a moderate paresis of the arm.

On 21 December 1960, he experienced a severe pain at the back of the head, vomited repeatedly, and became drowsy.

Admission to the Department of Medicine, Cantonal Hospital, Schaffhausen (22 December 1960).

FINDINGS. The patient had severe meningism. His head was held in the opisthotonic position. He was mentally clear, and the fundi were normal. The right hemiparesis was somewhat deeper than it had been previously.

Lumbar Puncture. Pressure 20 cm. The fluid was blood-stained, and was shown to be xanthochromic after centrifugation. The patient recovered satisfactorily.

COURSE. On 28 January 1961, he suffered a further sudden attack of headache and vomiting, from which he recovered within two days. On 1 February 1961 similar attacks recurred.

Re-admission to the Department of Medicine, Cantonal Hospital, Schaffhausen (1 February 1961).

FINDINGS. The patient was conscious, but mentally slowed, and had definite meningism. He again recovered.

COURSE. In the same year the patient commenced an apprenticeship as a draftsman. At the last follow-up examination, at the end of October 1963, the hemiparesis was still moderately severe in the arm, but scarcely detectable in the leg. Light hypaesthesia and hypalgesia were present in the right arm, and the right corneal reflex was depressed. The patient himself had no complaints.

PROGRESS (to August 1966). The boy's condition has remained unchanged. He has experienced no attacks, and is employed full-time as a draftsman.

CASE 11

L.M., born 22 August 1935.

FAMILY HISTORY. Nil relevant.

PREVIOUS HISTORY. Nil relevant. Tonsillectomy in 1945, after repeated tonsillitis. A bright pupil.

PRESENT ILLNESS. At the beginning of December 1950, when the patient was 15 years old, she experienced a sudden attack of severe headache, vomiting and unconsciousness. On 5 January 1951, she experienced another similar attack, remaining unconscious for $2\frac{1}{2}$ hours, vomiting continuously for a further 8 hours, experiencing headache for 3 days, and then recovering from all her symptoms. She had no neck stiffness.

On 12 January 1951, she experienced another sudden attack of right-sided headache, vomiting and unconsciousness which lasted for 10 minutes; clonic (?) movements commenced in the right arm, and then spread to involve the right leg as well. She had a continuous severe frontal headache, but no meningism.

Admission to the Department of Neurosurgery, University Hospital, Zurich (13 January 1951).

FINDINGS ON ADMISSION. The pupils were unequal, with the right one more widely dilated and responding to light. Mild left facial palsy was present. Otherwise there were no physical signs, and in particular no neck stiffness. Blood pressure 120/70 mm. Leucocytes 5300. ESR 4/9 mm.

EEG. A moderately severe abnormality was shown, bilaterally, in the postcentral regions. There was a continuous delta focus in the temporo-occipital part of the right hemisphere. *Right Carotid Angiogram.* There was slight stretching of the branches of the middle cerebral artery.

On 15 January 1951, a very severe attack of right-sided headache suddenly occurred, followed shortly afterwards by unconsciousness and disturbances of extrapyramidal function (choreatic) in the right extremities.

Ventriculography (16 January 1951). There was considerable displacement of the ventricular system to the left side, with indentation of the middle segment of the right lateral ventricle. The fluid was under pressure, but clear.

OPERATION. Right temporo-occipital craniotomy. A small acute subdural haematoma was found over the temporal lobe. The temporal convolutions were markedly widened, and there were findings of inflammatory cerebral oedema.

Post-operatively, the girl showed an acute exogenous type of reaction. Two attacks occurred, one shortly after the other, of athetoid movements in the right limbs, unconsciousness (initially with a fixed dilated right pupil) and of complete flaccid left-sided hemiplegia. The child recovered within days, and the limb paralysis completely regressed. A left homonymous upper quadrant hemianopia was noted.

Lumbar Puncture. The fluid was clear and normal!

Right Carotid Angiogram (2 February 1951). A pea-sized saccular aneurysm was demonstrated on the internal carotid artery near the origin of the middle cerebral artery. Some arteries were unusually thin (Fig. 12).

OPERATION (9 February 1951). Left frontal craniotomy. A thrombosed saccular aneurysm was identified on the right middle cerebral artery, and also a haemorrhagic cavity, about the size of a marble, on the medial aspect of the right temporal lobe and the insula. The haemorrhage was evacuated, and the aneurysm sac wrapped with muscle (the neck of the aneurysm was not visualised).

COURSE. A few months after the operation, frequent attacks of a psychomotor type developed, shown on the EEG to be arising from an epileptogenic focus in the right temporal region. Suppression of the attacks by anticonvulsant treatment proved difficult. The patient completed a commercial course successfully, and started work as an office clerk; however, she appeared unable to remain in one job for long. At the most recent clinical follow-up examination (November 1965, at the Department of Neurosurgery, University of Zurich), the left homonymous upper quadrant hemianopia was still shown to be present; otherwise, the neurological examination was negative. The organic psychosyndrome was thought to be negligible.

CASE 12

W.H., born 10 August 1936.

FAMILY HISTORY. Nil relevant.

PREVIOUS HISTORY. Measles, chickenpox and whooping cough as a small child, all without complications. A good pupil at school.

PRESENT ILLNESS. One evening in the middle of July 1948, after prolonged sunbathing, an attack of nausea, severe headache and vomiting occurred, with a temperature of 40°C. These symptoms had all disappeared by the next morning. At the end of July 1948, the boy bumped his head lightly in the bath, and immediately experienced severe headache, particularly frontal. Neck stiffness then appeared, with recurrent vomiting and fever.

Admission to the Civic Hospital, Solothurn (28 July-20 August 1948).

FINDINGS ON ADMISSION. The patient was mentally normal. He had slight neck stiffness, but no neurological deficit was observed. Left papilloedema was developing.

Lumbar Puncture. The fluid was uniformly blood-stained, with a pressure of 15 cm.

The headache and neck stiffness completely disappeared. However, on 19 August the boy experienced a sudden attack of shooting pain in the head, followed by deep unconsciousness, and focal convulsions in all extremities; these gradually faded away in the course of about 12 hours.

Admission to the Department of Neurosurgery, University Hospital, Zurich (20 August-2 October 1948).

FINDINGS ON ADMISSION. The patient was very drowsy; he reacted to painful stimuli, but not to commands. He had flaccid incomplete hemiparesis, which was marked in the arm and slight in the leg, and a mild central facial palsy. A right Babinski response was elicited. The right knee jerk was absent, but both ankle jerks were present. The boy had severe neck stiffness. Leucocytes 12,300. ESR 56/68 mm.

Left Carotid Angiogram. A saccular aneurysm was demonstrated at the termination of the left internal carotid artery, immediately before its bifurcation (Fig. 13).

OPERATION. The left common, internal and external carotid arteries were ligated.

COURSE. Upon discharge 5 weeks after ligation, the child still exhibited considerable motor and mild sensory aphasia; moderate hemiparesis was also present, with developing spasticity and hyper-reflexia.

Follow-up outpatient examination in February 1951 revealed a residual central facial palsy. The patient complained of difficulties with writing. He was being taught privately at home.

PROGRESS (Until August 1966). The patient entered a secondary school and afterwards successfully completed 3 years at a technical institution. During various visits abroad, he became fluent in a foreign language. He is now a prominent business man. The hemiparesis has disappeared completely, except for a slight disturbance of sensation in the right hand (to touch and temperature). Manual dexterity is completely normal. The patient has no subjective complaints, and no epileptic attacks have occurred.

CASE 13

J.J., born 13 December 1961 (7312/62).

FAMILY HISTORY. Oldest brother a case of cerebral palsy, due to birth trauma. Nil else relevant.

PREVIOUS HISTORY. Pregnancy normal. Normal birth at term. Birth weight 4570g, length 52cm; baby healthy. Psychomotor development normal (laughing at 5 weeks, sitting at 6 months, crawling at 10 months, walking at 12 months).

PRESENT ILLNESS. The patient had had a naevus vasculosus on the left side of her forehead since birth. At the beginning of December 1962, she suffered an attack of catarrhal rhinitis and a mild cough, but was afebrile. On 19 December she vomited once and slept longer than usual. On the morning of 20 December she was tearful, and in the afternoon she was found unconscious on her bed. Shortly afterwards, clonic convulsions developed in the right arm, accompanied by conjugate deviation of the eyes to the right side. The hemiconvulsions lasted about 1 hour.

Admission to the Children's Hospital, Zurich (20 December 1962-3 January 1963).

FINDINGS ON ADMISSION. The patient was unconscious, with clonic hemiconvulsions involving the right extremities, and conjugate deviation of the eyes to the right side. The convulsions were brought under control with amytal. The child was affected with acute tonsillopharyngitis, with bilaterally enlarged cervical lymph glands. Bacteriology: haemolytic streptococcus A. Temperature 38°C. Leucocytes 6850, juvenile forms 5.5. per cent, mature forms 54.5 per cent.

Lumbar Puncture. Fluid normal to all tests.

On 21 December, the child had regained consciousness completely; she showed a flaccid incomplete right hemiplegia with diminished tendon jerks.

EEG (20 December 1962). There was gross depression of the posterior regions of the left hemisphere.

EEG (24 December 1962). The depression was less marked.

Left Carotid Angiogram (21 December 1962). The arterial phase was normal. In the venous phase, an abnormal collection of veins was demonstrated in the central and fronto-precentral regions (Fig. 14a).

Pneumoencephalogram (28 December 1962). There was a slight displacement of the ventricular system to the right side. The right lateral ventricle was shown to be wider than the left one, with a slightly more deeply placed body of the lateral ventricle (cella media) (Fig. 14b).

COURSE. Until the patient's discharge at the beginning of January 1963, the hemiparesis appeared to be improving. In the course of weeks or months, however, the patient developed a spasticity which caused considerable functional limitation of hand movements, and a talipes equinus which affected the gait. Surprisingly, intellectual development was not significantly affected (history until August 1966). With regular anticonvulsant therapy,

no more attacks have occurred since January 1962.

EEG (27 October 1965). There were no significant abnormal findings.

The child is followed-up regularly in the outpatient clinic for cerebral palsied children. There is slight underdevelopment of the right arm and leg, but mental development is considered to be normal.

CASE 14

S.F., born 20 February 1957 (3314/57, 7977/59, 2988/61).

FAMILY HISTORY. One sister with a congenital cavernous haemangioma of the neck. Five maternal aunts died early in childhood, one of epilepsy. Parents and five sisters healthy.

PREVIOUS HISTORY. Somewhat difficult birth at term; a blue asphyxiated baby. The skin over the face, neck and chest contained multiple flat capillary haemangiomas. The newborn infant made a good recovery, and developed normally up to the ninth month of life. In September 1957, whooping cough. At the end of October 1957, bronchopneumonia, followed by a complete recovery.

PRESENT ILLNESS. On 20 November 1957, the child, at the age of 9 months, exhibited without warning a status epilepticus with right-sided hemiconvulsions and a loss of consciousness; the attack lasted 6 hours, and was accompanied by fever. Despite massive doses of drugs, the hemiconvulsions recurred sporadically during the succeeding two days.

Admission to the Children's Hospital, Zurich (23 November-18 December 1957).

FINDINGS ON ADMISSION. The patient exhibited a flaccid hemiplegia, with paralysis of the right arm, incomplete paralysis of the right leg, and a mild facial palsy. The tendon reflexes could not be elicited with certainty in either upper extremity: in both lower extremities they were increased without any definite lateralisation. There was conjugate deviation of the eyes and the head to the left side, and an inequality of the pupils, with the left one reacting well to light. The fundi were normal. The child was drowsy. There were no signs of meningism. The skin over the forehead, upper lids, ears, cheeks, shoulders and chest contained numerous poorly defined capillary haemangiomas of varying size; when the child cried they turned

219

bluish-red in colour, and when he was quiet they had a rosy appearance. The upper lid and the entire right arm appeared swollen, although the appearance did not suggest oedema. No further abnormalities were detected on routine physical examination, in particular the heart and lungs appeared normal.

Laboratory Findings. Blood: Hb 88 per cent; erythrocytes 6 million; leucocytes 7050, juvenile forms 4 per cent, mature forms 16 per cent; eosinophils 6.5 per cent; basophils 1 per cent; monocytes 8 per cent; lymphocytes 64.5 per cent. ESR 3/6/15 mm. Pulse 110/min and regular. The child was afebrile.

Lumbar Puncture. Protein 78 per cent (Kafka), cells 3⅔, colloidal gold reaction negative.

EEG (23 November 1957). A severe disturbance was demonstrated over the left hemisphere, with polymorphic delta activity; this disturbance was maximal in the parieto-temporal region. The right hemisphere was only moderately disturbed. During the recording, the patient experienced a brief attack, and his gaze travelled upwards and to the left side, without clonic manifestations. During the attack, synchronous spike and slow wave complexes were demonstrated over both occipital lobes, occurring sometimes alone, and sometimes in bursts; on the left side they spread out synchronously into the postcentral region, but on the right side only the slow waves spread postcentrally, not the spikes. Over the anterior part of the left hemisphere, only weak irregular delta activity was present, while on the other side it was mixed with theta waves. Following this sudden attack, the child fell asleep, and the activity initially recorded then reappeared.

Left Carotid Angiogram (26 November 1957) (repeated 14 December 1957). The arterial phase showed excellent opacification of the internal carotid, anterior and middle cerebral arteries. In the venous phase, an avascular area was demonstrated in the vicinity of the internal cerebral vein, the vein of Galen and the basilar vein. A second serial angiogram made late in the venous phase revealed a vascular mass with tortuous dilated components occupying the avascular area previously demonstrated. It opacified only about 8-10 seconds after injection of the contrast medium (Fig. 15).

Pneumoencephalogram (26 November 1957). There was a slight enlargement of all parts of both lateral ventricles and the third ventricle, which were normal in shape and position. In the brow-up view, the left thalamus was shown to be lying at a higher level than the right one (Fig. 16).

COURSE. The flaccid hemiparesis improved slightly up to the time of discharge on 18 December 1957; thereafter, it improved slowly, the arm being most severely affected. Psychomotor development ceased. With continuous medical treatment, it was possible to prevent all but two generalised convulsions; in August 1958 and again in February 1959, the patient had attacks of pneumonia with high fever, and on both occasions generalised convulsions occurred. Since the Summer of 1959, development has regressed further.

Second Admission to the Children's Hospital, Zurich (22 August-16 October 1959)

FINDINGS ON ADMISSION. The patient, a 2½-year-old boy, had severe erethitic oligophrenia, was not speaking, and had severe flaccid paralysis of the right arm. The muscles of the right leg were hypotonic, but moving. Tendon reflexes were normal in the upper extremities, and increased in the lower limbs, without any lateralising difference. Babinski and Rossolimo responses were absent. The child was unable to sit up unaided. The capillary haemangioma of the skin was unaltered in appearance.

EEG (8 September 1959). There was a slight depression in the left central-postcentral area with diffuse polymorphic delta activity of moderate severity mainly on the left side. An irregular background rhythm of 5/7 sec was shown in the right postcentral region. No epilepsy potentials were observed.

Left Carotid Angiogram (25 September 1959). The previous findings were unaltered: the vascular mass again opacified only late in the venous phase.

Right Carotid Angiogram (25 September 1959). The arterial and capillary phases were normal, with good filling of the internal carotid and anterior and middle cerebral arteries. In the early venous phase, an unusually large, corkscrew-like vein was demonstrated in the lateral parietal region, communicating with the deeply situated venous masses. This vein represented a drainage pathway, since it emptied earlier.

Pneumoencephalogram (6 October 1959). The left lateral ventricle was now markedly enlarged, compared with its previous appearance, and the ventricular system was slightly displaced to the left side. There was pooling of air over the surface of the left hemisphere.

Third Admission to the Children's Hospital, Zurich (20 June-15 July 1961).

At the age of 4 years, the child had learned to walk. He still did not speak, but understood simple commands. With continuous medical treatment, no further epileptic attacks had occurred.

FINDINGS ON ADMISSION. The boy, now aged 4 years and 4 months, was an erethitic idiot. The right arm was now definitely underdeveloped, and the flaccid paralysis was unaltered. The other extremities showed normal tone and movement. Tendon reflexes in the upper extremities were normal, and in the lower extremities they were increased, but no clonic component or lateralising difference could be demonstrated. Babinski and Rossolimo responses were absent. The fundi and pupils were normal. The haemangioma now involved the skin of the right arm and leg, as well as the lumbar region; the lesions previously present were unaltered in appearance. When the child cried, the naevi became bluish-red in colour.

Pneumoencephalogram (24 June 1961). All parts of both lateral ventricles and the third ventricle were now enlarged, particularly on the left side. The ventricular system was slightly displaced to the left side. There was a non-significant cortical distribution of air (Fig 16). *CSF.* Protein 30 mg per cent; cells 2⅓, colloidal gold reaction negative.

Routine clinical examination again revealed no evidence of a cardiac lesion.

COURSE (until August 1966). The boy is an erethitic idiot. Despite large doses of anticonvulsants, in various combinations, grand mal epileptic seizures have recurred. The patient is being nursed at home.

CASE 15

S.K., born 5 November 1959 (5123/62, 5987/65).

FAMILY HISTORY. Nil relevant.

PREVIOUS HISTORY. A capillary haemangioma, lying to the right of the mid-line on the forehead, was noted at birth; it extended from the root of the nose to the hair-line, and sharply delineated on the mid-line (Fig. 17*b*). Development was normal.

PRESENT ILLNESS. Late on the evening of 32 March 1962, the little girl, then 2 years 4 months old, and up to that time completely healthy, was found weeping in her bed, fully conscious, with a left-sided hemiplegia. On the way to hospital, she vomited twice.

Admission to the Children's Hospital Zurich.

FINDINGS. On admission, 2 hours after the attack, the left arm was spastic, flexed at the elbow, and held tight against the chest. The left leg was outstretched, and the left angle of the mouth paralysed. There was inconstant conjugate deviation of the head and eyes to the right side. The left limbs did not move; the right limbs showed normal movements. The left knee jerk was increased; a left Babinski response was present; all other reflexes were normal. Auscultation revealed no murmurs over the skull. There were no signs of meningism, and the child was conscious. Blood pressure 100/60 mm Hg. Pulse 84/min and regular. Afebrile. Blood: Hb 78 per cent; leucocytes 9800, with normal differential count. ESR 1/2/5 mm.

Lumbar Puncture. The fluid was clear, with a normal cell count. Protein, glucose and chloride content were normal. Colloidal gold reaction negative.

A few hours later, there was a sudden onset of clonic convulsions; these were at first confined to the left arm, and then spread to involve the right arm and leg as well, but not the left leg. The attack was accompanied by a loss of consciousness. The convulsions were controlled by amytal.

On 24 March 1962, the patient was still affected by a moderate hypotonic hemiparesis, which involved the face as well. Tendon reflexes were now symmetrical and normal. A left Babinski response was still present. The conjugate deviation had disappeared. On 26 March 1962, she suffered a second attack with clonic convulsions involving first the left extremities, and then, shortly afterwards, the right arm as well.

EEG (27 March 1962). There was a marked depression with polymorphic delta activity over the posterior parts of the right cerebral hemisphere. Epilepsy potentials were confined to the medial postcentral part of the right hemisphere. Background activity on the left side showed a fairly marked disturbance (slowing).

Right Carotid Angiogram (29 March 1962). Serial angiography revealed normal appearances in the arterial and capillary phases. In the early venous phase, however, a large abnormal vascular mass was demonstrated in the region of the right pulvinar and caudate nucleus, with wide draining veins leading to the internal cerebral vein, the vein of Galen, and the lateral veins (Fig. 17*a*).

Pneumoencephalogram (30 March 1962). The third ventricle and the central parts of both lateral ventricles were slightly displaced to the left side. Apart from this abnormality, the size and shape of the ventricular system showed normal appearances (Fig. 17*b*).

Within 2 weeks, the hemiparesis had disappeared, and when the patient was discharged from hospital on 13 April 1962 no neurological signs remained.

COURSE. Early in 1963, despite phenobarbitone treatment (100 mg/day), the patient began experiencing occasional small attacks of less than 1 second duration. She would suddenly fling her arms (or only the left one) outwards, often turning the head vigorously to the left side, but only rarely would she lose her balance, and she never suffered from a loss of consciousness. The disturbance was regarded as a 'tremor'. In October 1963, a flaccid paralysis of the left leg suddenly appeared, unaccompanied by epileptic features or any associated signs; this paralysis disappeared after one hour.

EEG (23 July 1963). The recording was made under phenobarbitone sedation. A symmetrical recording was made, with a predominance of 4-5 rhythms/second, with an amplitude of up to 100 microvolts in the left parieto-occipital region.

Routine following neurological examinations (19 November 1963-21 January 1964) revealed no abnormal findings; no cranial murmur could be detected.

Second Admission to the Children's Hospital, Zurich (27 January-20 February 1965).

The patient was admitted for therapeutic stabilisation, on account of numerous attacks; most of these took the form of a sudden weakness in the left leg, followed by twitching movements in the extremities, and clouding of consciousness. In January 1965, she experienced two grand mal seizures within the space of a week. Neurological examination revealed only a left Babinski response, and brisker reflexes in the left leg than in the right one.

EEG. There was a non-specific disturbance, of moderate severity, over the left hemisphere, without epilepsy potentials.

Pneumoencephalogram. No changes were observed, compared with the appearances in March 1962.

Third Admission to the Children's Hospital, Zurich (1 October-9 November 1965)

The attacks were no longer responding to treatment, and the neurological state was unaltered. On examination, the girl showed marked inco-ordination and unsteadiness, and clung to the nurse.

FINDINGS

EEG. The recording showed intermittent generalised epilepsy potentials in the form of abortive spike and wave complexes. Apart from this finding, the mild disturbance over, the left hemisphere was unaltered.

Psychiatric Examination. The child had an organic cerebral psychosyndrome, with markedly reduced intelligence (IQ 73, in the Schweitzer test).

PROGRESS (up to August 1966). No change has occurred in the patient's condition. Despite many drug combinations, numerous small attacks (up to 4 a day), and occasionally also grand mal attacks lasting up to 1 minute, have persisted.

CASE 16

M.M., born 19 April 1949 (9688/56).

FAMILY HISTORY. Homocystinuria was diagnosed in a 19-year-old sister in 1966. She presented the same body habitus as this patient, and a similar dislocated lens (1431/66). The parents and 4 other sisters were normal.

PREVIOUS HISTORY. Pregnancy and birth normal. Birth weight 3500g. Development normal: sitting-up unaided at 7 months, walking unaided at 15 months, speaking first words at 18 months. From the outset the boy was physically weak, with a strong tendency to develop colds. At the age of 5 years, a congenital ectopia of the lens was noted.

PRESENT ILLNESS. In October 1955, when the child was 6½ years old, he complained of attacks of headache, mainly over the left forehead.

Once, during a bout of fever, he exhibited marked weakness in both legs. In March 1956, he experienced a very severe attack of headache and vomiting, with neck stiffness and a temperature of 40°C. This attack lasted for 4-5 days, and recovery was complete within 10 days. At the end of May 1956, a similar type of illness was again present for 10 days, and this time the child was left with continuous lassitude. On 5 July 1956, when the child was 7 years 2 months old, he was out for a walk when his leg suddenly became hemiparetic. On the following day, the weakness had spread to involve the right arm as well, and on the 7 July 1956 a complete right hemiplegia was present. The child did not lose consciousness, nor was the attack accompanied by vomiting, fever or convulsions.

Admission to the Children's Hospital, Zurich (7 July 1956).

FINDINGS ON ADMISSION. The patient had a complete flaccid hemiplegia, including a central facial palsy. Moderately increased reflexes were elicited in all extremities, without any definite lateralising difference; bilateral Babinski responses were present; only the left abdominal reflexes could be elicited. The child was apathetic, and responded with difficulty to questions, although he understood them. Bilateral drug-induced myosis and subluxed lenses were not visible. Testing for sensory deficits was not possible. Unusually prominent veins were visible in the skin of the right temporal region.

The physical appearance of the child was unusual: he had an abnormally large and doliocephalic skull (circumference 56.5 cm), and his extremities, especially his toes, were long and tapering. His height was 129 cm (90th percentile), and his weight was 22.1 kg (25th-50th percentile). There was marked muscular hypotonia in the non-paralysed extremities. Physical examination revealed no further abnormalities, in particular no defect of the cardiovascular apparatus.

Laboratory Findings. Afebrile. Blood: Hb 99 per cent; leucocytes 10,600, juvenile forms 1 per cent, mature forms 55 per cent; monocytes 11 per cent; lymphocytes 23 per cent. Platelets showed normal appearances. ESR 17/43 mm.

Lumbar Puncture. Pressure normal, fluid clear. Cells 1/3. Protein 30 mg per cent. Colloidal gold reaction negative. Glucose 52 mg per cent. Bacteriologically sterile. Serological tests for syphilis negative in the blood.

EEG. The recording showed a massive, diffuse and deep-seated cerebral disturbance, with depression of the background activity. The left hemisphere was more severely involved than the right one. No epilepsy potentials were shown.

On the morning of 10 July 1956, the child vomited, and then was unable to speak.

Admission to the Department of Neurosurgery, University Hospital, Zurich (10 July 1956).

FINDINGS ON ADMISSION. The child was weak, passive and unco-operative. Definite flexion spasticity was present in the right arm, in addition to the complete flaccid right hemiplegia. Generalised hyper-reflexia was present, with right patellar and ankle clonus, and bilateral Babinski responses. No sensory deficit was found. Both carotid pulses were normally palpable.

Left Carotid Angiogram (under intubation anaesthesia). At the second attempt, percutaneous puncture of the artery was successful. When an attempt was made to advance the needle and its stilette up the lumen, resistance was encountered within a short distance. A contrast injection (Urografin 60 per cent) was made, but no intracranial opacification occurred. The carotid was therefore re-punctured about 2 cm lower in the neck, without technical difficulty. An occlusion of the internal carotid artery, just distal to its origin in the common carotid, was demonstrated.

Left Vertebral Angiogram. During the initial attempt to puncture the carotid artery, the needle entered the left vertebral artery. Contrast injection led to good visualisation of the vertebro-basilar tree, which was shown to be normal. The left middle and anterior cerebral arteries also opacified, through the left posterior communicating artery and collateral channels from the posterior cerebral artery; however, the carotid siphon did not opacify (Fig. 18).

COURSE. The child did not wake up from the anaesthetic. After 2 hours he reacted to pain stimuli. Meanwhile tachypnoea developed. During the night, his condition worsened, with repeated focal seizures and attacks of hyperthermia (up to a temperature of 40.7°C), and he died several hours later.

AUTOPSY. (Institute of Pathology, University of Zurich, 1074/56). The patient was found to have a thrombotic occlusion of the left internal carotid artery, from its origin to the carotid siphon. The thrombus extended like a pencil for 3 cm down the common carotid as well. The left cavernous sinus, left middle cerebral vein and several leptomeningeal veins were thrombosed. The arteries at the base of the brain were soft and normally developed. The thoracic and abdominal parts of the aorta were 3 cm in circumference, and the intima was soft.

The patient had massive cerebral oedema (weight of brain 1650g), with flattened gyri and completely obliterated sulci. On section, numerous small haemorrhagic foci were found scattered throughout the cortex and white matter. The left frontal, temporal and parietal lobes were markedly swollen and bluish-violet in colour. Both cerebellar tonsils were herniated into the foramen magnum. There were no abnormal cardiac findings, apart from dilatation of the right chambers, and some fatty degeneration of the myocardium.

Histology. The internal carotid artery showed a normal wall, with intact elastic fibres in sections taken near its origin. More distally, however, an area of complete rupture of the intima, and two-thirds of the thickness of the media was found. At this level, the elastic fibres were completely deficient. The muscle cells had lost their nuclei and contained eosinophils. This thrombus could be traced for a long distance in the lumen, without any connection to the intima being demonstrable (Fig. 19).

CASE 17

A.H., born 25 December 1944.

FAMILY HISTORY. Nil relevant.

PREVIOUS HISTORY. Nil relevant.

PRESENT ILLNESS. In the Autumn of 1958, the boy experienced an episode of morning headaches, which disappeared completely. On 10 December 1958, while at school, he suffered a sudden attack of giddiness and severe pain, which was centered in the neck and radiated into the eyes. During the following 2 weeks, the patient's parents noted a transient left facial palsy and ptosis on three occasions. Transient double vision and a disturbance of sensation of the left arm were both noted, with simultaneous vomiting and a general state of lassitude.

Admission to the Department of Neurosurgery, University Hospital, Zurich (29 December 1958-15 January 1959).

FINDINGS ON ADMISSION. Findings included chronic bilateral papilloedema, mild motor paresis of the left arm, a left Babinski response, and mild right sixth cranial nerve paresis. There were no disturbances of sensation, and the visual fields were intact.

Lumbar Puncture (performed in another hospital). Pressure was above 30 cm, and the fluid was xanthochromic. The cell count was normal, and there was a negative Pandy reaction.

EEG. A gross focal abnormality was shown in the right occipital region.

Right Carotid Angiogram. A space-occupying process was demonstrated in the postcentral occipital region of the hemisphere, with splayed opercular vessels, and stretched and bowed middle cerebral branches. There was no pathological circulation.

The patient was afebrile. Leucocytes 6200; Hb 95 per cent; ESR 4/7 mm. Blood pressure 110/70.

OPERATION (5 January 1959). A subcortical haematoma, the size of a hen's egg, was evacuated from the parieto-occipital region of the right hemisphere. The haematoma capsule was excised for histological study.

Histological Examination. (Institute of Pathology, University of Zurich) revealed an arteriovenous aneurysm (Fig. 20).

COURSE. The patient completely recovered, with no after effects, within a few weeks. Follow-up examination in April 1959 revealed an intact neurological system. The boy had no complaints.

PROGRESS (until August 1966). The patient has been completely healthy and trouble-free. He is a cadet in an officer's training school.

CASE 18

T.J., born 2 February 1967 (2408/69, 3152/69).

FAMILY HISTORY. Nil relevant.

PREVIOUS HISTORY. Pregnancy normal. Delivery normal and child healthy; birth weight 3340g. Normal milestones. Occasional upper respiratory tract infections, without complications.

PRESENT ILLNESS. On 7 June 1969, when the patient was 2 years 4 months old, she suddenly cried out while playing on the floor. She then stood up and walked to her room, and went to lie on the bed. Moments later, her mother found her limp, apathetic and unresponsive. The child vomited twice.

Admission to the Children's Hospital, Zurich
(7 June-24 October 1969).

FINDINGS. On admission, about 2 hours after the attack, the child was semi-conscious, and did react to painful stimuli. She had flaccid left-sided hemiplegia, which included the face. Tendon jerks were increased in the left limbs, and a left Babinski response was present. The left(!) pupil was dilated by a normal light reflex. There was no neck rigidity. Blood pressure 125/85 mm Hg. Pulse 96/min.

Lumbar Puncture. Pressure 15 cm. The fluid was grossly blood-stained and xanthochromic after centrifugation.

Skull Radiographs. Normal.

Right Carotid Angiogram. A microangioma was demonstrated in the arterial phase, in the mid-temporal region. A wideswept pericallosal artery was also noted, but otherwise the angiogram showed normal appearances (Fig. 21).

Admission to the Department of Neurosurgery, University Hospital, Zurich

OPERATION. Right temporal craniotomy. An angioma (1 x 1 cm) was resected from the wall of the temporal horn and trigone. The haemorrhage had been mainly into the ventricular cavity.

COURSE. A few hours after the operation, the patient was fully conscious. Apart from the flaccid hemiparesis, which was subtotal in the lower limb, a left hemianopia and a slight deviation of the tongue to the left side were present.

EEG (19 February 1969). There was a marked depression in the posterior region of the right hemisphere.

EEG (23 October 1969). The depression was still present, but it was of a lesser degree. There were intermittent bursts of generalised epileptic activity.

COURSE. Despite intensive physiotherapy, the hemiparesis failed to improve to any extent. At the time of discharge, on 23 October 1969, the patient was able to walk with aid, but remained unable to use the left hand and arm. No spasticity was present, but the left-sided hyperreflexia and Babinski response remained. The hemianopia and the left 12th nerve palsy remained unaltered. There was no gross sensory deficit, but refined testing was not possible. Mentally, the child showed satisfactory development. Anticonvulsant treatment with phenobarbitone was commenced.

Follow-up examination, in May 1970, revealed that, despite continuous physiotherapy, no improvement in the hemiparesis and hemianopia had occurred. The left extremities were already reduced in length. There was no speech disorder, apart from a slight defect in articulation due to persistent paralysis of the left 12th nerve. There was no obvious behaviour disorder.

EEG (27 April 1970). An epileptic focus was demonstrated in the right temporal region, with slight intermittent disturbances (increase in slow waves in both posterior regions).

No seizures have occurred to date under regular anticonvulsant treatment.

CASE 19

J.U., born 5 February 1950 (8011/55, 9417/56).

FAMILY HISTORY. Parents and two younger brothers normal.

PREVIOUS HISTORY. Pregnancy, birth and early development normal. Apart from frequent sore throats, no illnesses; no history of significant head injury.

PRESENT ILLNESS. On 22 November 1955, the parents noticed that the patient, then a little girl aged 5 years 9 months, was behaving unusually, without showing signs of illness; she continued to do this for several days. On 26 November, she complained of severe headache and unusual sensitivity to noise, vomited repeatedly, and had a temperature of 39°C. On 28 November, the family doctor was called, and he found slight neck stiffness, and redness of the pharyngeal mucosa.

Lumbar Puncture (29 November 1955). The CSF was colourless, with 243 mono-nuclear and 24 polymorphonuclear cells. The patient had a temperature of 38-39°C.

She was referred to hospital on 30 November, with the suspected diagnosis of non-paralytic poliomyelitis.

Admission to the Children's Hospital, Zurich
(30 November 1955).

FINDINGS. On admission there were no abnormal findings, apart from a temperature of 39°C; the girl's appearance was lively, and she seemed to be symptom free.

On 2 December 1955, she complained of severe frontal headache; the temperature was

39.7°C. A mild expressive right facial palsy now developed, accompanied by an inequality of the pupils—the left one being dilated. The fundi were normal.

Blood picture (2 December 1955). Hb 81 per cent; leucocytes 7100, with normal differential count, apart from eosinophilia. ESR 2/4 mm.

Lumbar Puncture. Surprisingly, the fluid was uniformly blood-stained, with about 6000 red cells/ml, and was shown to be xanthochromic after centrifugation.

EEG (2 December 1955). The recording showed a severe diffuse disturbance, with intermittent rhythmic 2-3 second bursts; there was a marked maximum over the left postcentral region. Suspicious epilepsy potentials were seen confined to the left fronto-temporal region.

On 4 December 1955, the child showed some speech difficulty; she appeared unable to find the correct words. During the night of 5 December 1955, she experienced her first epileptic attack, in the form of clonic hemiconvulsions of the right side of the body, and conjugate deviation to the right side. The seizure commenced in the right hand. The attack was brought under control within minutes by intravenous injection of amytal. After recovery of consciousness, a complete aphasia developed, which was now receptive as well. Tendon jerks were increased on the right side, but no paralysis was present. In the course of the day, the child vomited repeatedly, and developed severe meningism with a simultaneous fall in body temperature.

Left Carotid Angiogram (6 December 1955). The carotid siphon was markedly elongated, and the entire Sylvian group was elevated from the temporal fossa. The anterior cerebral artery remained in the mid-line (Fig. 22).

Transfer to the Department of Neurosurgery, University Hospital, Zurich.

OPERATION (8 December 1955). A walnut-sized subcortical haematoma was removed from the pole of the temporal lobe; there was softening of the surrounding brain substance.

Histological Examination (Pathological Institute, Cantonal Hospital, Zurich). There was evidence of an inflammatory process in the margins of the haematoma.

COURSE. The patient made a gradual but satisfactory recovery, and was left, after some months, with only a slight difficulty in finding the correct word and a relative weakness of concentration.

She developed measles at the beginning of June 1956, and on the third day of the rash she was found unconscious in bed, having been incontinent of faeces.

Emergency Admission to the Children's Hospital Zurich.

FINDINGS ON ADMISSION. The child was not responding to commands, but resisted examination. The only neurological finding was a left Babinski response. CSF was clear, with normal pressure; 16 monocytes, protein 30 mg per cent.

During the following two days, she experienced anxiety convulsions of sudden onset on two occasions, and also repeated visual hallucinations; her body temperature was normal. Again, she exhibited a marked transient dysphasia. In the course of a few days, the patient recovered to her pre-measles state. Unfortunately, no EEG was performed.

Soon after she commenced school at the age of 7 years, she began experiencing considerable difficulty in expression. She was obliged to repeat a year, and eventually was placed in the second class.

Follow-up EEG (7 December 1961). An active epileptic focus was shown in the left temporal lobe, accompanied by irregular bilaterally synchronous bursts of epilepsy potentials. The phenobarbitone treatment prescribed was not carried out, and in the Summer of 1963 seizure-like disturbances began, which were characterised by the sudden onset of a pressure feeling in the head, and acoustic hallucinations; however, no typical epileptic attacks occurred.

At the time of the last outpatient follow-up examination on 21 April 1964 the findings were, apart from a partial nominal dysphasia, an infantile organic psychosyndrome with a marked disturbance of memory. The girl is at present in the eighth special class; according to the parents, she is well integrated, and is causing no teaching problem. She is receiving regular anticonvulsant treatment.

CASE 20

W.F., born 31 October 1940.

FAMILY HISTORY. Nil relevant.

PREVIOUS HISTORY. Nil relevant.

PRESENT ILLNESS. In August 1956 this girl started experiencing frequent headaches. She felt completely well on 17 September 1956, and did her work as a trainee housekeeper. On the following morning, she was found on the floor beside her bed, with complete aphasia and a right-sided weakness.

Admission to the Department of Neurosurgery, University Hospital, Zurich (18 September–27 October 1956).

FINDINGS ON ADMISSION. The patient was slightly drowsy, with complete flaccid right-sided hemiplegia including the face, complete receptive aphasia, diminution of the right tendon jerks, a right Babinski response, and moderate neck stiffness. The right visual field was constricted to confrontation. Blood pressure 120/70. Leucocytes 6000. ESR 23/27 mm. Hb 98 per cent.

Lumbar Puncture. Slight xanthochromia, $1\frac{2}{3}$ monocytes, 18 erythrocytes, protein 54 mg per cent.

Left Carotid Angiogram. The opercular vessels were stretched and bowed, and there was slight downward displacement of the main branches of the middle cerebral artery. No pathological vessels were seen (Fig. 23).

Pneumoencephalogram. There was a moderate displacement of the ventricular system to the right side (Fig. 23).

OPERATION (24 September 1956). A plum-sized haematoma was evacuated from the white matter of the left hemisphere; it was found lying under the central region, and at the base of the third frontal convolution. A very haemorrhagic focus of blood vessels was found, which was excised for histological examination at the Pathological Institute, University of Zurich.

Histology. Examination showed a cavernous angioma (Fig. 24).

COURSE. At the time of the patient's discharge on 27 October 1956, a spastic right arm weakness of moderate severity, a slight weakness of the right leg and a partial motor aphasia were present. Visual fields were normal.

On 18 January 1957, the patient experienced her first epileptic (? generalised) seizure with a loss of consciousness. A second attack occurred 4 months later, and thereafter they were prevented with anticonvulsant therapy. Physical rehabilitation continued for 1 year.

EEG (18 November 1957). The recording showed a left temporal epileptic focus, and also a non-specific disturbance in the left precentral region.

Pneumoencephalogram (29 November 1957). The body of the left lateral ventricle was slightly enlarged (Fig. 23).

Left Carotid Angiogram (26 November 1957). Findings were normal (Fig. 23).

COURSE (until July 1966). The spastic right arm weakness persisted, with severe disturbances of hand function and minimal weakness of the leg. No speech disturbance remains. Despite withdrawal of medication, no further attacks have occurred. The patient married early in 1965, and her first healthy child was born early in 1966. The patient does all her own housework.

CASE 21

E.E., born 27 July 1952 (8251/56, 7944/55, 5241/54, 7291/59).

FAMILY HISTORY. Nil relevant.

PREVIOUS HISTORY. Mother developed albuminuria during pregnancy. Birth normal; birth weight 4320g; child healthy. Normal development. No previous illnesses.

PRESENT ILLNESS. The patient, a little girl, was perfectly healthy until 30 November 1954 (age 2 years 4 months) when she experienced nausea, generalised headache and neck pain, and ran a subfebrile temperature. A sudden rise in the temperature to 40°C then occurred, and the family doctor was called. He found a marked swelling of the lymph node at the right angle of the jaw, and a mild middle ear infection. Rapid improvement followed treatment with Elkosin. By 21 November 1954, the fever had disappeared; the child was lively, and went to bed without complaint. At 10.45 p.m., the parents heard the child cough, and found her whining in bed, with deviated eyes. She was motionless and unrousable, and had blood-stained saliva over her mouth, face and bedclothes. She had been incontinent of faeces; the stool had a normal colour. Shortly afterwards, she vomited a mass of blood-stained material.

Admission to the Children's Hospital, Zurich.

FINDINGS. On admission 2 hours later, the girl, who was normally developed for her age, was confused, unrousable and extremely pallid. Blood-stained saliva was issuing from her mouth, and her face, neck, chest and hands were soiled with caked blood. No source of the bleeding could be found on careful examination, and in particular there was no evidence of bite wounds on the tongue or lips. The carotid pulses were equal and normal on both sides. The patient was afebrile. Blood pressure 85/50 mm. Pulse 140/min and regular. The girl showed spontaneous symmetrical movements, and normal muscle tone. Tendon jerks were symmetrical and somewhat diminished. Babinski and Rossolimo responses were absent. No significant lymphadenopathy was detected; this included an absence of lymph nodes in the right angle of the jaw. Both ear-drums were normal.

Two hours after admission to hospital, the patient awoke, and about 15 minutes later exhibited tonic and clonic convulsions in the left arm and the left side of the face. She then lapsed into unconsciousness, and a complete flaccid paralysis of the left extremities and the left side of the mouth was observed. Despite liberal doses of phenobarbitone, further attacks of clonic seizures of the left arm occurred, without any change in the level of consciousness. During the course of the succeeding few days, a minor degree of voluntary movement returned in the left leg (movements on the right side of the body were normal), and the child regained consciousness completely. Apart from a strongly positive left Babinski response, no lateralising differences in the reflexes could be observed. The child repeatedly vomited black blood-stained material, and for 2 days the stools contained a large amount of altered blood.

Laboratory Findings on Admission. Blood: Hb 58 per cent; erythrocytes 2.91 million per mm³; leucocytes 24,800, juvenile forms 48.5 per cent, mature forms 31.5 per cent, eosinophils 1 per cent; basophils 0.5 per cent; monocytes 3.5 per cent; lymphocytes 14 per cent; 1 metamyelocyte; platelets 320,000. ESR 125/140 mm. Bleeding time, coagulation time, retraction time and coagulation factors all normal. Cold agglutination negative. Throat swab for haemolytic streptococci, pneumoccoci and haemophilus influenzae negative.

Lumbar Puncture. Pressure normal, fluid clear; 52⅔ erythrocytes, 3 monocytes, protein 21 mg per cent (Kafka).

Right Carotid Angiogram (22 November 1954). A percutaneous puncture was successful upon the second attempt under general anaesthesia. The proximal part of the internal carotid artery in the neck, immediately adjacent to the bifurcation of the common carotid, showed a narrowing of its lumen, which was maximal immediately before the artery entered the skull base. Directly distal to this point, a small out-pouching of the lumen was present, while the segment of the artery extending from the carotid canal to the intracranial bifurcation showed normal appearances. Only a few markedly thinned sylvian branches of the middle cerebral artery opacified, including the proximal half of the posterior temporal branch, the lumen of which was reduced to a thread; the anterior and posterior cerebral arteries and their branches were also present, the latter poorly opacified. In the next film of the series, the posterior temporal branch opacified well, as did the cerebral veins (internal cerebral vein, ascending cortical veins). The antero-posterior series showed similar appearances (Figs. 25 and 26).

EEG (22 November 1954). There was a marked depression of cerebral activity over the entire right side, and a moderate disturbance with slowed background activity over the left hemisphere; no epilepsy potentials were observed.

Follow-up Right Carotid Angiogram (24 November 1954). The internal carotid artery showed similar appearances to those of the first angiogram, although the narrowing was less marked; the out-pouching of the lumen immediately distal to the narrowed segment now appeared to be more severe. The middle cerebral artery was now better opacified, with the exception of the insular group which remained very narrow (Fig. 25).

Pneumoencephalogram (29 November 1954). Both lateral ventricles and the third ventricle were shown to be displaced about 1 cm to the left side, and the septum and the third ventricle were angled towards the left. Apart from a minor degree of enlargement of the third ventricle, their shape and size appeared normal. The basal cisterns were normal. Normal filling of cortical channels over the left hemisphere occurred, while there was no filling over the right hemisphere (Fig. 27).

CSF (29 November 1954). The fluid was mildly xanthochromic; bilirubin 0.54 mg per cent, colloidal gold reaction negative. No erythrocytes, 1 monocyte. Protein 27 mg per cent.

COURSE. The hemiplegia improved within a few weeks. After three weeks, only a spasticity with increased reflexes was still present, the arm being most severely involved. Upon discharge on 23 March 1955, the child was able to clench her fist, but was unable to extend her fingers. During walking, she slightly circumducted her left leg. The left expressive facial palsy persisted. Her initial mental recovery was good, and upon discharge she appeared to be perfectly normal. No further epileptic attacks occurred during the patient's stay in hospital.

EEG. A persistent depression of cerebral activity was revealed in the right precentral-central region; bilateral synchronous potentials, hinting of epilepsy, were observed for the first time on 18 February 1955. The anaemia and inflammatory changes in the blood returned completely to normal.

From March 1955, the child began to complain every few days of attacks of headache lasting about 30 minutes. She experienced attacks of 30-60 seconds duration 2-3 times a week, during which she became unresponsive, and developed a fixed gaze but no motor signs.

Second Admission to the Children's Hospital, Zurich (21 November-15 December 1955; 5 January-9 January 1956).

FINDINGS ON ADMISSION. The left spastic hemiparesis had markedly improved with intensive physiotherapy. Both carotid pulses appeared equally and normally palpable. No abnormality could be demonstrated either on inspection or palpation of the right angle of the jaw. Examination under anaesthetic of the epipharynx (Department of Otolaryngology, University Hospital, Zurich; 13 January 1956) revealed the presence of a small mid-line adenoidal pad, but no abnormal findings; in particular there was no identation or aneurysmal dilatation on the right side.

Follow-up Right Carotid Angiogram (12 December 1955). An aneurysmal sac 2 cm in diameter was demonstrated on the internal carotid artery, immediately before its entry into the base of the skull. Apart from the aneurysm, the course and calibre of the artery were completely normal. All the sylvian branches of the middle cerebral group appeared unusually thin, with the exception of the angular and posterior temporal arteries, which were well opacified. The anterior cerebral vessels, which were well shown, were displaced to the right side. In the venous phase of the antero-posterior series, the ascending cortical veins appeared to be displaced downwards from the cranial vault (Figs. 25 and 26).

Pneumoencephalogram (29 November 1955). Both lateral ventricles and the third ventricle were displaced to the right side, and the septum pellucidum and the third ventricle were angled towards the right. Both anterior horns and the cellae mediae, as well as the third ventricle, were enlarged, the right lateral ventricle more markedly so than the left (Fig. 27).

CSF (29 November 1955). Normal findings.

OPERATION (Department of Neurosurgery, University Hospital, Zurich; 12 January 1956). The right common and internal carotid arteries were exposed, but it proved impossible to free the aneurysm. The internal carotid was therefore ligated, and a segment excised.

Histological Examination (Institute of Pathology, University of Zurich). The arterial wall was normal, and there was no evidence of inflammatory changes or of a dissecting aneurysm.

Right Precentral and Parietal Burr-holes (16 January 1956). A cerebral cyst adjacent to the cortex, containing clear fluid, was demonstrated through the parietal burr-holes.

Histological Examination of the Cyst Wall (Institute of Pathology, University of Zurich). Meningo-encephalic cicatrical tissue was found.

COURSE. The spastic hemiparesis remained unaltered, following carotid ligation. However, some improvement occurred with prolonged intensive physiotherapy.

Pneumoencephalogram (23 May 1959). The right lateral ventricle was moderately dilatated, and the left lateral ventricle was normal in size. There was marked displacement of the ventricular system to the right side, just as had been demonstrated at previous examinations (Fig. 27).

In the course of 1956, an infantile organic psychosyndrome made its appearance, characterised by defective concentration, rapid exhaustion, increased irritability and depression. The IQ (Terman-Merrill) on 4 March 1964 was 74, and on 25 November 1965 (Biäsch) 67. The patient at $13\frac{1}{2}$ years of age exhibited an intellect corresponding to that of a normal 9-year-old, and had the speech of a 10-year-old.

With regular drug treatment, no epileptic attacks occurred from the Summer of 1955 to the Autumn of 1966, although an EEG on 19 September 1958 contained numerous generalised seizure complexes. Five subsequent follow-up EEGs (1959-1966) were performed, and no further epilepsy potentials were demonstrated, although a disturbance persisted in the posterior part of the right hemisphere; this disturbance took the form of delta groups, which were partially rhythmic and partially polymorphic, apparently arising from the brain stem. Cerebral activity over the left hemisphere remained within the limits of normal.

Findings in July 1966. Permanent spastic left hemiparesis was present, with a marked loss of function of the hand and a moderate disturbance of gait. There was shortening and wasting of the left arm; this was less marked in the leg. There were no gross disturbances of sensation. The infantile organic psychosyndrome was unaltered. The patient was still free from attacks with drug treatment.

CASE 22

M.E., born 19 December 1946 (1572/57, 2551/66).

FAMILY HISTORY. Nil relevant.

PREVIOUS HISTORY. Pregnancy uneventful. Birth at term, birth weight 2250g. Development in the first two years of life was somewhat retarded. Mumps and measles as a small child.

PRESENT ILLNESS. On 5 March 1957, when the child was 10 years 3 months old, she developed scarlet fever. After some weeks, a right otitis media appeared with right cervical lymphadenitis and stomatitis. After apparent improvement, a massive haemorrhage occurred from the nose and mouth on 23 March 1957, and the child vomited a mass of dark blood. During the course of the day, she became progressively more confused and drowsy.

Admission to the Children's Hospital, Zurich (23 March 1957).

FINDINGS ON ADMISSION. The patient exhibited flaccid incomplete left hemiplegia, with a left Babinski response and symmetrically diminished tendon jerks in all extremities. She was unrousable and drowsy, with a purulent perforated right otitis media and haemorrhagic stomatopharyngitis. There was an enlarged lymph node at the right angle of the jaw, which was painful to pressure and about the size of

a date. The fundi and pupils were normal. There was extensive fine desquamation of the skin.

Laboratory Findings. Blood: Hb 81 per cent; erythrocytes 4 million, leucocytes 19,250, juvenile forms 23 per cent, mature forms 58 per cent; basophils 1 per cent; monocytes 4 per cent; lymphocytes 14 per cent; platelets normal. ESR 120/132 mm. Temperature 35.2°C. Blood pressure 115/80 mm. Pulse 80/min, and regular.

Lumbar Puncture. Pressure 15 cm, fluid clear; 8 cells ($7\frac{1}{3}$ monocytes, $\frac{2}{3}$ segmented). Protein 30 mg per cent (Kafka); colloidal gold reaction normal; glucose 74 mg per cent. Bacteriological culture sterile. A throat swab and pus from the right external auditory canal showed haemolytic streptococci group A, and coagulase positive staphylococcus aureus haemolyticus.

EEG (24 March 1957). A severe extensive disturbance was shown over the right hemisphere with a massive depression.

Admission to the Department of Otorhinolaryngology, University Hospital, Zurich (24 March 1957).
The child was admitted on suspicion of an otogenic intracranial complication.

FINDINGS ON ADMISSION.
Right mastoidectomy (24 March 1957). A disappointing finding was a thickened mucosa with scanty exudate and no intracranial extension; a puncture of the dural sinus revealed blood-stained fluid.

While the drowsiness diminished, the hemiparesis increased to a complete hemiplegia by 26 March 1957.

Right Carotid Angiogram (26 March 1957). The cervical carotid artery opacified normally for the proximal 3 cm of its course; at this point the lumen narrowed in a conical manner, and all flow stopped proximal to the skull base. Retrograde filling of the vertebral artery occurred via the common carotid, and the basilar artery and several of its branches were weakly visualised (Fig. 28).

Pneumoencephalogram (4 April 1957). The ventricular system was normal in size shape and position (Fig. 29).

CSF. Clear; protein 22 mg per cent; 17 monocytes; colloidal gold and mastix tests normal. Bacteriological culture sterile.

Intensive therapy with vasodilators (Ronicol i.v.) exerted no effect on the flaccid hemiplegia. Both the otitis media and the stomatopharyngitis responded to antibiotics, and the patient's general condition improved markedly.

OPERATION (12 April 1957). Resection of the left stellate ganglion, *i.e.* contralateral to the side of the carotid thrombosis.

COURSE. The first voluntary movements returned 1 day after stellectomy, and on 15 April 1957 they appeared in the left arm. On 24 April 1957, the little girl was able to walk with support, and two weeks later unaided. However, a considerable degree of spastic hemiparesis remained, including a severe loss of function of the hand, and a lesser disturbance of gait. A very marked infantile organic psychosyndrome developed. Previously the girl had been a good pupil and had managed to pass beyond the 8th primary school class, but now she failed to progress further. She spent one year as a trainee housekeeper, then began to learn dressmaking. In 1963 she had to be admitted to a closed institution because of her uncontrollable temper. No epileptic attacks had been observed.

Second Admission to the Children's Hospital, Zurich (24 August-7 September 1964).

FINDINGS ON ADMISSION. On admission the patient had a marked spastic left-sided hemiparesis, with complete loss of function of the hand, and a mild disturbance of gait. There was some shortening of the left extremities (forearm and hand by 1½ cm, leg by 1 cm). Dysaesthesia was present in the left half of the body, but deep sensitivity and pain sensitivity were retained. The cranial nerves were intact, apart from definite expressive facial palsy; there was no sign of Horner's syndrome. *EEG.* A discrete non-specific disturbance was demonstrated over the middle and posterior temporal regions of the right hemisphere. No epilepsy potentials were observed.

Pneumoencephalogram. The ventricular system was considerably displaced to the right side. The right lateral ventricle was moderately enlarged (Fig. 29).

Psychiatric Examination. A moderately severe psychosyndrome was present, but the child's intelligence was average (IQ about 100 according to Hamburg, Wechsler and Terman). Her mental processes were markedly slowed during performance of the test. She was easily tired (exercise curve according to Kraepelin), and showed marked affective lability.

COURSE (until Autumn 1966). The weakness has persisted unaltered, but the patient is otherwise free from complaints. A rehabilitation programme was unsuccessful, partly due to the patient's failure to co-operate. At present she is confined, because of mental instability, to a closed institution, where she helps with the housework and in the garden.

CASE 23*
R.G. born 5 July 1956 (3417/59)

FAMILY HISTORY. Nil relevant.

PREVIOUS HISTORY. Normal pregnancy. Delivery at term, healthy baby; birth weight 2500g. Development normal. Repeated affect spasms following painful minor injuries, during the first and second years of life.

PRESENT ILLNESS. On 13 and 14 April 1959, the child, who was then 2 years and 9 months old, seemed unusually tired, and frequently interrupted her play to go and rest. She had no fever, and showed no signs of any infection.

On 15 April 1959, she awoke normally, but at about 8.30 a.m. she suddenly collapsed unconscious beside her mother, and was incontinent of urine. When she was picked up, her limbs fell flaccid to her sides. About one hour later, a complete right-sided hemiplegia was noted, accompanied by a loss of speech and asymmetry of the mouth. The girl vomited repeatedly, and was incontinent of urine and faeces.

Admission to the Department of Paediatrics, University Hospital, Berne (18 April-18 June 1959).

FINDINGS ON ADMISSION. Complete flaccid right hemiplegia was present, with central facial and hypoglossal palsy, as well as aphasia. There was a diminution of tendon jerks, particularly on the right, and a left Babinski response was elicited. There were no signs of meningism. Clinical examination was negative in respect of any focal infection, and the cardiovascular system was normal. Blood pressure 100/70 mm Hg. Pulse 70/min, and full. The patient was afebrile. Blood: Hb 15.5 g per cent; leucocytes 8100, with normal differential count. ESR 31/58 mm. Haemolytic staphylococci were isolated in a throat swab.

*This case is included by kind permission of Professor E. Rossi, Director, Department of Paediatrics, University Hospital, Berne.

231

Lumbar Puncture. Pressure 14 cm; fluid clear; 2⅓ cells; protein 24 mg per cent (Kafka); glucose 75 mg per cent (Hagedorn).

EEG. A marked delta focus was demonstrated over the left hemisphere, with a maximum in the temporo-occipital region. No epilepsy potentials were present.

Left Carotid Angiogram (21 April 1959). The internal carotid artery opacified normally as far as the siphon, its calibre being regular and normal. In the terminal part of the internal carotid, two indentations were demonstrated, and similar deformities were shown in the trunk of the middle cerebral artery; in the antero-posterior projection, the vessels looked like a string of pearls. Only three main branches of the middle cerebral artery filled well; many smaller arteries appeared unusually thin, and a number of the insular branches did not opacify at all. The anterior cerebral artery failed to fill. A circumscribed and weak contrast shadow was demonstrated around one opercular branch (? extravasation) (Fig. 30a).

Follow-up Left Carotid Angiogram (28 April 1959). The appearances were virtually unchanged, with numerous indentations occupying the same sites as before. Again, there was a paucity of middle cerebral branches, and an absence of the insular twigs. The anterior cerebral group again failed to fill (Ronicol and novocaine were injected during the angiogram, but had no effect) (Fig. 30b).

Right Carotid Angiogram (5 May 1959). Findings were normal, with complete visualisation of the entire arterial tree. The left anterior cerebral artery opacified via the anterior communicating artery. The trunk of the internal carotid was shown to be considerably larger than the left one.

Pneumoencephalogram (18 June 1959). There was widening of the body and trigone of the left lateral ventricle.

COURSE. Voluntary movements were observed in the right leg after two weeks. In the course of the succeeding weeks, a distal weakness with very little spasticity developed, involving the arm more severely than the leg. Speech recovered completely within 6 months, and at the same time the central facial palsy disappeared. Bladder and anal sphincter function returned within weeks.

In 1961 epileptic attacks of a Jacksonian type commenced, which were gradually brought under medical control.

PROGRESS (until Autumn 1966). The girl was attending the primary school, and managing after a fashion, although she tired easily, and showed spells of severe lack of concentration. She was severely unstable of mood, but her speech was only slightly abnormal. The spastic hemiparesis persisted, despite regular physiotherapy, giving the child a marked limitation of hand movements, and a slight disturbance of gait. There has been no shortening of the paralysed limb to date, and the patient has been free from attacks since the beginning of 1964.

CASE 24

F.D., born 2 September 1964 (5363/65, 5418/65, 1569/70).

FAMILY HISTORY. A brother with a vascular naevus on the scrotum, and a sister with a vascular naevus on the buttocks.

PREVIOUS HISTORY. Pregnancy and birth normal; healthy baby; birth weight 3700 g. Psychomotor development slightly delayed (laughing at 6 weeks, sitting unsteadily at 9½ months). Left ptosis since birth.

On 18 June 1965, the child was knocked over in her baby carriage by a drunken motor cyclist, but she was not injured. She cried for a short while, but did not lose consciousness, and did not vomit. Immediately after the incident she behaved quite normally.

PRESENT ILLNESS. On 20 June 1965, two days after the accident, the child, then 9 months old, exhibited for the first time clonic convulsions of the right arm and leg. These convulsions lasted a few seconds, and recurred 2-3 times in the succeeding four days. At the same time a flaccid paralysis of the right arm was present, which recovered spontaneously.

On 12 July 1965, the child, who had been perfectly healthy on the previous day, awoke with a flaccid weakness of the right extremities; this weakness was complete in the arm and partial in the leg. She began to vomit.

Admission to the Cantonal Hospital, Chur.

FINDINGS ON ADMISSION. Fontanelle puncture revealed normal CSF, and no subdural collections. Coagulation factors were normal.

Admission to the Children's Hospital, Zurich 15 July-26 August 1965).

232

FINDINGS ON ADMISSION. The child was fully conscious, with flaccid right-sided hemiparesis including the face. The fundi were normal. The anterior fontanelle was soft; skull radiographs were normal. No vascular lesions were seen in the skin.

EEG. A depression was revealed over the entire left hemisphere. Intermittent subclinical discharge phenomena which were arising from the left central region were rapidly spreading bilaterally.

Pneumoencephalogram. The left lateral ventricle was slightly enlarged. There was no mid-line displacement of the ventricular system. The roof of the right lateral ventricle appeared to be depressed (Fig. 31a).

OPERATION (20 July 1965). Three burr-holes were made on the right side and one on the left. Findings were normal, with no evidence of a subdural haematoma.

Left Carotid Angiogram (20 July 1965). The internal carotid artery was normal, but localised stenosis was demonstrated at the carotid bifurcation. The middle cerebral artery and the branches and the trunk of the anterior cerebral artery were normal. However, there was marked narrowing of the branches distal to the origin of the anterior communicating artery. The posterior communicating artery was supplying the trunk and branches of the posterior cerebral artery. In the arterial phase, a fine vessel network opacified from the anterior and posterior choroidal arteries and from the perforating branches in the region of the basal ganglia. Meningeal branches arising from the ophthalmic artery were markedly hypertrophied (Fig. 31a).

Follow-up Left Carotid Angiogram (13 August 1965). There were no significant changes. A further network of pathological vessels was demonstrated to opacify by transdural anastomoses (external carotid—middle meningeal artery), which was now better visualised (Fig. 31a).

Right Carotid Angiogram (13 August 1965). A mirror image was obtained, in that the origin of the middle cerebral artery showed a circumscribed area of focal narrowing similar to that on the left side; however, the sylvian branches opacified well. The anterior cerebral group was somewhat better seen than on the left side. The trunk of the posterior communicating artery was unusually large, and was supplying the posterior cerebral artery and its branches. A network of fine pathological vessels opacified from the perforating vessels in the region of the basal ganglia, and from the anterior and posterior choroidal arteries.

COURSE. The hemiparesis gradually disappeared within two months, after which time a hyper-reflexia involving the right leg and bilateral Babinski responses were present. By the time of the patient's discharge at the end of August 1965, no definite lateralising signs could be demonstrated. Early on the morning of 12 September 1965, the child awoke and cried out that she was unable to move her limbs. She then went into a deep sleep and, when she awoke 2½ hours later, no motor deficit remained. On 15 September, a flaccid weakness of the left side of the body suddenly appeared, accompanied by clonic movements of the right hand. The child appeared to be in a dream-like state, with her eyes open, but showing no response to commands.

Admission to the Children's Hospital, Zurich (16 September-28 October 1965).

FINDINGS ON ADMISSION. The child was fully conscious, and was found to have complete flaccid left-sided hemiplegia, including the face. There was spasticity of the right arm, the fist being held in a clenched position. The reflexes were symmetrical and normal. Bilateral Babinski responses were elicited. A general physical examination gave normal findings. Shortly after admission, an attack lasting 2 minutes occurred, consisting of conjugate deviation to the left side, clonic movements of the right leg, cyanosis and unconsciousness.

Lumbar Puncture. Normal Findings.

EEG. Significant low amplitude waves were present over both hemispheres, but were more marked on the left side. No epilepsy potentials were present.

COURSE. In the course of three weeks the patient developed a spasticity of the left extremities, particularly of the arm, with paresis of the leg. In November 1965, she suffered attacks of recurrent seizures, despite regular anticonvulsant treatment. These attacks took the form of sudden unconsciousness and conjugate deviation of the eyes to the right side, but there were no convulsions. Following these episodes the child remained stuporose for 6 months. However, she gradually began to respond, showing grasp movements with the right hand.

Despite regular physiotherapy, the child remained severely incapacitated and bedridden, due to bilateral spastic hemiparesis. No seizures have occurred since November 1965.

Follow-up Examination at the Children's Hospital, Zurich (2-4 April 1970).

FINDINGS. The child, now 6½ years old, is severely mentally defective. She understands simple commands, and speaks a few poorly vocalised words. She has severe bilateral spastic hemiparesis, which is more marked on the left side, and cannot sit up without support.

Repeat Left Carotid Angiogram (3 April 1970). There was complete occlusion of the distal end of the internal carotid, including the trunk of the anterior and middle cerebral arteries. A dense collateral network of perforating vessels was demonstrated in the region of the basal ganglia, supplying blood to the occluded vascular territories. The posterior communicating arteries were supplying the trunk and branches of the posterior cerebral artery. Large transdural anastomoses opacified from the middle meningeal artery. There was another collateral network from a hypertrophied ophthalmic artery (Fig. 31b).

Repeat Right Carotid Angiogram (3 April 1970). There was an occlusion of the distal carotid bifurcation. An extensive collateral network had been formed by perforating arteries and the anterior and posterior choroidal arteries. A large posterior communicating artery was supplying the posterior cerebral artery. Transdural anastomoses, opacifying from the middle meningeal artery, were less developed than on the left side. An ophthalmic artery was contributing to the meningeal collateral network (Fig. 31b).

Left Vertebral Angiogram (3 April 1970). The left vertebral, basilar and posterior cerebral arteries opacified normally. There was an extensive supply to the collateral network from the posterior choroidal artery. Another collateral pathway was demonstrated by transdural anastomoses which opacified from the occipital meningeal artery (Fig. 31b).

CASE 25

H.B., born 16 August 1962 (2159/69, 1613/70).

FAMILY HISTORY. Nil relevant.

PREVIOUS HISTORY. Pregnancy and birth normal; birth weight 2500g; body length 46 cm.

Placenta contained several calcified infarcts. Baby healthy.

On the second day of life, the girl underwent an uneventful operation for duodenal atresia (Children's Hospital, Zurich). At the age of 4 months she underwent an operation for mechanical ileus. Moderate psychomotor retardation. Frequent upper respiratory tract infections without complications. A left-handed child.

PRESENT ILLNESS. In April 1969, the girl, who was 6½ years old, presented for the first time with episodic speech difficulties (unable to find certain words). On 20 May, following a mild upper respiratory tract infection, she showed unusual fatigue and refused to go to school. On the following morning, a facial palsy was present, and a few hours later a flaccid paralysis of the left arm suddenly developed, accompanied by intermittent left-sided clonic spasms involving the face and arm. The patient remained fully conscious.

Admission to the Department of Paediatrics, Cantonal Hospital, Winterthur.

FINDINGS ON ADMISSION. The child, who was obviously mentally retarded, was fully conscious, with flaccid left-sided paralysis involving the arm and face (including the forehead) but not the lower limb. Intermittent clonic spasms of the paralysed parts occurred. Other symptoms were rhinitis, a reddening of the left ear drum, a tender left mastoid, and coughing. The patient was afebrile.

Lumbar Puncture. Pressure 16 cm; fluid normal.
Skull and Chest Radiographs. Normal.
Admission to Children's Hospital, Zurich (21 May-3 June 1969).

FINDINGS ON ADMISSION. Eight hours after the onset of the illness, only a left facial palsy still remained. Muscle tone and tendon jerks were normal in all extremities, and there was no Babinski response on either side. The patient was afebrile. Blood: Hb 13.8 g per cent; leucocytes 6000, with a shift to the left (30 per cent bands). Micro-ESR 2/5/11 mm. Tests for syphilis and toxoplasmosis were negative. Amino-acid chromatography in urine gave normal results.

EEG. Focal epileptic activity was shown in the parietal areas on both sides, with a slight depression over the right parietal region.

Right Carotid Angiogram (23 May 1969). The internal carotid artery was normal, but there was an occlusion of the trunk of the middle cerebral artery. There was an extensive collateral network of perforating branches in the region of the basal ganglia, which opacified a few branches of the middle cerebral artery. The anterior cerebral artery and its branches were normal: the pericallosal artery was surrounded by a tuft of fine vessels. The large posterior communicating artery was supplying the posterior artery and its branches; there was a stenosis of the mid-point of the trunk of the posterior cerebral artery. A net-like vascular pattern was seen in its vicinity. A venogram was normal (Fig. 32).

Left Carotid Angiogram (30 May 1969). Findings were normal, except that the anterior cerebral artery and its branches only faintly opacified (the main supply came from the right internal carotid via the anterior communicating artery). The large posterior communicating artery was supplying the posterior cerebral artery. No abnormal collaterals were seen.

COURSE. On the day following admission, the neurological deficit of the face and extremities disappeared. At the time of discharge, the child's parents considered her to be fully recovered, although her retarded mental condition was unaltered. During the succeeding weeks, she began to use her right hand more and more. She was kept on regular anticonvulsant therapy, and no seizures occurred. In the Spring of 1970 she was enrolled in a special school for the mentally handicapped.

Second Admission to the Children's Hospital, Zurich (5-11 April 1970).

FINDINGS ON ADMISSION. The child's mental status was unaltered. Neurological findings were normal.

EEG. Focal epileptic activity was demonstrated over both parietal regions, and particularly on the right side. There were signs of slightly depressed activity over the right hemisphere.

Repeat Right Carotid Angiogram (6 April 1970). The appearances of the occluded middle cerebral trunk and the collateral network from the perforating branches were unaltered. The tuft of vessels surrounding the pericallosal artery was also unchanged. The main distal branch of the posterior cerebral artery was completely occluded. The posterior choroidal collateral channels were hypertrophied (Fig. 32). In the antero-posterior projection, both anterior cerebral arteries and their branches opacified well. There was a good supply to the left (!) middle cerebral artery across the anterior communicating artery.

Repeat Left Carotid Angiogram (6 April 1970). Appearances were unaltered from the previous year. No abnormal collateral network was seen.

Left Vertebral Angiogram (8 April 1970). Catheterisation from the femoral artery revealed an occlusion of the narrowed left vertebral artery near the mouth of its posterior inferior cerebellar branch; the latter vessel opacified normally. No abnormal collateral channels were seen (Fig. 32).

Right Vertebral Angiogram (8 April 1970). The injection was made with the catheter tip in the right subclavian artery. The right vertebral and basilar arteries opacified normally. The main supply to the right posterior cerebral artery occurred via the right carotid and posterior communicating arteries. The right posterior inferior cerebellar artery was not visualised. No abnormal collateral channels opacified from the vertebro-basilar system (Fig. 32).

CASE 26

S.E. born 16 April 1950 (5065/51, 7786/63).

FAMILY HISTORY. Nil relevant.

PREVIOUS HISTORY. Pregnancy, birth and development normal. Meningococcal meningitis at the age of 13 months, with complete recovery (admitted to the Children's Hospital, Zurich for 4½ weeks). Measles, mumps, chickenpox and whooping cough as a child, without complications. No other serious illnesses. No significant head injuries.

PRESENT ILLNESS. On 13 February 1963, the patient, then a girl aged 12 years 10 months, went sledging with the family. On the way home she fell off the sledge and, when asked, admitted to a mild headache. In the evening she was bright, and free from complaints. In the course of the following morning, her father noticed that she was somewhat listless during skating. After the mid-day meal she complained of severe headache, and refused to go out skiing with the family, going to lie on her bed instead. During the afternoon she vomited repeatedly, and felt dizzy. In the night her parents heard her groan and go to the toilet, but found nothing wrong. The following morning she failed to wake up normally, and was found to have passed urine in her bed. When awoken, she could not speak, and indicated that she had a headache. The family doctor was called, and he found her in a 'comatose state', with her pupils widely dilated and reacting poorly to light; all knee jerks were absent.

Urgent Admission to the Children's Hospital, Zurich (15 February 1963).

FINDINGS ON ADMISSION AT 12.30 p.m. The patient was stuporose, and lay quietly in a supine position, raising her hand (? side) every now and then to her head. Initially she responded slowly but correctly to shouted questions (her name), and simple commands (*e.g.* put out the tongue, press the hand). She moved all four extremities voluntarily, and in response to pain stimulation, without any obvious lateralising differences. Muscle tone was generally reduced. Tendon jerks were normal and symmetrical; definite right, and possible left, Babinski responses were elicited. The left pupil was more widely dilated than the right one, and both reacted slowly to light. The fundi were normal. There were no signs of meningism, and no signs of external trauma. Skull radiographs were normal, and respiration was regular. Blood pressure 140/80 mm Hg. Pulse 66/min, and regular.

Laboratory Findings. Blood: Hb 88 per cent; erythrocytes 4.34 million; leucocytes 7300, juvenile forms 50.5 per cent, mature forms 25.5 per cent; eosinophils 0.5 per cent; basophils 0.5 per cent; monocytes 2.5 per cent; lymphocytes 20.5 per cent; platelets normal. Temperature 33.8°C.

EEG (15 February 1965). At 1 p.m., a moderately diffuse disturbance with a focal maximum was seen in the left postcentral region (polymorphic delta waves). Intermittent bilateral fronto-precentral spindle-shape wave complexes were observed, each lasting for 13-14 seconds. There was some reduction of the fast low amplitude waves in the left parietooccipital region.

At 1.45 p.m., the child passed into a deep coma; both her pupils were widely dilated and unreactive to light. Her pulse was 140/min, and her respiration regular. She was incontinent of urine.

Transfer to the Department of Neurosurgery, University Hospital, Zurich.

OPERATION. Immediate intubation was performed in preparation for burr-holes, but the respiration then became irregular and the blood pressure dropped to 60/40 mm Hg. Artificial respiration was then commenced. Burr-hole investigation (bilateral temporal and left frontal) gave negative results, and it was found impossible to enter the ventricles.

A Left Carotid Angiogram was then performed. The internal carotid artery appeared normal to the level of the siphon, but the middle cerebral artery did not opacify. Short segments of both anterior cerebral arteries, and the anterior communicating artery were demonstrated; the ophthalmic artery was also seen, and there was retrograde filling of the basilar artery via the posterior communicating artery. Three series were made, and they all showed the same appearances (Fig. 33).

Lumbar Puncture (after burr-hole examination). The fluid was moderately blood-stained, and there was a trace of xanthochromia upon centrifugation. A bacteriological culture was sterile, and virus studies (cell culture on monkey kidney, as well as intracerebral and subcutaneous innoculation in mice) were negative.

COURSE. The patient remained in a deep coma, with a temperature of 32-34°C. Pulse 90/40 min; blood pressure no longer measurable. Artificial respiration was continuously necessary, and, despite intravenous infusion of urea and papaverine, the child died at 11 p.m. on 16 February 1963.

AUTOPSY (Institute of Pathology, University of Zurich). There was thrombosis of the left internal carotid artery in the distal knee of the carotid siphon, and also of the right internal carotid artery in the carotid siphon. Extensive recent haemorrhagic softening of the white matter, with perifocal oedema, was found in the left cerebral hemisphere. The circle of Willis was patent, and arterial walls were normal. The right middle cerebral artery from the internal carotid bifurcation was reduplicated. There was a hyperplastic left posterior cerebral artery between the basilar and posterior communicating arteries.

Histology. Histological examination revealed old splitting and fragmentation of the internal elastic laminar, with intimal plaque formation over the defects in both carotid siphons (Figs. 34*a* and *b*).

236

CASE 27

A.R., born 6 October 1955 (2458/64)

FAMILY HISTORY. Nil relevant.

PREVIOUS HISTORY. Prone to upper respiratory tract infections, leading to tonsillectomy in the Autumn of 1962. Left handed. A bed-wetter until the age of 7 years.

PRESENT ILLNESS. From the early part of 1964, the child experienced occasional attacks of headache and nocturia. On the morning of 10 August 1964, he developed a left-sided hemiparesis, first in the leg, and spreading after a few hours to involve the arm. Simultaneously, mental changes occurred, accompanied by marked slowing, but with no loss of consciousness or convulsions. The boy vomited repeatedly, and had a severe frontal headache.

Admission to the Cantonal Hospital, St. Gallen (11 August 1964).

FINDINGS ON ADMISSION. The patient had incomplete left-sided motor and sensory hemiparesis, including the face, mild papilloedema, and hypertension (225/160 mm Hg).

Transfer to the Department of Neurosurgery, University Hospital, Zurich (11 August 1964).

FINDINGS ON ADMISSION. A flaccid left hemiparesis was present, with a left Babinski response and increased reflexes in the left leg; reflexes were absent in the left arm. There was an absence of movement sensitivity in the left arm and foot. Left homonymous hemianopia was present.

Right Carotid Angiogram. No gross abnormality was demonstrated; a solitary insular artery appeared thinned (Fig. 35).

CSF. Normal pressure; fluid clear; one cell; protein 48.4 per cent (Kafka); colloidal gold reaction 5222211111.

Pneumoencephalogram. A technical failure occurred.

Admission to the Children's Hospital, Zurich (12 August-29 August 1964).

FINDINGS. The boy was drowsy, and the hemiparesis was unaltered.

Ophthalmological Examination (Department of Ophthalmology, University Hospital, Zurich). The fundi on both sides were angiospastic, with severe grades of papilloedema. Blood pressure levels in the arms were 210/150, and in the legs 260/190.

Heart. The beat of the apex was in the normal position, with the second sound increased.

Electrocardiography revealed a sinus rhythm, and some early left ventricular hypertrophy.

Urine. Specific gravity 1033, later constantly 1010. Constant albuminuria; bacteriologically sterile: no deposits.

Creatinine Clearance. Normal (76 ml/min).

Serum Chemistry. Normal values for urea and electrolytes, pH 7.5. Base excess: + 3.5 m val.

EEG (14 August 1964). A severe disturbance was shown over the right hemisphere, in the form of continuous polymorphic delta activity. The left hemisphere was moderately disturbed.

The blood picture was normal, and the child was afebrile. ESR 5/15 mm.

Caval Catheterisation. The left kidney was grossly enlarged, with chronic pyelonephritic changes. The right kidney was not visualised.

Retrograde Aortography. The right kidney was aplastic; also demonstrated was a hypoplastic left renal artery, with malformation of the lower pole, and good function of the upper pole.

COURSE. A good recovery was made from the hemisyndrome within three weeks, under treatment with hypotensive and vasodilator drugs (papaverine).

PROGRESS (until August 1966). No neurological deficit remains. The child is in the fourth grade in the primary school, and has no difficulties. The hypertension has been satisfactorily controlled by drugs. No further attacks have occurred.

CASE 28

G.M., born 22 August 1950 (5513/63)

FAMILY HISTORY. Father with renal hypertension, leading to left nephrectomy in 1959.

PREVIOUS HISTORY. Pregnancy, birth and development normal. Left-handed. Up to the Summer of 1963, the boy was healthy and free from complaints. In the middle of July he had a two day attack of nausea, headache and vomiting, but recovered completely. A similar attack occurred at the beginning of August, accompanied by a transient fever of 38°C.

PRESENT ILLNESS. On the morning of 21 August 1963 the boy, who was then 13 years old, was cycling to school when he was suddenly overcome and lost consciousness. This attack was accompanied by foaming at the mouth, and was followed immediately by clonic seizures in both (?) arms lasting for 10 minutes. A few minutes later, a brief similar attack occurred, with conjugate deviation of the eyes to the right side. The patient was given 200 mg of phenobarbitone intramuscularly. Upon awakening, he vomited copiously for a short while, and complained of severe headache.

Emergency Admission to the Children's Hospital, Zurich (21 August 1963).

FINDINGS ON ADMISSION. The boy was somnolent and confused, and responded with difficulty. He had marked expressive (but not receptive) aphasia. Flaccid right-sided hemiparesis was present; it was most marked in the leg and discrete around the right angle of the mouth. Reflexes were increased in all limbs. A right Babinski response was elicited; the left abdominal reflexes were diminished. There were signs of severe meningism, accompanied by marked acute bilateral papilloedema with fundal haemorrhages on the right side.

Clinical examination revealed the presence of a severe aortic isthmus stenosis. Blood pressure in the arms varied between 160/100 and 200/140 mm Hg, and in the legs it was around 110/70 mm Hg.

Lumbar Puncture. The fluid was uniformly blood-stained, and was shown to be xanthochromic after centrifugation. It was bacteriologically sterile.

Bilateral Carotid Angiogram (22 August 1963). Injection of the left side produced good filling of the internal carotid and middle cerebral artery and its branches. The anterior cerebral artery was not visualised (Fig. 36).

Upon right-sided injection, both anterior cerebral arteries and their branches opacified, although their calibre was unusually thin. No abnormal vessels or malformations were demonstrated (Fig. 36).

EEG (21 August 1963). A moderate diffuse and non-specific disturbance was demonstrated with a questionable depression in the left central region. No epilepsy potentials were present.

Laboratory Findings. The patient was afebrile on admission. Blood: Hb 95 per cent; leucocytes 11600, juvenile forms 41.5 per cent, mature forms 50.5 per cent; monocytes 2.5 per cent; lymphocytes 5.5 per cent. Macro-ESR 5/15 mm.

COURSE. The hemiparesis regressed within 3 days, apart from the expressive aphasia which took 2 weeks to completely disappear. On 1 September 1963, 11 days after the first attack, a further subarachnoid haemorrhage occurred,

on this occasion with a massive motor deficit. A bout of fever lasting 3-5 days after the first haemorrhage was followed by a second bout lasting nearly one week after the second attack. The boy gradually recovered. Psychiatric examination on 7 October 1963, seven weeks after the initial haemorrhage, revealed an organic psychosyndrome of slight to moderate severity, characterised by weakness of visual and auditory memory, and emotional lability.

OPERATION (9 October 1963). An operative correction of the aortic isthmus was undertaken with a dacron prosthesis. The child made an uneventful recovery, and on discharge from hospital on 30 October 1963, the blood pressure levels and femoral pulses had returned to normal.

EEG (7 March 1964). A slight diffuse nonspecific disturbance was detected, but the findings were marginal.

Follow-up Examination (2 March 1964). According to the boy's teacher, he was doing well at school, and early in the year he had been promoted to the sixth grade in the secondary school. Subjectively, he was free from symptoms, although physically he was not very active, on the advice of his own doctor. The only remaining neurological deficit appeared to be some clumsiness of the right hand.

COURSE (until August 1966). The patient has remained free from complaints, and no longer exhibits any neurological signs. No epileptic attacks have occurred, although no prophylactic drug treatment was undertaken. The boy completed his secondary school education satisfactorily, and is at present a trainee draftsman.

CASE 29

P.F., born 16 July 1959 (8092, 8251/63).

FAMILY HISTORY. Nil relevant.

PREVIOUS HISTORY. Pregnancy birth and development normal. Prone to upper respiratory tract infections, but no serious illnesses.

PRESENT ILLNESS. On 10 August 1962 the patient, then 3 years old, fell with a glass pipette in his mouth, and bumped his head on the floor. The pipette broke, and moderately severe bleeding commenced from the mouth. Within seconds, the soft tissues at the left angle of the jaw began to swell up. Within minutes, the child collapsed and became pulseless and pale. Following immediate blood transfusion, he recovered within half an hour, and three hours later could speak and move his arms normally and stand on his legs. Fourteen hours after the accident, sudden tonic convulsions of the entire left (!) side of the body, including the face, occurred; these recurred at intervals over the next twelve hours. Immediately after the seizures, a flaccid right hemiplegia, complete in the arm, partial in the leg, and involving the face, was present. There was a complete expressive aphasia, but no receptive deficit. The child remained drowsy for 8 days.

Within several weeks, during physiotherapeutic rehabilitation, a severe spastic hemiparesis developed, involving particularly the right arm. Speech returned over several months, at first slowly, and then rapidly, and 7 months after the accident no residual disturbance could be detected.

Six and a half months after the accident, epileptiform attacks commenced; these attacks gradually increased in frequency until, finally, they occurred every 30 minutes; they were accompanied by a loss of consciousness, lasting a few seconds, a tonic movement of the head to the right, and elevation of the right arm. The child occasionally fell backwards.

Admission to the Children's Hospital, Zurich (22 March–10 April 1963).

FINDINGS ON ADMISSION. A moderately spastic right hemiparesis was present; there was a loss of function of the right hand, a moderate disturbance of gait, and a mild facial palsy. There was no definite loss of sensation and no speech disturbance. The right forearm was shortened by 0.5 cm.

EEG. An active epileptogenic focus was detected in the left mid-temporal region. There was a moderate depression of background activity over the entire left hemisphere.

Left Carotid Angiogram. A thrombotic occlusion was demonstrated in the internal carotid artery at the base of the skull (Fig. 37).

CASE 30

R.H., born 29 August 1952.

PRESENT ILLNESS. This 6-year-old boy experienced recurrent subarachnoid haemorrhages from an arteriovenous malformation on a posterior-inferior cerebellar artery. This aspect of the case has been discussed in detail on page 13.

The cause of the recurrent subarachnoid haemorrhage was demonstrated by angiography.

Bilateral Carotid Angiography (22 September 1958). The right side showed normal appearances. The left carotid angiogram failed because of technical difficulties. At the first attempt, the needle was placed in the external carotid artery at the level of its lingual branch, and the internal carotid tree was not visualised. At the second attempt, only poor opacification of the internal carotid and its branches occurred.

Follow-up Left Carotid Angiogram (13 October 1958). Performed immediately prior to operative removal of the arteriovenous malformation from the cerebellum, angiography revealed excellent filling of the entire carotid tree. The only unusual feature was narrowing of the distal part of the carotid siphon, in comparison with the calibre of the proximal segments of the middle cerebral artery (Fig. 38).

OPERATION (Department of Neurosurgery, University Hospital, Zurich). *See above.*

After satisfactory post-operative recovery, the patient suddenly developed, on 1 January 1959, a speech disturbance, followed (on 5 January) by a weakness in the right arm and a difficulty with swallowing. Physical examination on 9 January revealed the presence of severe flaccid right-sided hemiplegia, with diminished tendon jerks in both upper limbs and increased jerks in the right leg, a right Babinski response, marked central right-sided facial palsy, and dysarthria without expressive dysphasia. The tongue was deviated to the right side. Mental slowing was also observed.

Re-admission to the Department of Neurosurgery, University Hospital, Zurich (13-25 January 1959).

FINDINGS ON ADMISSION. The child's condition was unaltered.

EEG. A marked extensive disturbance (maximal in the lateral postcentral region) was shown over the entire left hemisphere.

Left Carotid Angiogram. There was marked narrowing of the calibre of the trunk of the middle cerebral artery, with non-filling of the majority of its sylvian branches. The calibre of the internal carotid artery, including its siphon, was normal (Fig. 38).

COURSE. A partial thrombosis of the middle cerebral artery was diagnosed, and drug treatment (Marcumar) commenced. Within a week, the hemiparesis showed some regression. On 23 January 1959, severe convulsions suddenly and unexpectedly recurred, consisting partly of disturbances of extrapyramidal movements involving mainly the right side, and partly of focal seizures. The child became increasingly comatose, and died on 21 January 1959 in hyperthermia.

BRAIN EXAMINATION (Research Division, Department of Neurology, University of Zurich). A dissecting aneurysm was present in the left internal carotid artery, extending into the branches of the middle cerebral artery (the proximal segments of the carotid artery were not examined). There was long-standing cerebral softening in the basal ganglia and left internal capsule. Recent softening with oedema was found in the right insular cortex, extending into the putamen as far as the globus pallidus. Internal hydrocephalus was also present (Figs. 39 and 40).

CASE 31

A.E., born 25 November 1954 (7437/66).

FAMILY HISTORY. Nil relevant.

PREVIOUS HISTORY. Pregnancy, birth and development normal. Always somewhat underweight. Whooping cough, measles and chickenpox as a small child, no complications. Tonsillectomy at the beginning of February 1964.

PRESENT ILLNESS. The patient was well until 23 March 1964, when, at the age of 9 years 4 months, he complained of tiredness. The next morning, he refused to go to school because he felt unwell, and remained in bed. No fever was present. At 11.30 a.m. his mother found him with a complete right-sided weakness and a distorted face. He could not speak clearly, but was conscious, and understood what was said to him. He vomited, and appeared to have a headache.

Admission to Cairo Hospital.

FINDINGS ON ADMISSION. The flaccid right sided hemiplegia was confirmed. The boy was febrile and had neck stiffness.

Lumbar Puncture showed 'cloudy fluid and numerous pus cells'.

The patient was treated for meningoencephalitis with antibiotics and sulphonamides.

In the course of 2 weeks, the speech disability largely disappeared, and the hemiplegia became less dense. One month later a further bout of fever occurred, without any worsening of the neurological signs.

Admission to the Children's Hospital, Zurich (9 February 1966).

FINDINGS. Severe spastic right-sided hemiplegia was present, with complete loss of function of the hand, and an abnormal gait with foot drop and circumduction of the limb. A central facial palsy was also present. The child's speech was intact, and his intellectual ability was not obviously diminished.

EEG (11 February 1966). Minor non-specific disturbances were shown over the posterior part of the right hemisphere.

Pneumoencephalogram. There was slight enlargement of the left lateral ventricle (Fig. 41).

Finger clubbing and cyanosis prompted detailed investigation. Blood: Hb 13.8 per cent; haematocrit 48 per cent; erythrocytes 6.44 million; mean corpuscular volume $74.5 \mu m^3$ (reduced). Oxygen saturation in the right radial artery 82 per cent.

Chest Radiograph. The cardiac outline was normal. A bullet-shaped shadow was noted in the right costophrenic angle overlying the diaphragm.

Electrocardiogram. Normal. No pathological murmurs.

Angiocardiography. An arteriovenous malformation was demonstrated in the right lung field, arising from a pulmonary artery, with broad drainage into the left auricle (Fig. 42).

After the diagnosis had been made, a soft murmur synchronous with the pulse was heard over the posterior wall of the chest in the vicinity of the malformation.

OPERATION (Department of Surgery, University Hospital, Zurich). The arteriovenous malformation was resected from the antero-basal segment of the right lower lobe. The postoperative course was uneventful.

CASE 32

R.A., born 5 April 1949 (6408/55).

FAMILY HISTORY. Nil relevant.

PREVIOUS HISTORY. Pregnancy, birth and development normal. Scarlet fever as a small child.

PRESENT ILLNESS. Towards the end of December 1951, the patient experienced a mild influenzal infection with coughing for two weeks, and then recovered completely. Two weeks later, on 23 January 1952, a sudden heart attack occurred, with irregular rhythm, palpitations, vomiting, abdominal pain, and spikes of fever up to 39°C; recovery took place within three weeks. On 18 February 1952, in the course of only two hours, generalised oedema appeared, with only a trace of albumin in the urine. Two days later, the child went into a sudden coma, and complete left-sided hemiplegia developed. A diagnosis of cerebral embolism was made in a foreign hospital. In June 1952 more attacks of paroxysmal tachycardia occurred, with pulse rates up to 260/minute. Auricular fibrillation was confirmed by electrocardiography.

Admission to the Children's Hospital, Zurich (25 April-2 August 1955).

FINDINGS. Severe spastic left motor hemiparesis was present, with a complete loss of function of the hand, and a considerable disturbance of gait. Central facial palsy was present, and there was a definite organic psychosyndrome.

Pneumoencephalogram. There was marked atrophy of the right hemisphere (Fig. 43).

EEG. An active epileptogenic focus was shown in the right temporal region.

Electrocardiogram. Normal.

Chest Radiograph. The cardiac contour was normal, and there was no evidence of congestion.

COURSE (until December 1966). The permanent spastic hemiparesis remained, with a complete functional loss of the hand, and atrophy. No epileptic attacks have been observed to date. The patient has been successfully rehabilitated by training as a book-keeper.

CASE 33

A.I., born 7 August 1952 (2795/64, 3632/65).

FAMILY HISTORY. Nil relevant.

PREVIOUS HISTORY. Measles and chicken pox as a small child. Tonsillectomy in 1955 following repeated attacks.

PRESENT ILLNESS. At 11 a.m. one day at the beginning of August 1964, the child experienced a sudden attack of dizziness (veering towards the left) for about ten minutes. Two similar attacks occurred the following day, but there were no further complaints.

In the night of 22 August 1964, a frontal headache suddenly appeared. On the following morning the child felt nauseated, vomited, and again experienced an attack of ataxia towards the left side. Admission to another hospital resulted in the removal of a normal appendix (afebrile, leucocytes 12,100). Following convalescence, she remained completely free of symptoms. On 4 September 1964, she experienced a sudden attack of left fronto-temporal headache; this was accompanied by a loss of sensation in the left side of the face and the left half of the tongue, diplopia with double vision, dizziness with a tendency to veer to the left side, unsteadiness on standing, and vomiting.

Neurological Findings (9 September 1964). Horizontal and vertical nystagmus; dysaesthesia in the left trigeminal distribution and in the left part of the oral cavity; ataxia of the left extremities; muscular hypotonia.

Neurological Findings (15 September 1964). The nystagmus had increased, and there was evidence of diplopia on looking to the right side; hypaesthesia was present in the second and third divisions of the left trigeminal nerve and there was a suspicion of right facial palsy; there was ataxia of the left extremities and truncal ataxia with a tendency to veer towards the right side.

Lumbar Puncture. Protein 43 mg per cent, cells normal; Mastix test 5566433333.

EEG. Normal.

Admission to the Children's Hospital, Zurich (21 September-12 October 1964).

FINDINGS ON ADMISSION. Horizontal nystagmus to the left side, inconstant diplopia with superimposed images on upward and downward gaze, diminished left corneal reflex, diminished sensation in the distribution of the second division of the trigeminal nerve on the left, diminished sensation to pain over the left half of the tongue, ataxia of the left extremities with muscular hypotonia. There were no other neurological findings and the physical examination was otherwise normal. Afebrile. Blood count: leucocytes 7300, immature forms 21 per cent, segmented forms $47\frac{1}{2}$ per cent; ESR 16/38 mm.

Lumbar Puncture. Protein 46 mg per cent; $6\frac{1}{3}$ monocytes, 1 segmented; colloidal gold reaction 1122221111.

EEG. Normal findings.

241

Pneumoencephalogram. The ventricular system, including the fourth ventricle, was normal (Fig. 45).

Left Vertebral Angiogram (28 September 1964). With the patient under general anaesthesia, direct puncture of the artery in the neck was performed without difficulty. The cervical part of the vertebral artery and its posterior inferior cerebellar branch opacified normally, while the basilar artery failed to do so. An identical appearance was obtained following a second injection made for stereoscopic angiograms (Fig. 45).

COURSE. Within a few weeks the patient had improved to the extent that she was subjectively free from symptoms. By the time of her discharge from hospital, a partial regression of the neurological signs had also taken place. On 3 January 1965 she suddenly developed paraesthesiae over the left half of the face and the left hand; she exhibited clumsiness in the use of the left hand, unsteadiness on standing and walking, and nausea.

Second Admission to the Children's Hospital, Zurich (3-11 January 1965).

FINDINGS ON ADMISSION. The patient was mentally clear, and her IQ (Standford-Luckert) was at least 106 (the test was influenced by subjective complaints). She was found to have horizontal nystagmus (more marked to the left side), hypaesthesia and hypalgesia in the first and second divisions of the left trigeminal nerves, and moderate ataxia of the left limbs. Romberg's sign was present, without any specific pattern in the girl's tendency to fall, and her gait was ataxic.

Lumbar Puncture. A traumatic puncture, with the fluid at first blood-stained, but then clear. Protein 71 mg per cent; erythrocytes 5000. Monocytes 40; segmented cells 7. Colloidal gold reaction negative.

EEG. Normal findings.

Follow-up Left Vertebral Angiogram (4 January 1965). Appearances were similar to those demonstrated on 28 September 1964, although on this occasion the basilar artery and its branches opacified weakly (Fig. 45).

Left Carotid Angiogram (4 January 1965). Normal appearances were demonstrated. The posterior communicating artery did not opacify.

Routine clinical examination revealed no abnormality. The patient was afebrile. Leucocytes 6100, juvenile forms 26 per cent, mature forms 13 per cent, eosinophils 7 per cent. Micro-ESR 3/8/13 mm. Cardiovascular system normal. Blood pressure 105/75 mm Hg. *Electrocardiogram* normal.

COURSE. Considerable subjective improvement occurred within one week. Until August 1966 the child remained subjectively free from complaints, and was doing well in the first grade of the secondary school. Her mother observed that periodically the left side of her face became very red.

CASE 34

B.H., born 16 March 1962 (1356/64)

FAMILY HISTORY. Nil relevant.

PREVIOUS HISTORY. Pregnancy, birth and development normal. Chickenpox at the beginning of 1963, followed by whooping cough. No complications. No history of head injury. On 5 April 1964 the patient vomited for no apparent reason, and became pale. However, she recovered promptly and was again lively and cheerful.

PRESENT ILLNESS. At 10 a.m. on 13 April 1964 the patient, then two years old, suddenly began to weep, became pallid and fell asleep. Upon awakening several hours later, she tried to get up, but her left side fell away under her, and she appeared not to have the strength to lift herself up. On being picked up, she immediately fell over again. A facial asymmetry was noted 'as if the left cheek was swollen'. Only on the following morning did the parents notice that the child was not using her left arm during play. Mentally, she became listless and passive, which was in striking contrast to her normal behaviour. No epileptic attacks were observed.

On 15 April 1964 the paediatrician noted a left central facial palsy and a muscular hypotonia, with increased tendon jerks and a Babinski response in the left extremities; she had a staggering gait.

Admission to the Children's Hospital, Zurich (16 April 1964).

FINDINGS ON ADMISSION. Slight flaccid left-sided hemiparesis was present (maximal in the arm). Increased reflexes were elicited in the left leg, and there was a positive Babinski response. Abdominal reflexes were absent on the left side. Detailed testing of sensation was not possible. The girl only showed slight uncertainty on walking, the left leg being dragged slightly. She held her left hand prone during writing, and showed an inability to extend her fingers completely or to abduct the thumb. The cranial nerves were intact, apart from the central left facial palsy. The fundi were normal.

Laboratory Examination. The patient was afebrile. ESR 8/22 mm. Blood: Hb 78 per cent; reticulocytes 7 per thousand; leucocytes 7150, juvenile forms 14 per cent, mature forms 31.5 per cent; eosinophils 0.5 per cent; basophils 0.5 per cent; monocytes 7 per cent; lymphocytes 46 per cent; plasmocytes 0.5 per cent. Platelets 417,000.

Skull radiographs. Normal.

EEG (18 April 1964). There was slowing of the background activity over the right hemisphere, accompanied by a marked increase in polymorphic delta activity (with a maximum in the centro-parietal region.) Photostimulation demonstrated the presence of rhythmic $2\frac{1}{2}$-second, high amplitude waves over the parieto-occipital region of the right hemisphere. No epilepsy potentials were recorded. A sleep tracing revealed asymmetry of the sleep spindle, as well as increased potentials unfavourable to the right hemisphere.

Right Carotid Angiogram (17 April 1964). The contrast column ended abruptly at the level of the carotid siphon, and only a few thin insular arteries opacified. The posterior cerebral artery and two of its branches opacified through the posterior communicating artery. Neither the anterior nor the middle cerebral artery was seen (Fig. 46).

Follow-up Angiogram (4 May 1964). Appearances remained unchanged.

COURSE (until August 1966). Slight improvement of the spastic hemiparesis occurred following regular physiotherapy, but the child did not use her left hand voluntarily and walked with a definite limp. She was an educational problem, but suffered no further attacks.

CASE 35*

H.B., born 17 July 1954.

FAMILY HISTORY. A healthy farming family; four older and four younger sisters.

*This case was made available by Dr. W. Pulver, Chief, Department of Medicine, Cantonal Hospital, Lucerne, to whom thanks are expressed.

PREVIOUS HISTORY. Pregnancy, birth and development normal. No history of significant illnesses or attacks. Occasional uncomplicated sore throats. No complaints on physical exercise.

PRESENT ILLNESS. The patient was completely well until 12 January 1966, on which day, aged $11\frac{1}{2}$ years, she overtaxed herself physically. The journey home from school during the mid-day break took far longer than the usual 30 minutes, because of a fresh fall of snow. After a large midday meal the girl hastened back to school without resting, in the company of an older sister. They arrived late, and on the schoolhouse steps she was overcome with nausea; shortly afterwards she experienced a severe headache in the right fronto-temporal region. She wanted to open a window to get some fresh air, and in doing so staggered and then fell unconscious down the steps, without injuring herself further. She regained consciousness after about 10 minutes and then exhibited a left-sided weakness. She vomited repeatedly, but was able, with a little help, to get into a motor car to be taken to a doctor.

The doctor and the child's parents established the following: the child's mouth was displaced to the right side; she stuttered during speech; she had flaccid paralysis of the left arm with minor involvement of the left leg, and reduced tactile sensation over the left half of the body; she was drowsy, but her body temperature was normal. She continued to complain of severe frontal headache and nausea.

Over the next few days the hemiplegia regressed somewhat. Piercing headaches occurred intermittently over the right temporal region. During the night of 17 January 1966 there was a sudden increase in the intensity of the right-sided fronto-temporal headache, and the child felt nauseous and vomited repeatedly. She complained of the sensation of formication over the right (?) side of the head and the right (?) arm, followed by a feeling of heaviness in the left extremities. The next morning a complete paralysis of the left half of the body was present, with full preservation of consciousness. The body temperature remained normal.

Admission to the Department of Medicine, Cantonal Hospital, Lucerne (19 January 1966).

FINDINGS ON ADMISSION. Incomplete spastic left-sided hemiplegia (including the face) was present. Left tendon jerks were increased, and

243

a left Babinski response was elicited. There were signs of left hemi-hypaesthesia, but deep sensibility was preserved. The skin temperature was lower over the left extremities than over the right ones. Bilateral abdominal reflexes were present. The fundi and visual fields were intact.

Laboratory Findings. Afebrile, ESR 7/14 min. Blood: leucocytes 4500, with a marked shift to the left, otherwise a normal differential count; Hb 12.9 per cent; haematocrit 39 per cent; quick test 76 per cent. Platelets 201,000. Blood cultures (24 and 26 January 1966) negative. Throat swab bacteriologically sterile. Antistreptolysin titre 166 (repeat examination 2½ weeks later: unaltered). Urine normal. Blood pressure 135/40 mm Hg.

Electrocardiogram. There was evidence of left ventricular strain. A phonocardiogram indicated a high-frequency, ejection-type, protomesosystolic murmur. The carotid pulse curve was normal.

Chest Radiograph. The heart was of normal size and position, but a definite left ventricular configuration was present. Pulmonary vascular markings were normal and there was no evidence of congestion.

EEG (20 January 1966). A massive diffuse disturbance with depression of the background rhythm was demonstrated over the entire left hemisphere. There were marked, predominantly right-sided, signs of brain-stem disturbance in the form of high amplitude delta rhythms.

Lumbar Puncture. Pressure 13 cm, fluid clear. 3 monocytes/μl. Total protein (Kafka) 36 mg per cent. Colloidal gold reaction negative. Sugar (Hagedorn-Jensen) 84 mg per cent. Chloride 776 mg per cent.

Skull Radiographs (antero-posterior and lateral projections). Normal.

Right Carotid Angiogram (21 January 1966). There was good and regular filling of the internal carotid artery as far as the siphon. Immediately distal to the siphon, the lumen was shown to be reduced to a thread-like calibre, and beyond this point irregularly narrowed. Proximal to the bifurcation, the lumen again widened, opacified well, and was shown to possess smooth walls. The trunk of the middle cerebral artery opacified moderately well and appeared normal, while its branches were only very poorly visualised. The anterior cerebral artery was not seen at all; the terminal part of the internal carotid artery opposite the mouth

of the anterior cerebral artery possessed smooth walls (Fig. 47).

Left Carotid Angiogram (22 January 1966). The entire internal carotid tree, including the anterior and middle cerebral arteries, opacified normally. The right anterior cerebral artery filled through the anterior communicating artery; its proximal part also filled by retrograde flow almost to the intracranial carotid bifurcation (Fig. 48).

Follow-up Right Carotid Angiogram (4 February 1966). The internal carotid and anterior and middle cerebral arteries and their branches opacified excellently. The lumen in the segments shown previously to be narrowed or occluded now possessed smooth walls of normal calibre (Fig. 48).

COURSE. After the second attack, 5 days after the first apoplectiform insult, the hemiplegia gradually began to recede with regular physiotherapy. On 23 May 1966 the patient was transferred to a rehabilitation centre, still with a considerable degree of spastic hemiparesis.

CASE 36*

H.M., born 17 April 1945.

FAMILY HISTORY. Maternal grandmother successfully underwent pituitary operation at the age of 53 years. Nil else relevant.

PREVIOUS HISTORY. Pregnancy, birth and development normal. Pneumonia at 9 months. Measles, whooping cough, chickenpox, mumps and scarlet fever as a small child, without complications. Appendicectomy at the age of 7 years. Fractured arm at 11 years.

PRESENT ILLNESS. On 1 March 1959 the patient, then a boy aged 14 years, attended church service, and upon standing up in church suddenly experienced a severe pain in the right frontal region, and a numb feeling in the left leg ('like a rubber leg'). On returning home with his bicycle, he found his left leg was powerless, and he arrived home dragging it; his speech was slurred, his face was asymmetrical, and he vomited. Within 3 hours all these symptoms had disappeared completely, first the leg weakness and then the speech defect.

*Case previously published in Krayenbühl (1960) 'Beitrag zur Frage des cerebralen angiospastischen Insults.' *Schweiz. med. Wschr.,* 90, 961.

Admission to the Department of Neurosurgery, University Hospital, Zurich (5-6 March 1959).

FINDINGS ON ADMISSION. The patient was subjectively free from complaints. Neurological examination gave negative results, except for a slight increase in reflexes in the left leg. The cardiovascular system was normal. Blood pressure 120/60 mm. Afebrile. Leucocytes 4800. ESR 5/10 mm.

Right Carotid Angiogram. There was severe narrowing of the anterior cerebral artery and its terminal branches. The sylvian vessels opacified well (Fig. 49). Reversed collateral opacification of the anterior cerebral artery from the middle cerebral branches was well demonstrated.

COURSE. The patient remained completely free from symptoms. He was treated for two months with dihydroergotamine (10 drops, three times a day).

Follow-up Right Carotid Angiogram (6 July 1960). There was severe stenosis of the proximal part of the anterior cerebral artery, but the more distal parts were better opacified (Fig. 49).

COURSE (until August 1966). The patient, who has remained free from symptoms and is without disability, successfully completed a course in a commercial school. He participates in sports.

CASE 37

N.R., born 2 March 1950 (6130/55, 9461/60, 2893/64).

FAMILY HISTORY. Nil relevant.

PREVIOUS HISTORY. Pregnancy, birth and development normal. No minor illnesses.

PRESENT ILLNESS. On 12 March 1955 the patient, a 5-year-old girl, was found lying on the floor crying and fully conscious. She had been incontinent of urine. A few moments previously she had been playing happily. There was no history of previous illness, nor any preceding episodes. She was picked up by her aunt and put on her bed, where flaccid weakness of the left extremities and an asymmetrical face were noted. The family doctor arrived shortly afterwards, and confirmed the presence of an incomplete flaccid left-sided hemiparesis, which was more dense in the arm than in the leg. The child was able to limp about unaided, and no evidence of injury could be found. Her

body temperature was normal. Her condition remained unaltered; she was kept in bed, but had no complaints, and her speech was normal. On the following day she was confined to the house, limping about by herself; she was noted to use both arms when greeting her mother. Saliva was lost from the paralysed corner of the mouth. However, on the morning of 14 March 1955, the left arm was completely paralysed; the asymmetrical face and the limping gait remained unaltered.

Admission to the Children's Hospital, Zurich (15 March-27 April 1955).

FINDINGS. A flaccid left-sided hemiparesis was present, with complete paralysis of the arm, and partial paralysis of the leg and left side of the face excluding the forehead. The tongue was deviated to the left side. Tendon jerks were normal, and there were no definite lateralising differences. A left Babinski response was present, and left abdominal reflexes were absent. There was no definite disturbance of superficial or deep sensitivity. The fundi were normal, and visual acuity and fields remained intact. Slight dysarthria was noted, but the child appeared to be mentally normal. No other abnormal findings were detected on clinical examination; in particular there was no evidence of head injury, infection or heart disease. The girl was afebrile on admission.

Laboratory Findings. Blood: Hb 93 per cent; leucocytes 5900, juvenile forms 1.5 per cent, mature forms 43.5 per cent; eosinophils 6.5 per cent; monocytes 6 per cent; lymphocytes 41 per cent; plasma cells 1.5 per cent; platelets abundant. ESR 7/21 mm. Blood pressure 100/50 mm Hg. Pulse about 80/minute, and regular.

Lumbar Puncture. Pressure 16 cm water. Fluid clear. 17 monocytes, 4 segmented; $\frac{1}{3}$ erythrocytes; protein 30 mg per cent (Kafka). Colloidal gold reaction negative. Glucose 50 mg per cent.

EEG (16 March 1955). There was a moderate diffuse disturbance of cerebral activity with generalised slowing of the background activity, but, surprisingly, no lateralising differences and no abnormal focus were seen. No epilepsy potentials were present.

Right Carotid Angiogram (31 March 1955). The internal carotid artery was shown to be normal in its entire course. Only the anterior and middle opercular and insular branches of the middle cerebral artery were well opacified, while the posterior temporal and angular branches appeared very thin and poorly opacified. These branches and the parietal opercular arteries appeared only in the second radiograph of the series, opacifying from the pericallosal artery through a collateral circulation. The anterior and posterior cerebral vessels, on the other hand, opacified well and completely in the arteriographic phase. The venous phase showed normal appearances (Fig. 50).

Follow-up Lumbar Puncture (13 April 1955). Pressure normal; fluid clear; 7 monocytes. Protein 32 mg per cent. Colloidal gold reaction negative.

COURSE. On the second day after admission to hospital (16 March 1955), a bout of fever commenced which lasted 7 days, and which proved resilient to penicillin; the temperature reached 39.8°C. No focus of local infection could be found, and the blood tests remained negative. After the temperature had returned to normal on 23 March 1955, the proximal muscles of the paralysed arm showed some active movement for the first time. On 31 March 1955, the tendon jerks were found to be increased in the left extremities. By the time of discharge from hospital on 27 April 1955, the spastic hemiparesis had definitely improved, although finger movements were still grossly impaired, and movements of opening and closing the fist were regularly accompanied by associated movements of the mouth. The left leg was circumducted during walking. The facial palsy had improved only slightly. With prolonged physiotherapy, the hemiparesis gradually showed further regression. No epileptic attacks were observed. Now and then the patient complained of left-sided (!) frontal headache.

Second Admission to the Children's Hospital, Zurich (28 September-1 October 1960).

FINDINGS. The patient was admitted for a follow-up examination. The mild spastic left-sided hemiparesis was still present, involving mainly the distal part of the left arm; the leg involvement was scarcely noticeable; the facial muscles were also involved, although symmetrical movements were present. Left tendon jerks were increased, but there was no clonus or Babinski response. Detailed re-examination now revealed definite wasting of the muscles of the left arm and leg. There was a difference of 1 cm between the lengths of the two hands and the two feet, and the left middle finger was 0.5 cm shorter than the right. Mentally the child was completely normal.

Right Carotid Angiogram (29 September 1960). The internal carotid artery opacified normally to the level of the siphon, but neither the anterior nor the middle cerebral artery was shown. The posterior cerebral artery was well seen, and a reversed collateral circulation was present from its terminal branches to the rostral opercular and insular branches of the middle cerebral artery, which opacified in the second radiograph of the angiographic series (Fig. 50).

Left Carotid Angiogram (29 September 1960). Both anterior cerebral arteries and their branches filled from the left internal carotid artery. A rich collateral circulation was shown between the terminal branches of the right anterior cerebral artery and the territory of the middle cerebral artery, which was not itself opacified (Fig. 50).

EEG (28 September 1960). Normal, with no lateralising differences.

COURSE. The patient's condition remained unaltered until one morning in September 1964, when she experienced a sudden attack of frontal headache and unsteadiness. No other symptoms were observed, and these complaints disappeared spontaneously within a few minutes.

Third Admission to the Children's Hospital, Zurich (4-6 October 1964).

FINDINGS. The low-grade distal hemiparesis remained unaltered, with minimal spasticity in the arm, a moderate limitation of hand movements, and an inability to make fine finger movements. There was a slight weakness of dorsal flexors in the foot, but no facial palsy. The left arm and leg were definitely shortened, the arm by 3 cm, the foot by 1½ cm; the circumference of the upper arm was reduced by 2 cm, the forearm by 1 cm, the thigh by 0.5 cm, and the calf by 0.5 cm.

The child was mentally normal. She was a pupil at a commercial school and had no scholastic difficulties.

EEG. Focal epilepsy potentials were present on both sides, precentrally, although they were definitely more frequent on the left side. No other abnormality or asymmetry was shown.

COURSE (until August 1966). The patient has been treated with anticonvulsants since October 1964, and has experienced no attacks. She completed her commercial course successfully, and has remained completely free from symptoms. Physical examination in February 1966 revealed that the hemiparesis was static. *EEG* (14 February 1966). There was a suspicion of epilepsy potentials on both sides in the precentral region (more marked on the left). No other abnormality was noted.

CASE 38

S.F., born 16 March 1940.

FAMILY HISTORY. Nil relevant.

PREVIOUS HISTORY. Nil relevant. No serious illnesses. In the summer of 1954 the child complained of tinnitus (? side) for one day, which disappeared spontaneously.

PRESENT ILLNESS. On 2 November 1954 the patient, a 14½-year-old boy, went to school as usual, feeling completely well. During the 9 a.m. break he developed a severe right temporal headache, followed immediately by a feeling of pressure in the right knee. Seconds later he collapsed fully conscious on the steps, and was unable to move his left limbs. A doctor was called, who confirmed the presence of a left hemiplegia (involving the arm completely and the leg incompletely), as well as facial and hypoglossal palsy and abnormally brisk left knee and ankle jerks. The child vomited repeatedly.

Emergency Admission to the Department of Neurosurgery, Insel Hospital, Berne.

FINDINGS ON ADMISSION. On admission, at 11.30 a.m., the patient was pale, slightly confused and drowsy, but fully conscious. Severe spastic hemiparesis was present, with increased reflexes and a Babinski response on the left side. The arm was more severely affected than the leg; the left facial and hypoglossal nerves were also involved. There was blurring of the left optic disc, and the boy had difficulty with looking towards the left side. There were no other abnormal findings on physical examination. Blood pressure 135/80 mm Hg. Pulse 72/min, and regular. Afebrile. ESR 2/4 mm. Blood: Hb 100 per cent; leucocytes 5900, juvenile forms 5.5 per cent, mature forms 73 per cent; eosinophils 2 per cent; lymphocytes 4 per cent; monocytes 5.5 per cent.

Lumbar Puncture. Pressure 15 cm; fluid clear; 2⅓ monocytes. Protein 30 mg per cent (Kjeldahl); colloidal gold reaction 0012211000. *Right Carotid Angiogram* (2 November 1954). A percutaneous puncture was made. The extern-

al carotid opacified normally, but the internal carotid was visualised only as far as the base of the skull, where its outline was lost in the overlying bone structure. The calibre of the artery appeared narrow and regular; its intracranial portion was not visualised at all. *Right Carotid Angiogram* (4 November 1954). Following surgical exposure, the common carotid artery was punctured. On this occasion the internal carotid was visualised to the level of the siphon. The lumen up to 3 cm proximal to the siphon appeared to be regular and well filled, but beyond this point the calibre was slightly but definitely narrower, and there was some irregularity of the walls. From the commencement of the siphon, the lumen again showed normal appearances, until just proximal to its end where it tapered, and the contrast column was abruptly cut off. None of the large cerebral arteries was visualised. There was good filling of the external carotid artery and its branches (Fig. 51a).*

COURSE. Within a day the hemiparesis began to regress, and on 4 November 1954 the first active movements in the fingers and hand were noted, even before treatment was commenced with vasodilators (Nicon acid), anticoagulants and stellate ganglion blocking (alternating left and right). Slow improvement continued until 13 November 1954. During the night of 14 November 1954, the patient experienced a heavy feeling in the left extremities, and on the following morning a complete spastic paralysis of the arm returned, and a severe disturbance of the leg was confirmed; the facial palsy was unaltered. The lower limb weakness rapidly recovered, but the arm remained completely paralysed until the end of November. Upon discharge from hospital on 20 December 1954, the patient was able to walk unaided, by circumducting his left leg; a severe spastic weakness of the arm with hyper-reflexia remained, with only a mild degree of facial palsy. The patient had been afebrile throughout, apart from exhibiting a mild fever at the time of the angiogram.

In December 1955 the patient experienced several brief attacks of 'tearing and pulling' sensations in the left arm. On 3 January 1956 he had his first epileptic attack. It commenced

*The angiograms were kindly made available by Professor H. Markwalder, Department of Neurosurgery, University Hospital, Berne.

with clonic seizures in the left arm, and then became generalised, with a loss of consciousness lasting for 10 minutes; lassitude and headache lasted for one day, but there was no increase in the paralysis. A second similar attack occurred at the end of January 1956.

Admission to the Department of Neurosurgery, University Hospital, Zurich (9-14 February 1956).

FINDINGS. Severe spastic left hemiplegia was present; the arm was more severely involved than the leg, and there was no facial involvement. The muscles of the paralysed limbs were moderately atrophied. There was no sensory impairment, and the optic fundi were normal. Blood pressure 110/45 mm Hg.

EEG (9 February 1956). A depression was demonstrated over the right hemisphere, with intermittent rhythmic 3/second waves over the right lateral precentral and postcentral regions. No epilepsy potentials were observed.

Right Carotid Angiogram (10 February 1956). The internal carotid artery was well visualised, as was the middle cerebral artery with its posterior temporal, angular and opercular branches. The insular arteries appeared to be narrow, and the anterior cerebral artery and its branches failed to opacify. The capillary and venous phases were normal (Fig. 51*a*).

Vertebral Angiogram (10 February 1956). The right vertebral artery and the basilar artery and its branches were well visualised. Some flow through the posterior communicating artery resulted in poor opacification of the middle cerebral group.

Pneumoencephalogram (11 February 1956). The left lateral ventricle was moderately enlarged, particularly the cella media (body) and the trigone. There was no displacement of the ventricular system (Fig. 51*b*).

CSF. Pressure normal; fluid clear. Cells 10⅔. Protein 22 mg per cent. Colloidal gold and Mastix reactions normal. Serological tests for syphilis in the blood and in the CSF were negative.

COURSE. No further attacks occurred with regular anti-epileptic treatment. The severe spastic hemiparesis remained unaltered, despite continuous physiotherapy. The patient experienced transient difficulties with walking during an influenzal infection in the Autumn of 1957. A sudden brief attack of weakness in the left leg occurred one morning in April 1958.

The patient failed to complete his secondary school studies; on the other hand, he was able to complete an apprenticeship in banking, and at the end of December 1961 he passed his driving test.

PROGRESS (until August 1966). The left hand remained functionally useless, and showed no active movements. Only a slight limp was present on walking, and the gait was not significantly affected. No further progress has occurred during the past few years, despite continued physiotherapy. No further epileptic attacks have occurred with regular anticonvulsant treatment. The patient is in full-time employment as a bank clerk, and is subjectively well.

CASE 39
S.K., born 27 May 1938.

FAMILY HISTORY. Nil relevant.

PREVIOUS HISTORY. Birth and development normal. Measles as a small child. Conjunctivitis of the right eye in 1954.

PRESENT ILLNESS. On 8 May 1955 the patient, then a healthy boy aged 17 years, ate his lunch normally and then went to the toilet because he felt unwell and dizzy. He experienced a severe right frontal headache, and then developed, without any loss of consciousness, a flaccid left-sided hemiparesis. He vomited repeatedly.

Admission to the Cantonal Hospital, Münsterlingen (8-31 May 1955).

FINDINGS ON ADMISSION. The patient was drowsy and reacted slowly, but he was orientated for time and place. Flaccid left-sided hemiplegia was present, with facial and hypoglossal nerve involvement. Tendon jerks were absent in the left arm, and increased in the left leg. A left Babinski response was elicited. The left corneal response was absent. Temperature 37°C. Blood pressure 120/80 mm Hg. Pulse 64/minute. ESR 3/7 mm. White cell count 9600.

Lumbar Puncture (10 May 1955). Pressure 95 mm; fluid lightly xanthochromic, and clear; 1 cell; protein 26.4 per cent; Mastix and colloidal gold reactions negative.

Neurological Examination (12 May 1955). Flaccid right-sided hemiplegia was present, with incomplete involvement of the leg; the left reflexes, including the abdominal and cremasteric reflexes, were absent. There was a reduced sensation to pain over the entire left half of the body, and an absence of sensation of movement in the left extremities, with anaesthesia of the entire left leg. The left corneal reflex was absent. There was no meningism.

Admission to the Department of Neurosurgery, University Hospital, Zurich (31 May-10 June 1955).

FINDINGS ON ADMISSION. The patient was mentally clear. He had severe left-sided hemiparesis, which was almost complete in the arm and of moderate severity in the leg; central left facial palsy was present. Tendon jerks on the left side were increased, and a left Babinski response was elicited. All sensation was reduced over the left half of the body. There was a disturbance of movement sensation in the left fingers. The left corneal reflex was absent. The left pupil was dilated; it reacted well to light. The optic fundi and visual fields (Bjerrum screen) were intact. The left hand was red, cold and swollen. The patient was afebrile. Blood: Hb 109 per cent; leucocytes 5200. ESR 10/14 mm. Blood pressure 120/80-130/65 mm Hg.

EEG (1 June 1955). There was a depression over the right cerebral hemisphere, in the form of polymorphic delta activity which was seldom rhythmical. No epilepsy potentials were seen.

Right Carotid Angiogram (9 June 1955). The middle cerebral artery and its branches failed to opacify, only the internal carotid and the anterior cerebral arteries being visualised. No collateral circulation was demonstrated (Fig. 52 *a*).

Pneumoencephalogram (3 June 1955). There was a mild degree of enlargement of the body of the right lateral ventricle. In other respects the ventricular system was normal in size and position (Fig. 52*b*).

Lumbar Puncture. Pressure normal; fluid clear; cells 2⅔; protein 19.8 mg per cent (Kafka); colloidal gold and Mastix reactions normal. Serological tests for syphilis in the blood and CSF were negative.

General Physical Examination (Medical Outpatient Department, University Hospital, Zurich; 9 June 1955). There was no evidence of any circulatory disorder, particularly Buerger's disease. An electrocardiogram was normal.

COURSE. Between May and October 1956, the patient experienced three epileptic attacks.

Shortly before the onset of each attack he had a warning sign and then felt a seizure of the left hand, before becoming unconscious. After each attack there was transient worsening of the hemiparesis.

Admission to the Department of Neurosurgery, University Hospital, Zurich (16-18 October 1956).

FINDINGS ON ADMISSION. The spastic left hemiparesis was maximal in the arm, slight in the leg, and did not involve the face. No sensory disturbances were noted.

EEG (17 October 1956). A marked depression with theta and delta activity was observed over the right central and temporo-occipital region. No epilepsy potentials were present.

Pneumoencephalogram (17 October 1956). The right lateral ventricle was enlarged (particularly the cella media and the anterior horn). There was moderate displacement of the ventricular system to the right side (Fig. 52 *b*).

CSF. Cells 2; protein 13.2 per cent; colloidal gold reaction negative.

With phenobarbitone (100-150 mg/day) the patient remained free from attacks. However, when he ceased to take his tablets after about 6 weeks, he experienced further epileptic attacks which were suppressed by resumption of drug treatment.

EEG (25 March 1960). There was a moderate depression, with intermittently absent background activity and mixed theta and delta activity, over the entire right hemisphere. No epilepsy potentials were observed.

Outpatient Follow-up Examination in the Department of Neurosurgery, University Hospital, Zurich (15 May 1962).

FINDINGS. The patient had moderately severe spastic left hemiparesis, which was maximal in the arm, and slight in the leg, with discrete facial palsy. Left tendon jerks were increased, and a left Babinski response was elicited. Mentally, the patient made a somewhat depressing impression. He was working full time as a storeman. He had experienced no epileptic attacks, with regular phenobarbitone treatment.

COURSE (until August 1966). The spastic hemiparesis remained unaltered. The left hand was functionally useless, with no active movements in the fingers. The gait was only slightly disturbed. The patient continued to work as a labourer, but in recent years had taken to drink. He had abandoned his regular drug medication, but denied any further attacks.

CASE 40

U.H., born 21 October 1953.

FAMILY HISTORY. Older brother died at the age of 8 weeks from a traumatic cerebral haemorrhage.

PREVIOUS HISTORY. A baby of short gestation (seventh month of pregnancy); birth weight 2000g. The child developed normally, but remained delicate up to about the fourth year. Thrush at 18 months, measles at 7 years, chickenpox at 8 years, all without complications.

PRESENT ILLNESS. At the beginning of November 1962 the patient, a 9-year-old girl, had an accident with her scooter, and broke off half of one of her upper incisor teeth. She got up at once, and was only sent home when she volunteered that she had a slight headache. She did not vomit, and was soon free from complaints. On 23 November 1962 the child stated, on her return from school, that she had been unable to do gymnastics because of a headache. Her mother noticed that she appeared tired, but in the afternoon she was brighter, and went out sledging. On the following day the child complained of tiredness, and carried out her chores more slowly than usual; however, later on she participated in games in a lively fashion.

On 25 November 1962 she was free from complaints, and spent the entire afternoon sledging with her brothers and sisters. She had no accidents. However, when she set out to return home at 6.30 p.m., she suddenly collapsed. She got up immediately, unaided, but then collapsed again, and could not move because her right side was paralysed. When she tried to call out to her brothers and sisters, she found that she was unable to speak, although she could still shout and had not lost consciousness. She was carried home, and referred to hospital as an emergency.

Admission to the Department of Surgery, Cantonal Hospital, St. Gallen.

FINDINGS. On admission at 9 p.m., the patient was awake and reacting, and could understand words, but was unable to speak. Complete flaccid right-sided hemiplegia was present, with reflex responses to pain stimuli in the right arm and leg. The child had central right facial palsy and hypoglossal nerve paralysis. Knee and ankle jerks were abnormally brisk on both sides. A right Babinski response was present, and abdominal reflexes were present only on the left side. The right pupil was enlarged, and reacted more slowly to light than the left one. Repeated reflex yawning was noted. Blood pressure 125/60 mm Hg. Pulse 84/minute. Her respiration was normal.

Lumbar Puncture. Fluid clear (no laboratory examination).

Referral to the Department of Medicine, Cantonal Hospital, St. Gallen (26 November 1962).

FINDINGS. The clinical findings of the previous day were largely unaltered. The pupils were now equal and both reacted well to light. Both fundi were normal. The right tendon jerks were brisker than the left ones. The patient was reacting more sharply to movement than to pain stimuli over the right side of the body. Both carotid pulses were normally palpable, but the left one was markedly tender to pressure. Cardiac auscultation revealed a metasystolic murmur in the left parasternal region, but there was no supporting evidence of organic heart disease. The remainder of the clinical examination was normal. Blood pressure 125/80 mm Hg. Pulse 108/min. Temperature 37.4°C. Blood: Hb 91 per cent; erythrocytes 4.7 million; leucocytes 8300, juvenile forms 28 per cent, mature forms 29 per cent; eosinophils 23 per cent; basophils 1 per cent; monocytes 8 per cent; lymphocytes 30 per cent; plasmocytes 1 per cent. Platelets showed normal appearances. ESR 13/25 mm.

EEG (26 November 1962). There was a diffuse and significant disturbance of the left hemisphere compared with the right side; this disturbance took the form of continuous polymorphic delta activity which contrasted with the reduced background activity; a maximum was present in the parieto-occipital region of the hemisphere. Only minimal functional disturbances were present over the right hemisphere.

Admission to the Department of Neurosurgery, University Hospital, Zurich (4 December 1962).

FINDINGS ON ADMISSION. Findings were unaltered from those of 26 November 1962.

EEG (5 December 1962). A severe disturbance was found over the entire left hemisphere, with continuous delta activity of 2-3/sec frequency, which was more rhythmical in the temporo-occipital region, and more irregular and slower in the lateral and paramedian regions; no maximum could be demonstrated. Only mild abnormalities were shown on the right side, with an occipital maximum. Irregular delta waves were interspersed with the rich background activity, at a frequency of 10/sec.

Left Carotid Angiogram (5 December 1962). The internal carotid opacified normally to the level of the distal end of the siphon. The middle cerebral artery, immediately beyond its origin from the carotid, showed a 1 cm cuff of severe stenosis. The ascending fronto-polar and the posterior temporal branches were not shown, and the insular arteries were unusually thin and incomplete. The anterior cerebral artery was poorly visible in the antero-posterior series, lying in its normal mid-line position. The second and third radiographs of the angiographic series showed unusually good contrast opacification in the parietal and opercular regions (Fig. 53).

OPERATIVE EXPLORATION OF THE LEFT PARIETAL LOBE (7 December 1962). The cerebral convolutions appeared widened and pale. A small incision was made into the cortex, and oedematous tissues were demonstrated in the subcortical white matter. Biopsy from this region revealed the typical appearances of cerebral softening.

COURSE. In mid-December 1962 the girl began to speak again, and towards the end of the month she was using sentences; at the same time, slight voluntary movement returned in the leg. At the beginning of January 1963, she was able to walk with support, and towards the end of the month she was able to walk unaided, although with difficulty. At this stage, she first began to move the upper arm. It was now possible to demonstrate a definite reduction in pain and temperature sensitivity in the right extremities. In the Spring of 1963 she returned to school, joining one class lower (the third grade of the primary school), and learned quite successfully to write with her left hand. Since the Autumn of 1963 she has been covering the 45 minute journey to school on foot by herself. Examination in the middle of January 1964 revealed the presence of a severe residual spastic hemiparesis, the right hand being virtually useless, and a Heidelberg spring

being necessary for walking. No speech disturbances could be observed, and no epileptic attacks had occurred. Occasionally, the child suffered from headaches.

PROGRESS (until August 1966). The paralysis remained stationary. No further attacks occurred. The child had difficulty at school, repeating the fifth grade.

CASE 41

G.E., born 31 January 1954 (9331/56, 8877/66).

FAMILY HISTORY. Nil relevant.

PREVIOUS HISTORY. Pregnancy, birth and development normal. Acute tonsillitis in July 1955, with a recurrence in October complicated by left otitis media.

PRESENT ILLNESS. At the beginning of May 1956, the patient experienced an acute rhinotracheo-bronchitis, with a temperature of 40°C, which was cured by sulphonamides within two weeks. After breakfast on 21 May 1956, she experienced a sudden loss of consciousness with urinary incontinence. Consciousness returned within one minute, and a complete flaccid left-sided hemiplegia, including the face, was then present. No convulsions occurred.

Admission to the Children's Hospital, Zurich (21 May-26 October 1956).

FINDINGS ON ADMISSION. On admission three hours after the attack, the patient was drowsy, and did not answer questions. Complete flaccid left-sided hemiplegia was present, with central left facial palsy, and conjugate deviation of the head and eyes to the right side. Tendon jerks were present on both sides, with no definite lateralising differences. A left Babinski response was elicited, and abdominal reflexes were absent.

Heart. There was a harsh systolic murmur over the apex.

Chest Radiograph. The cardiac outline was enlarged to the left side, with a rounded apex, and there were signs of right heart failure (Fig. 55).

Electrocardiogram. A protodiastolic gallop was present; there was a slightly reduced ST segment, and a negative T-wave.

Laboratory Findings. Blood pressure 95/65 mm Hg. Pulse 160/min. Temperature 38.5°C. Blood: Hb 60 per cent; erythrocytes 3.8 million; leucocytes 15,000, juvenile forms 25.5 per cent, mature forms 40.5 per cent; micro-ESR 5/15/27 mm. Blood culture negative. Urine: albumin (+), a few red and white cells in the deposit. Culture negative. Throat swab: normal flora.

Lumbar Puncture. Pressure normal; 248 monocytes and 121 segmented cells/µl; protein 120 mg per cent; glucose 64 mg per cent; colloidal gold reaction 13344443331. Bacteriological culture sterile.

EEG. A depression was shown over the right hemisphere, with a maximum over the posterior and lateral parts. No epilepsy potentials were observed.

Right Carotid Angiogram (22 May 1956). The middle cerebral artery was sub-totally occluded close to its origin from the internal carotid. There was retrograde filling of the sylvian branches from the pericallosal artery. (These pictures were unfortunately lost, and the description was taken from the case notes).

COURSE. The fever promptly disappeared with antibiotic treatment. In the course of a week, the level of consciousness returned to normal, and the child began to speak again. Within 6-8 weeks, the hemiparesis developed a spastic component in the trunk and limbs, while the facial palsy virtually disappeared.

The electrocardiogram returned to normal within a few days, while the abnormal cardiac murmur remained variable for a long time, and only finally disappeared in 1958. A chest radiograph made on 25 July 1956 showed a normal cardiac contour (Fig. 55).

Pneumoencephalogram (11 July 1956). The right lateral ventricle was slightly enlarged (Fig. 54 *a*).

EEG (18 June 1956). Generalised paroxysmal discharges were present, as well as marked depression over the entire right hemisphere.

EEG (17 July 1959). In addition to the generalised changes, focal epileptic discharges were demonstrated over the right central-precentral region.

Despite parental objection to anti-epileptic treatment, the patient has experienced only one definite attack, in July 1965. This attack was provoked by sleep deprivation, and took the form of a Jacksonian attack which rapidly became a generalised seizure.

Second Admission to the Children's Hospital, Zurich (8-9 August 1966).

FINDINGS. Severe spastic left-sided hemiparesis was present, with a complete loss of function in the hand (which could not be voluntarily opened), and a marked circumductory gait. There was wasting and shortening of the paralysed extremities (the leg and foot were 2 cm shorter). There was no facial palsy, and superficial and deep sensibility was intact.

The child exhibited a definite organic psychosyndrome. She was 12½ years old before she reached the fourth grade in a school for mentally backward children.

EEG. Intermittent paroxysmal epileptic discharges were recorded over the anterior part of the right hemisphere, with a sporadic spread to the opposite side. An asymmetry unfavourable to the right hemisphere was present, without actual depression.

Electrocardiogram. Normal.

Chest Radiograph. Normal.

Right Carotid Angiogram (8 August 1966). The sub-total occlusion of the middle cerebral artery which had been demonstrated in 1956 had disappeared, and all branches were now normally visualised. Moderate displacement of the anterior cerebral artery to the left side was shown (Fig. 54).

CASE 42

G.M., born 29 July 1960.

FAMILY HISTORY. Nil relevant.

PREVIOUS HISTORY. Pregnancy and birth normal. Birth weight 2580g; healthy child. Development normal (sitting at 6 months, walking at 12 months, first words before 1 year). Chickenpox and German measles without complications.

PRESENT ILLNESS. At the beginning of October 1961, the child had a slight cold without coughing; the temperature was not recorded. On 6 October, the right leg was noticed to collapse under the child on two occasions in the course of the day. On awakening the following morning, the child showed a paralysis of the right side of the body, but this regressed within hours. At 9.30 a.m. she began moving about, and a slight limp of the right leg was then noticed. In the afternoon, the parents observed clonic seizures (localisation?) and some drowsiness. The child's temperature was 37.4°C. At 5 p.m. she developed a complete hemiplegia of the right side.

Admission to the Department of Paediatrics, University Hospital, Geneva (7-17 October 1961).

252

FINDINGS ON ADMISSION. The child was awake, and was found to have sub-total flaccid right-sided hemiplegia, with diminished reflexes, and a Babinski response. Central right facial palsy was present, but the remaining cranial nerves were intact. A general physical examination showed no other symptoms, in particular no evidence of a focal infection or a cardiovascular abnormality. The patient was afebrile. Blood: Hb 10.3 g per cent; leucocytes 6750, juvenile forms 3 per cent, mature forms 56 per cent.

Lumbar Puncture. Fluid clear; 25 monocytes; 5 polymorphs/μl; protein 10 mg per cent; sugar 58 mg per cent: chloride 730 mg per cent.
EEG. A depression was demonstrated over the left hemisphere, with polymorphic delta activity showing a maximum in the precentral region. There were non-specific disturbances of moderate severity over the right hemisphere.
Pneumoencephalogram. The right lateral ventricle was enlarged, and the entire ventricular system was somewhat displaced to the right side.
Laboratory Findings. Thromboelastogram (Hartert) normal. Prothrombin time (Quick) normal. Virus studies in the stools, CSF and throat washings, normal.

Admission to the Department of Neurosurgery, University Hospital, Zurich (17-20 October 1961).

FINDINGS ON ADMISSION. The patient was conscious, with sub-total flaccid right-sided hemiplegia. Right tendon jerks were mildly increased, and a right Babinski response was present. There was no definite disturbance of sensibility.
Left Carotid Angiogram. The middle cerebral artery was occluded at its origin from the internal carotid. There was a significant retrograde collateral circulation through the pericallosal artery, in the capillary phase (Fig. 56).

COURSE. With regular physiotherapy, the child made a remarkable recovery, and the spastic hemiplegia largely disappeared.

PROGRESS (until August 1966). The child showed a mild residual disturbance of function of the right hand, but was able to use it. She had no disturbance of gait, was mentally normal, and had no intellectual impairment. Early in 1966 she was admitted to an ordinary school. She has received continuous regular physiotherapy,

but no drug treatment, and has experienced no further attacks.

CASE 43
H.M., born 30 March 1944 (9858/60).
FAMILY HISTORY. A younger brother underwent craniotomy at the age of 1½ years for a large choroid plexus papilloma.
PREVIOUS HISTORY. Nil relevant.
PRESENT ILLNESS. The child suddenly experienced, at the age of 14 months, a flaccid left-sided hemiplegia during the course of a febrile illness lasting 5 days. Precise details of the illness are no longer available. A doctor, who was consulted two weeks after its onset, assumed the illness to have been poliomyelitis. At 17 months, the child was walking freely, although there was some difficulty with the left leg. Three years later she was submitted to an operation for lengthening of the Achilles tendon. At the age of 16 years, she was seen in hospital.

Admission to the Children's Hospital, Zurich (3 May-16 August 1960).

FINDINGS ON ADMISSION. A spastic left-sided hemiparesis of medium severity was present, and was most marked in the arm. For practical purposes, the hand was virtually useless, supination and pronation being almost impossible. A marked disturbance of gait was present (with circumduction), but the girl was able to support her weight on her left leg. The tendon jerks were markedly increased in the left arm, and only slightly increased in the left leg, and a left Babinski response was present. The left extremities were atrophic, the arm being shortened by about 2 cm and the leg by about 1 cm. No gross disturbance of superficial or deep sensibility could be demonstrated, although the patient appreciated movements of the left side of the body somewhat less well than on the opposite side. The fundi and visual fields were normal. On psychiatric examination, the patient showed debility, a tendency to depression, and feelings of inferiority and aggression. Clinical examination revealed no evidence of a heart lesion.
EEG (19 May 1960). Normal.
Right Carotid Angiogram (29 July 1960). There was excellent filling of the internal carotid artery to the level of the siphon. The anterior cerebral artery was not visualised. Only a few unusually thin branches of the middle cerebral

artery were demonstrated in the insular region; the lumen of the posterior temporal artery was reduced to thread-like dimensions, in contrast to the excellent filling of the posterior cerebral artery and its branches (Fig. 57a).

Left Carotid Angiogram (3 August 1960). The right anterior cerebral artery filled via the anterior communicating artery, and showed a well developed collateral network which supplied the right middle cerebral region (Fig. 57a).

Pneumoencephalogram (29 July 1960). Only the right lateral ventricle filled with gas, and showed a normal appearance and size. The septum pellucidum was in the mid-line (Fig. 57b).

CSF. Normal findings.

CASE 44

I.L., born 4 May 1956 (9784/66).

FAMILY HISTORY. A maternal uncle died in infancy from a heart defect; a maternal aunt died at the age of 6 years from pericarditis.

PREVIOUS HISTORY. Pregnancy, birth and early development normal. No significant illnesses.

PRESENT ILLNESS. On 7 October 1957 the child, a healthy 1½-year-old girl, became ill and was found by the family doctor to have left upper lobe pneumonia. She was severely ill, but recovered completely over the course of several days. On 26 October the child, who was then quite well, was sitting on the table when she suddenly and unaccountably fell off and bumped her head on the floor. She cried out, then vomited and was unable to speak; she did not lose consciousness. A doctor was called to examine her, and he found a flaccid paralysis of the right arm, which he thought due to a shoulder contusion and a mild head injury. In the course of a return visit 4 days later, however, he noted a flaccid paralysis of the right leg as well, and referred the patient to hospital.

Admission to the Department of Medicine, Cantonal Hospital, Münsterlingen (30 October 1957).

FINDINGS ON ADMISSION. Flaccid hemiparesis was present on the right side. A right Babinski response was elicited. Knee jerks were absent on both sides. Eye ground and pupillary responses were normal on both sides.

Laboratory Findings. Hb. 60 per cent; leucocytes 11,000; juvenile forms 2 per cent, mature forms 48 per cent; eosinophils 2 per cent; lymphocytes 35 per cent; plasmocytes 2 per cent.

Lumbar Puncture. Pressure above 35 cm H_2O (child was crying); fluid clear; cells 1⅓; protein 15.4 mg per cent (Kafka); colloidal reactions normal; bacteriological cultures sterile.

Admission to the Department of Neurosurgery, University Hospital, Zurich (13 November 1957).

The child was referred to this hospital on suspicion of brain injury.

FINDINGS ON ADMISSION. A sub-total flaccid right-sided hemiplegia was present; it was complete in the arm and severe in the leg, with a partial facial palsy which spared the forehead. Tongue motility was normal. The child was unable to speak, but could understand verbal commands and carried them out correctly. Reactions to pain stimuli were present on both sides of the body, including a definite withdrawal reflex in the right arm with movement of the thumb and shoulder. The right corneal reflex was perhaps diminished. The pupils and fundi were normal. Tendon jerks were increased on the right side, particularly in the leg. A right Babinski response was present.

Laboratory Investigations. Blood: Hb 68 per cent; erythrocytes 4.4 million; leucocytes 10,800, juvenile forms 6.5 per cent, mature forms 62 per cent; eosinophils 5 per cent; basophils 1 per cent; monocytes 8 per cent; lymphocytes 17.5 per cent. Platelets abundant. ESR 40 mm/hr. Blood pressure 120/80 mm Hg. Pulse 100/min. The heart and lungs were normal to percussion and auscultation.

Lumbar Puncture. Pressure normal; fluid clear; cells 2⅔; protein 22 mg per cent; colloidal gold reaction normal; serological reactions for syphilis negative. Antibody titre in the blood of influenzal virus A 64 (complement fixation), influenzal virus B 0; poliomyelitis types 1, 2 and 3 (neutralisation) negative.

Skull Radiographs (antero-posterior and lateral stereoscopic projections). Normal findings.

EEG (14 November 1957). There was a marked depression of background activity over the left hemisphere, particularly over the lateral regions. There were bursts of radiating discharges with a 3-3½/sec rhythm over the right side.

Pneumoencephalogram (14 November 1957). The left lateral ventricle showed a generalised slight enlargement. The ventricular system was displaced slightly to the left side. The cortical sulci were widened, particularly on the left side (Fig. 58*b*).

Left Carotid Angiogram (18 November 1957). The internal carotid and anterior cerebral artery were well visualised and normal. Flow through the posterior communicating artery resulted in equally good visualisation of the posterior cerebral artery, and also led to a retrograde flow into the basilar artery. The middle cerebral artery and its branches were not visible in the first phase of the serial angiogram, but they opacified during the second phase, and were even better visualised in the third one, through filling of many opercular and insular branches through collateral channels of the anterior cerebral group (Fig. 58*a*).

On 20 November 1957, the patient left the hospital, since her parents refused to permit prolonged hospitalisation for physiotherapy to be carried out.

Outpatient Examination at the Children's Hospital, Zurich (9 December 1963).

No reliable information was available covering the period from November 1957. It was stated that no epileptic attacks had been observed. Early in 1963, the patient was admitted to the first grade in the primary school, ostensibly with satisfactory results.

FINDINGS. Considerable spastic right-sided hemiparesis was found, with almost complete loss of function of the right hand. The leg was slightly less severely involved, and the child walked unaided with a circumductory gait. The paralysed extremities were markedly underdeveloped, the arm being 6 cm, and the leg 2 cm, shorter than those on the normal side. A minor facial palsy was also present. Her speech was normal. There were no visual field defects.

COURSE. At the beginning of November 1966, the patient experienced her first epileptic attack; she complained suddenly of dizziness, fell from her chair, and exhibited convulsive seizures of the right side of the body for 10 minutes, without definitely losing consciousness.

Admission to the Children's Hospital, Zurich (14 November-3 December 1966).

The severe spastic right-sided hemiparesis was unaltered. Supination of the forearm and extension of the hand and fingers were completely impossible. The patient was unable to lift the arm unaided to the horizontal position. A talipes equinus, amenable to treatment, was present, and the patient exhibited a typical limping gait with circumduction. Significant limb-shortening (arm—6 cm, leg—2 cm) and atrophy were present. The minimal right facial palsy remained. The patient showed markedly diminished sensation reaction to pin-prick and cotton wool over the entire right side of the body, including the trigeminal distribution, compared with the normal left side. Vibration was also reduced on the right side in the arm, leg and trunk, but it was not completely abolished. Movement sensation in the fingers and tendons was only slightly diminished, and two-point discrimination in the hand and the foot was not abnormal! Visual acuity and visual fields were intact. There was no speech disturbance. The patient's IQ (Hamburg-Wechsler test) was 62.

EEG (16 November 1966). No epilepsy potentials were present in the waking state. A mild intermittent disturbance (polymorphic slow waves) was shown over the left hemisphere; it was maximal in the precentral-temporal regions. There was marked asymmetry unfavourable to the left hemisphere, upon hyperventilation.

EEG (17 November 1966). This sleep recording showed a very active epileptogenic focus in the left mid-temporal region, with a step-wise spread into both occipital regions.

Left Carotid Angiogram (18 November 1966). Visualisation of the branches of the anterior and middle cerebral arteries was complete. The anterior cerebral artery lay considerably to the left of its normal mid-line position (Fig. 58*c*).

Pneumoencephalogram (18 November 1966). The ventricular system was markedly displaced to the left side; the left lateral ventricle only showed a minor degree of enlargement (Fig. 58*b*).

CSF. Normal in all respects.

CASE 45

M.M., born 29 August 1955 (1492/60, 3103/61, 735/64, 2929/64).

FAMILY HISTORY. Nil relevant.

255

PREVIOUS HISTORY. Pregnancy, birth and development normal. In the middle of November 1960, the child underwent tonsillectomy for recurrent tonsillitis. Almost immediately afterwards, she developed measles which passed off without complication. She soon rejoined her kindergarten class and felt quite well.

PRESENT ILLNESS. On 10 December 1960 the child, then 5 years and 3 months old, fell—according to the accounts of children who saw the incident—off a low wall; immediately afterwards, the kindergarten teacher could find nothing wrong with her. On the way home at 11.00 a.m. she suddenly collapsed, but the precise course of events is not clear, since it was not observed. A passer-by found the child in a limp and confused state, answering slowly and indistinctly, and carried her home where she vomited repeatedly. The family doctor found the child pallid and exhausted, with a paralysis of the left arm, and referred her immediately to hospital.

Admission to the Children's Hospital, Zurich (10 December 1960).

FINDINGS ON ADMISSION. On admission at 1.30 p.m., the child was suffering from flaccid right-sided hemiparesis; the upper arm was completely paralysed, but some movements were noted in the fingers and lower limbs. A left facial palsy was present, and the tongue was deviated to the left side. Both knee jerks were increased, but the remaining tendon jerks were normal and symmetrical. A left Babinski response was present, the left abdominal reflexes were absent, and the left corneal reflex was diminished. The pupils and fundi were normal. The head was held rotated to the right side, but the girl was able upon command to turn it to the left. There was no meningism. The child, who was drowsy, carried out simple commands correctly and was able to pronounce her own name weakly. General physical examination produced no evidence of localised infection or a cardiac defect. The tonsillectomy wounds appeared to have healed completely on both sides. A throat swab revealed bacteriologically normal flora. The patient was afebrile. Blood pressure 110/75 mm Hg. Pulse 96/min and regular.

Laboratory Investigations. Blood: Hb 80 per cent; erythrocytes 5.07 million; leucocytes 11,850, metamyelocytes $\frac{1}{2}$ per cent, juvenile forms 24 per cent, mature forms 59 per cent;

monocytes 5 per cent; lymphocytes 11.5 per cent; platelets normal in appearance. ESR 6/29 mm.

Lumbar Puncture. Bloody tap. Pressure 10 cm; fluid, after centrifugation, clear. Culture bacteriologically negative.

EEG (10 December 1960). A depression was shown over the right central-parietal region, in the form of polymorphic delta waves, with markedly diminished background activity. In addition, there were isolated paroxysmal generalised bursts of slow waves, some with bilaterally synchronous spikes. There was a background rhythm of 8-10/sec frequency, which was sparse, with a definitely reduced amplitude on the right side.

Right Carotid Angiogram (16 December 1960). There was good normal visualisation of the internal carotid, the anterior cerebral and the posterior cerebral arteries. Only the posterior temporal and the angular branches of the middle cerebral artery filled well, while most of the insular and opercular branches were absent in the arterial phase of the serial angiogram. They were visualised in the second capillary phase radiograph, opacifying by retrograde filling from branches of the anterior group of arteries (Fig. 59).

Follow-up Right Carotid Angiogram (10 January 1961). The previous findings were unaltered, with retrograde opacification of the insular and opercular branches from the anterior cerebral group of arteries (Fig. 59).

EEG (12 January 1961). No definite focus was now present. A moderate diffuse disturbance, with polymorphic delta waves, was demonstrated over the posterior parts of both hemispheres. Several paroxysmal, bilaterally synchronous spikes, with slow and diffuse after-deflections, were recorded.

COURSE. Treatment with vasodilator drugs (Ronicol, and later Papavydrin) was commenced soon after admission to hospital. On 29 December 1960, the child was able to move her whole arm, although power was much reduced. On 31 January 1961, a moderately severe hemiparesis, involving particularly the arm (which was spastic), was still present, accompanied by a left hyper-reflexia; a mild palsy still involved the left side of the mouth. In the course of January 1961, a very marked infantile psychosyndrome developed, with disinhibition, a lack of concentration, dis-

256

tractibility, and a depression of memory and thought. The child became extremely psycholabile and temperamental. No epileptic attacks were observed. She was discharged from hospital on 31 January 1961.

Second Admission to the Children's Hospital, Zurich (4-15 July 1961).

Regular anti-epileptic treatment and physiotherapy were now commenced. No attacks had been noted at home.

FINDINGS ON ADMISSION. There had been no change in the degree of hemiparesis since January 1961, but no marked spasticity or increase in reflexes were now present; a left Babinski response was still elicited.

EEG (6 July 1961). Very active generalised epilepsy potentials were shown, with bilaterally synchronous spike and wave complexes of 2-3/sec frequency. No focus and no asymmetry were present.

Pneumoencephalogram (10 July 1961). The ventricular system filled well. The right lateral ventricle was moderately enlarged, particularly the body and the trigones. The third ventricle was displaced to the left side and was angled. In the antero-posterior view, the right upper thalamic outline lay at a lower level than the left one.

CSF. Normal findings.

COURSE. Regular physiotherapy and anticonvulsant drug treatment were commenced, and no further attacks occurred. The hemiparesis remained stationary. However, educational problems increased, since the child was unusually excitable, and fought constantly with her brothers and sisters. She started school early in 1963, but her performance was poor and she was unable to concentrate.

Third Admission to the Children's Hospital, Zurich (6-14 February 1964).

FINDINGS ON ADMISSION. Marked spastic hemiparesis was still present, with left expressive facial palsy. The left hand was functionally useless, in that the fist was clenched and the thumb flexed within it. The lower limb was less severely involved, with a moderate paralysis of dorsiflexion of the foot and markedly diminished active tendon movements. Reflexes were brisk on the left side, and a left Babinski response was present. No disturbance of superficial or deep sensibility was detected. Significant trophic changes were present in the left arm, which was about 6 cm shorter than

the right arm; the legs were symmetrical. Psychiatric examination showed no change in the infantile organic psychosyndrome since 1961. The child's IQ (Terman-Merrill) was 91. *EEG* (under medication). Suspicious epilepsy potentials were present in both parietal regions in the sleep recording. Generalised, bilateral synchronous spike and wave complexes were present upon photic stimulation, as well as scattered discrete and irregular spike and wave complexes in both parieto-occipital regions.

Follow-up Right Carotid Angiogram (7 February 1964). In contrast to the earlier studies, a second anterior insular artery now opacified primarily (that is, not in a retrograde direction, as had been the case in an earlier angiogram); the posterior insular group again opacified in a retrograde direction through the pericallosal artery (Fig. 59).

Pneumoencephalogram. The right lateral ventricle was now definitely dilated, in contrast to the previous findings, and the ventricular system was displaced slightly to the right side.

Fourth Admission to the Children's Hospital, Zurich (6-21 October 1964).

The patient was admitted for intensive physiotherapy. Her condition remained unaltered.

COURSE (until August 1966). The spastic hemiparesis persisted unchanged. The child's performance in Class 4 (a special class for the mentally handicapped) was satisfactory. She remained free from attacks with regular anticonvulsant treatment. Educationally, she became more accessible.

CASE 46

C.L., born 15 March 1952 (9058/60).

FAMILY HISTORY. Nil relevant. Two younger siblings healthy.

PREVIOUS HISTORY. Pregnancy normal, without significant intercurrent illnesses. Fetal movements first felt during the 4th-5th months, and the mother remained healthy and normal up to the end of pregnancy; no abrupt abnormal movements were observed. Birth at term; spontaneous breech presentation; healthy child. On the fifth day of life, mild melaena developed without other significant symptoms (supervised by a paediatrician). Development normal (sitting at 6 months, walking at 15 months, first words before one year). No significant illnesses.

257

PRESENT ILLNESS. The parents noticed that the child, then 2 years old, preferred to use the right hand when at play, and later became aware of an inadequacy of the left hand. Early in 1959, the girl was seen to school by her father and later remembered nothing about it. During the same period, her teacher noticed an 'absence' in the child during a school class. She appeared suddenly to go into a trance, was then anxious, and appeared to speak as if she were at home. Recovery took place within minutes. On another day, the child suddenly became vacant during lunch, and could not remember what had been said during the conversation.

Admission to the Children's Hospital, Zurich (13-25 January 1960).

FINDINGS ON ADMISSION. Body height and weight, and the circumference of the head, were at the 50th percentile. A mild spastic left-sided hemiparesis was present, particularly in the left hand; it was less marked in the left foot. Tendon reflexes were brisk on the left side, and a left Babinski response was elicited. There was no facial palsy. The left extremities were definitely underdeveloped when compared with the opposite side; the upper arm was about 1 cm shorter, the forearm about $1\frac{1}{2}$ cm shorter, and the calf about $\frac{1}{2}$ cm shorter. Muscular atrophy was found, particularly in the forearm. Left-sided homonymous hemianopia was present. The gait was only slightly abnormal, and there was no definite disturbance of sensibility. Mental development was somewhat retarded.

EEG. A marked depression, with diminution of amplitude, was shown over the right parietal area. Focal epilepsy potentials were present in the right postcentral region, with wide dissemination.

Pneumoencephalogram. There was a gigantic defect in the right parietal, occipital and temporal lobes. The left lateral ventricle was of normal size, but was displaced to the right side with the third ventricle (Fig. 60a).

Right Carotid Angiogram. The internal carotid and anterior cerebral vessels filled well and were normal. Of the middle cerebral vessels, only the posterior insular branches opacified, the main trunk with its angular and posterior temporal branches being absent (Fig. 60b).

Laboratory Investigations. Tests for toxoplasmosis and syphilis were negative, and the CSF

was normal in all respects. A general clinical examination revealed no abnormal findings.

COURSE. With regular anticonvulsant treatment, the child remained free from attacks until the Summer of 1965, when she again experienced a transient confused state. Then, with the same drug dose, she was again free from attacks. She had difficulty at school, and early in 1966 completed the statutory 9 school years (at a farm school in a small village).

Outpatient Examination at the Children's Hospital, Zurich (5 August 1966).

FINDINGS. There was a moderately severe loss of function in the hand (finger spreading and splaying was impossible, but she was able to make a powerful fist). The child had a slight limp, without circumduction. She was able to walk on her toes and heels. The left extremities were underdeveloped; the forearm was about 3.5 cm shorter, and the calf and foot were about 2 cm shorter than the opposite side. The circumference of her hand was 3.5 cm. Tendon reflexes were increased on the left side, and a left Babinski response was present. Dysaesthesia was found over the left arm only, and movement sensibility (especially to vibration) was disturbed in the left upper limb only. Stereognosis was definitely reduced on the left side. Total left-sided homonymous hemianopia was present; the other cranial nerves were intact.

EEG. A marked depression was shown over the right hemisphere; however, an alpha rhythm of reduced amplitude remained over the right temporo-occipital region. Sporadic epilepsy potentials were found over both hemispheres; they were more marked over the right side, and had a positive amplitude. Visual evoked responses showed a somewhat reduced amplitude on the right side; however, they remained clearly present in the bipolar leads.

CASE 47

H.U., born 10 June 1963 (9694/63, 805/64).

FAMILY HISTORY. Nil relevant.

PREVIOUS HISTORY. The mother was healthy throughout the pregnancy, which was her first, and was medically examined at monthly intervals; she took no drugs. Birth at term; spontaneous and free from complication; child healthy; birth weight 2250g; body length 46 cm; head circumference microcephalic (29 cm),

258

which was immediately noted. Psychomotor development severely retarded.

Admission to the Children's Hospital, Zurich (30 September-24 October 1963).

FINDINGS ON ADMISSION. This 3½-month-old infant (length 57 cm, head circumference 35.5 cm) had spasticity of all extremities and non-lateralising hyper-reflexia. He demonstrated opisthotonus, and had poor control of his head. His primitive reflexes (symmetrical and asymmetrical tonic neck reflex, tonic labyrinthine reflex, tonic hand and foot grasp reflex) were symmetrical. He did not laugh, and did not focus his eyes with certainty.

Laboratory Investigations. Serological reaction for syphilis was negative in the mother. A Sabin-Feldmann test in the child was positive to 1:16 in the blood.

EEG (7 October 1963). Diffuse polymorphic theta and delta activity was observed in both parieto-occipital regions, with sharp waves arising at various points. The sleep tracing revealed paroxysmal, irregular, more or less generalised bursts of sharp waves. There were no significant lateralising differences.

Pneumoencephalogram (10 October 1963). Massive porencephaly was visualised in the right hemisphere; there was a wide communicating channel from the lateral ventricle into a cavity occupying the entire parietal lobe, with the exception of a narrow rim of the cortex, and encroaching on the occipital lobe and the upper portion of the temporal lobe. The right basal ganglia were considerably smaller than those on the left side (Fig. 61a).

CSF. Fluid clear; protein 26 mg per cent; cells 2⅔; colloidal gold reaction normal.

Right Carotid Angiogram (16 October 1963). The middle cerebral artery failed to fill, while the anterior and posterior cerebral arteries opacified well (Fig. 61b).

Skull Radiograph. The antero-posterior projection revealed the cranial vault to be markedly smaller on the right side than on the left.

Radiographs of the Forearms and Calves. Bone lengths and thicknesses were symmetrical and normal.

COURSE. In view of the epilepsy potential observed in the EEG, prophylactic drug treatment with phenobarbitone was commenced. Despite this treatment, the patient began exhibiting salaam spasms in the middle of January 1964 (at a rate of 4-15 a day).

Second Admission to the Children's Hospital, Zurich (16 February - 21 March 1964).

FINDINGS ON ADMISSION. The infant exhibited very severe psychomotor retardation. The extremities were hypertonic without lateralising differences! Reflexes were sluggish, but there were no lateralising differences. The patient was microcephalic, with a head circumference of 39 cm.

EEG. A typical picture of hypsarrhythmia was recorded.

The patient was treated with Hydroadreson and no further attacks occurred, although only a slight regression of the epileptic activity was shown upon EEG.

COURSE (Until August 1966). After the onset of epileptiform seizures at the age of 7 months, psychomotor development practically ceased. At the age of 2 years, the child is completely bedridden, unable to lift the head, and completely unaware of its surroundings. No further seizures have been observed following the start of phenobarbitone medication on admission to hospital.

CASE 48
F.M., born 12 August 1962 (9593/66).

FAMILY HISTORY. Nil relevant; one older and one younger sibling healthy.

PREVIOUS HISTORY. Pregnancy normal, no illnesses or accidents. Normal birth at term; birth weight 4200g; healthy child. Psychomotor development retarded (laughing after 2 months, sitting at 10-11 months, walking at 18 months, first words at 3 years). Febrile influenza at the age of 4 months, without complications. No other illnesses, and no accidents.

PRESENT ILLNESS. When the child was about 4 months old, the parents noticed a paucity of movement of the right arm and, somewhat later, of the right leg as well. No seizures had been witnessed.

Admission to the Children's Hospital, Zurich (24 October-16 November 1966).

FINDINGS ON ADMISSION. Severe spastic right-sided hemiparesis was present, particularly in the arm. Reflexes on the right side were increased, and a right Babinski response was present. The hand was functionally useless, and the forearm and arm could only be utilized for simple holding purposes. The child walked freely, with a typical steppage gait. The right extremities were definitely under-developed (difference in length—3 cm). No reliable test of sensibility was possible. Normal left carotid pulsation was absent, but the right carotid was normally palpable. The child was microcephalic (head circumference 46.5 cm = within the 3rd percentile), and his body size was 103 cm (between the 25th and 50th percentile). He appeared to be intellectually retarded, but no objective testing was possible because of language difficulties. Screening tests for oligophrenia in the urine, and tests for toxoplasmosis and syphilis, were negative. The CSF was normal in all respects.

EEG (25 October 1966). There was a marked depression of cerebral activity over the entire left hemisphere. Discrete epileptogenic foci were found in the left temporo-occipital region, with a tendency towards a generalised spread.

Pneumoencephalogram. The left cerebral hemisphere was massively atrophied, with a marked enlargement of the left lateral ventricle, and considerable displacement of the ventricular system to the left side (Fig. 62a).

Great Vessel Angiography. (Catheterisation of the aortic arch from the right brachial artery.) Appearances on the right side were normal, apart from an unusually large common carotid artery. On the left side, the common carotid artery was shown to have a strikingly thinner calibre from the level of its origin on the aortic arch. In its middle third, it gave origin to a thyroid artery of normal calibre. Distally, the lumen narrowed progressively, until the contrast column ceased at about the level of the normal carotid bifurcation. No internal carotid artery could be demonstrated. Both vertebral arteries opacified well and appeared to be normal (Fig. 62b).

CASE 49

D.A., born 23 February 1960 (2966/61, 5248/62).

FAMILY HISTORY. Nil relevant; parents and three older siblings healthy.

PREVIOUS HISTORY. The girl was born at term, after a normal pregnancy. Lively child; birth weight 3 kg. Physiological neonatal jaundice from 3rd to 7th days of life. Psychomotor development normal (sitting at 6 months, walking at 12 months, speaking a few words at 15 months).

PRESENT ILLNESS. On 9 June 1961, at the age of 15 months, the child was irritable and hoarse, but ran no temperature. The hoarseness persisted until 16 June 1961. On this day, the child was exposed to sharp sunlight for $1\frac{1}{2}$ hours, and then began to vomit repeatedly. She was put to bed by her mother, who noticed a weakness of the muscles and a fever of 39.5°C. Suddenly, $2\frac{1}{2}$ hours later, a status epilepticus commenced, with ostensibly generalised tonic and clonic convulsions and conjugate deviation of the head and eyes to the left side; this condition lasted on and off for 7 hours. After the last seizure, the child regained consciousness. The family doctor was called and found a flaccid left-sided hemiparesis to be present.

Emergency Admission to the Children's Hospital, Zurich (17 June-30 August 1961).

FINDINGS ON ADMISSION. The child was apathetic and scarcely rousable, with a complete flaccid weakness of the left arm, incomplete weakness of the left leg, and involvement of the facial nerve. Tendon jerks were indefinite on the left side, but normally elicited on the right side. A left Babinski response was present. Abdominal reflexes were bilaterally diminished. General clinical examination revealed no other abnormal findings, and no evidence of focal infection. The child's temperature on admission was normal, but one day later spiked to 39°C. She was then sub-febrile for several days.

Laboratory Investigations. Blood: Hb 85 per cent; erythrocytes 4.41 million; leucocytes 9400, juvenile forms 7 per cent, mature forms 24 per cent; eosinophils 0.5 per cent; basophils 1 per cent; monocytes 19 per cent; lymphocytes 45 per cent; plasmocytes 3.5 per cent; platelets appeared normal. ESR 13/25 mm. Serum calcium 9.5 mg per cent.

Lumbar Puncture. Fluid clear; protein 27 mg per cent; cells $\frac{2}{3}$; colloidal gold reaction normal; glucose 67 per cent. Bacteriological culture sterile. Throat swab: a few haemolytic streptococci, group A, also some streptococci and a few blastomyces. Faecal flora normal. Virus tests (repeated after 3 weeks): none detected in the stool. In the blood, complement fixation of Coxsackie B 1, 2, 3, 4 and 5 negative; adenovirus negative; neutralization of poliomyelitis types 1, 2, 3, negative.

EEG (22 June 1961). A severe, continuous and widespread disturbance was demonstrated over the right hemisphere, with polymorphic delta activity and a suspicion of depression in the central region. There was a mild disturbance over the left hemisphere, with mixed theta and delta activity, apart from a theta background rhythm. No epilepsy potentials were present.

Pneumoencephalogram (23 June 1961). The ventricular system showed a normal appearance and size (Fig. 64).

CSF: normal.

Right Carotid Angiogram (23 June 1961). A percutaneous puncture was made without difficulty under general anaesthesia. Three injections were made, two for lateral stereo-scopic series, and one for an antero-posterior series of angiograms. In the arterial phase of the first injection, the internal carotid artery opacified normally to the level of the siphon, except for an altered calibre in the vicinity of the carotid canal. The anterior cerebral artery and its branches opacified poorly. The middle cerebral group opacified incompletely in this phase, but was well demonstrated in the capillary phase; however, the various branches showed a markedly narrowed lumen. Good filling of the right vertebral artery and the vertebro-basilar tree was also present, through retro-grade channels via the common carotid artery. The venous phase appeared normal. The second injection revealed three spastic segments in the course of the internal carotid artery, the first about 2 cm in length situated proximal to the carotid canal, the second situated immediately proximal to the siphon, and the third situated immediately proximal to the knee of the siphon; at the latter level, the contrast column ended abruptly. Again, there was good retrograde filling of the vertebral and basilar arteries and their branches. In the capillary phase, laminar contrast filling of the internal carotid on either side of the carotid canal was present, and the carotid siphon opacified as well. The middle cerebral group was first seen in the capillary phase, and the calibre of these vessels remained unusually narrow. The anterior cerebral group was not visualised at all. The third injection (antero-posterior series) revealed good filling of the internal carotid artery to the level of the siphon in the arterial phase, but poor filling of the trunk of the middle cerebral artery which now had a normal calibre; the middle cerebral group filled well and normally in the capillary phase. The anterior cerebral group remained absent. As in the first two injections, the vertebro-basilar tree opacified well (Figs. 63a and b).

COURSE. The child made a gradual recovery. On admission to hospital she was given vasodilator drugs (Papavidrine), and treatment was continued for several weeks. On 6 July 1961, the first flicker of voluntary movement was noted in the arm. In the course of August, an increasing spasticity developed, and upon discharge from hospital at the end of the month a marked spastic hemiparesis, maximal in the arm, was present. At home, the child was taught to walk again, but she had a circum-ductory gait and an equinus deformity, which the physiotherapists were unable to correct.

EEG (18 July 1961). There was a definite depression of cerebral activity over the right hemisphere in the parieto-central region.

EEG (23 November 1961). Some slight asym-metry of the theta background rhythm (un-favourable to the right hemisphere) was still present, but no definite depression remained.

COURSE. During the winter of 1961-62, the child had whooping cough complicated by a purulent middle ear infection and a high fever; however, the hemiparesis was unaffected, and no epileptic attacks occurred. Development continued normally, her speech was normal for her age, and no personality changes were detected by the parents.

On 4 April 1962, when the child was 2 years 2 months old, she had an ordinary catarrhal infection. Two months later, on 4 June, she called out to her mother early in the morning and was found a few moments later to be unconscious and experiencing convulsions (over the entire body, with the exception of the left arm); she had been incontinent of urine. Similar attacks continued repeatedly for two hours.

Admission to the Children's Hospital, Zurich (6 April-15 November 1962).

FINDINGS ON ADMISSION. The child was un-conscious, with completely flaccid extremities, and areflexia. A left Babinski response was present. There was evidence of tonsillopharyn-gitis, with bilaterally enlarged lymph nodes. The girl had a temperature of 40°C. Blood: Hb 76 per cent; leucocytes 14,100, juvenile forms 29 per cent, mature forms 49.5 per cent; eosinophils 3.5 per cent; monocytes 10 per cent; lymphocytes 8 per cent. Platelets appeared normal. Micro-ESR 2/5/9 mm.

Lumbar Puncture. Pressure 16 cm; fluid clear; protein 22 mg per cent; cells $\frac{2}{3}$; colloidal gold reaction normal; glucose 112 mg per cent. Bacteriological culture sterile. Blood glucose 112 mg per cent. Throat swab: normal flora.

Chest Radiograph. There were signs of slightly accentuated parahilar shadowing.

EEG (18 April 1962). Several generalised disturbances, with diffuse polymorphic delta activity, were present on both sides; these were maximal over the fronto-precentral regions. No epilepsy potentials were present.

Pneumoencephalogram (16 April 1962). Both lateral ventricles were enlarged, the right more than the left. There was displacement of the ventricular system to the left side (Fig. 64). *CSF* was again normal in all respects.

COURSE. On 7 April 1962, the child was scarcely rousable and somnolent, and the muscular system was severely hypotonic; only the right ankle jerk was elicited weakly, and a left Babinski response was present. On 9 April 1962, after the fever had disappeared, the patient experienced a clonic convulsion, with seizures involving only the right arm and the right side of the face. On 10 April 1962, she experienced her last epileptic attack, which on this occasion involved the left leg as well. Both attacks were controlled within minutes with intravenous amytal. Following these attacks, the child's condition deteriorated severely. She showed no further recovery, and appeared to lose all contact with her surroundings. She was an erethetic idiot, and was unable to sit up, speak or understand anything. In the course of a single week, the original picture of spastic left-sided hemiparesis reappeared.

EEG (14 September 1962). A very active generalised epilepsy was demonstrated, with intermittent bilateral synchronous bursts of mixed spikes and sharp waves, partly polyspike and wave groups, separated by short flat intervals. In addition, multi-focal sharp waves were recorded.

Pneumoencephalogram (15 August 1962). The lateral ventricles and the third ventricle were massively and almost completely symmetrically enlarged. No definite displacement of the ventricular system was now present. There was gross 'pooling' of subarachnoid air, particularly over the left hemisphere, showing markedly enlarged cortical sulci (Fig. 64). *CSF* was again normal in all respects.

Right Carotid Angiogram (21 September 1962). The entire arterial tree was excellently visualised; apart from a somewhat bowed course of the pericallosal artery, no abnormality was demonstrated (Fig. 63b).

CASE 50

S.M., born 31 July 1954 (9631/56).

FAMILY HISTORY. No evidence of consanguinity. Mother hard of hearing since birth. Five siblings deaf and dumb; four siblings normal.

PREVIOUS HISTORY. Pregnancy and birth normal. Walking at 18 months, first words uttered about the same time. No significant illnesses.

PRESENT ILLNESS. At the beginning of June 1956, in the course of an intestinal infection, the child cried out at night, exhibited clonic right-sided hemiconvulsions, and became unconscious. The following morning she was drowsy, and presented with a right-sided hemiplegia. The weakness gradually improved, particularly in the leg.

Admission to the Children's Hospital, Zurich (29 June-28 July 1956).

FINDINGS ON ADMISSION. A severe right-sided hemiparesis was present which was virtually complete in the arm, and considerably less severe in the leg. The right arm was moderately spastic. The legs exhibited no definite differences in tone. Reflexes were increased on the paralysed side and a Babinski response was elicited. The child was moderately microcephalic (head circumference 49.5 cm). A general clinical examination revealed no further pathological findings, in particular no cardiovascular lesions.

EEG. An extensive and massive depression of cerebral activity was shown over the entire left hemisphere. Cerebral activity was normal over the right side. There were no epilepsy potentials.

Pneumoencephalogram (4 July 1956). Moderate hydrocephalus was present. The left lateral ventricle was slightly enlarged (Fig. 65b).

Left Carotid Angiogram (11 July 1956). The internal carotid artery showed a normal calibre and good filling. The anterior and middle cerebral arteries and their branches appeared unusually thin, particularly the middle cerebral group. On the antero-posterior series, the contralateral anterior cerebral artery was also demonstrated, and showed a somewhat wider lumen than the left one (Fig. 65a).

COURSE. There was no change in the neurological deficit at the time of discharge from hospital.

PROGRESS (until March 1964). The severe spastic hemiparesis remained, with a complete loss of function of the hand. The child walked unaided, with a marked circumductory gait. She was severely oligophrenic (at the age of 10 years she was still in the kindergarten class of an institution), with a severe degree of hearing loss, although she was not deaf and dumb. No further attacks were observed.

CASE 51

S.D., born 11 May 1956 (1554/57, 6158/58, 9293/60).

FAMILY HISTORY. Nil relevant.

PREVIOUS HISTORY. Pregnancy normal. Antepartum haemorrhage 4 days before birth. Born 2 weeks before term, no complications. Birth weight 2520g. Asphyxia? Delayed psychomotor development. Spastic symptoms of cerebral damage present within the first month.

PRESENT ILLNESS. At the age of 10 months the child ran a temperature of 40°C and exhibited clonic left-sided hemiconvulsions (involving particularly the arm) for 5 hours. For part of the time the patient was unconscious.

Admission to the Children's Hospital, Zurich (22 March-15 August 1957).

FINDINGS ON ADMISSION. The patient was examined after the hemiconvulsions had been brought under drug control. He was stuporose, with flaccid left hemiplegia including a facial palsy. Tendon jerks were increased on the left side. A few hours after admission a clonic left-sided hemiconvulsion occurred, with conjugate deviation of the eyes and head to the right side.

Right Carotid Angiogram (29 March 1957; after the disappearance of the fever and elimination of the acute infection). A percutaneous puncture was made under general anaesthesia, with no technical difficulty. Three injections were made for two lateral stereoscopic series and an antero-posterior series. After the first injection, the entire carotid tree was normally visualised, and the vessels were of normal calibre. The needle point lay in the common carotid artery (Fig. 66). The second injection was made after advancing the needle about 0.5 cm up the artery, and the

needle point was shown to lie in the internal carotid artery immediately above the carotid bifurcation. A similar picture of good opacification of the internal carotid (which showed a normal calibre) to the level of the carotid siphon was obtained. However, the anterior cerebral artery was no longer visualised, and the middle cerebral artery and its branches appeared narrower and considerably less well opacified than they had been with the first injection. Retrograde filling of the vertebrobasilar tree was noted (Fig. 66). The third injection was made after the needle had been withdrawn about 0.5 cm (antero-posterior series) and the internal carotid and anterior and middle cerebral arteries and their branches again filled well and showed a normal calibre. The needle point lay in the common carotid artery (Fig. 66).

Pneumoencephalogram (29 March 1957; following angiography). Both lateral ventricles were slightly and symmetrically enlarged, and the third ventricle was dilated.

CSF was normal in respect of cells, protein and colloidal gold reaction.

EEG (22 March 1957). There was a massive depression over the entire right hemisphere, with slow wave bursts which were maximal over the posterior segments. Sporadic epilepsy potentials were observed over this hemisphere as well. A less severe non-specific disturbance was seen over the left hemisphere, without epilepsy potentials.

EEG (29 March 1957; prior to angiography and pneumoencephalography). The massive depression over the right hemisphere and the severe non-specific disturbance over the left hemisphere were undiminished, but no epilepsy potentials were seen.

COURSE. Within two weeks the flaccid left-sided hemiplegia regressed, and a progressive spastic tetraparesis developed, which, initially, was more severe on the left side. All mental development ceased.

Follow-up EEGs were made in 1958 and 1960, when the child was admitted for infectious illnesses, and revealed a persistent depression over the right hemisphere; in addition there was mild dysrhythmia over the left hemisphere, but no epilepsy potentials were recorded.

PROGRESS (until August 1966). The child presented a nursing problem and was completely demented, with a spastic tetraplegia and frequent epileptic attacks, due to severe brain damage.

CASE 52

S.H., born 7 May 1946 (1354/53).

FAMILY HISTORY. Nil relevant. No history of migraine.

PREVIOUS HISTORY. Nil relevant. Right handed.

PRESENT ILLNESS. The child was bright and healthy until he was 7 years old. Then, at 10 a.m. on the morning of 2 August 1953, while enjoying a hot bath, he suddenly called out that he was unable to wash himself and could not move his right arm. His mother at first did not believe him, and lifted him onto his feet, whereupon he collapsed, fell over and burnt his arm on the boiler. He was unable to walk, and had to be carried to bed. He remained fully conscious, spoke normally, and had no subjective complaints. An hour later the family doctor examined the boy and found a complete flaccid right-sided hemiplegia with normal and symmetrical tendon jerks.

Admission to the Children's Hospital, Zurich (2-6 August 1953).

FINDINGS ON ADMISSION. On admission at 1 p.m., the boy was fully conscious, with complete flaccid paralysis of the right arm and sub-total paralysis of the right leg; active movements were, however, possible at the hip and knee joints. Tendon jerks were symmetrical and normal. A right Babinski response was present, and right abdominal reflexes were diminished. There was no sensory deficit, and no meningism. The cranial nerves were intact. The child was mentally normal and afebrile. Leucocytes 4800, with normal differential count. Cardiovascular system clinically normal.

Skull Radiographs (antero-posterior and lateral projections). Normal.

Lumbar Puncture. Pressure normal. CSF clear. Protein 26 mg per cent; $\frac{2}{3}$ monocytes; glucose 58 mg per cent; colloidal gold reaction negative.

COURSE. By 4 p.m. the hemiplegia had regressed to the point of recovery; the boy could walk without limping, and moved his right arm with increasing strength. Tendon jerks remained normal, but the right Babinski response was still present. On the following day the Babinski response was only questionably present, and by the time of discharge on 6 August no neurological deficit remained. The child's

parents refused permission for carotid angiography or pneumoencephalography.

EEG (3 August 1953). There were no abnormal findings, in particular no asymmetry and no abnormal foci; no epilepsy potentials were recorded.

PROGRESS (until August 1966). The patient has experienced no further disturbances, and no headaches. He is now a young man, a part-time student at a training college and a sports enthusiast.

CASE 53

B.G., born 20 April 1944*

FAMILY HISTORY. Nil relevant.

PREVIOUS HISTORY. Nil relevant.

PRESENT ILLNESS. The patient, a $13\frac{1}{2}$-year-old schoolboy, became ill in the middle of October 1957, with a bout of fever and shivering which lasted 2 days and left him with a feeling of lassitude and a loss of appetite. On 17 November 1957 he had a further bout of temperature (up to 39°C), which lasted 4-5 days with a sore throat and a cough. Treatment with sulphonamides produced an improvement, although the temperature remained sub-febrile. The boy vomited nearly every day, had persistent headaches, and felt tired. On 6 December 1957 the vomiting increased, the temperature rose to 38°C, and the boy became confused and stated that he could not see very well. During the night of 7 December he experienced repeated seizures of the right arm, with rotation of the head to the right side, and became increasingly drowsy and apathetic; he did not lose consciousness.

Emergency Admission to the Department of Neurosurgery, University Hospital, Zurich (7 December 1957).

FINDINGS ON ADMISSION. The boy was markedly drowsy and scarcely rousable, with a flaccid right-sided hemiparesis which was considerably more marked in the arm than in the leg. Reflexes were absent in the right arm, but were abnormally increased elsewhere; bilateral Babinski responses were elicited. There was a gross diminution of vision, the patient being unable to identify a finger held before his eyes, and only being able to distinguish light from

---

*Case previously published in Krayenbühl (1959) 'Die cerebral Venenthrombose.' *Schweiz. med. Wschr.*, 89, 191.

dark. Tonic and clonic seizures involving the right arm and the face (but not the right leg) and lasting about 2 minutes continued to occur at approximately hourly intervals; the boy did not lose consciousness. A general neurological and clinical examination revealed no further abnormal findings, and specialist otorhinolaryngological examination was negative. Temperature 38.5°C. Blood pressure 145/100 mm. Blood: Hb 78 per cent; leucocytes 12,600, juvenile forms 3 per cent, mature forms 72 per cent; eosinophils 1 per cent; basophils 1 per cent; monocytes 5.5 per cent; lymphocytes 17.5 per cent. Platelets appeared normal. Prothrombin time (Quick) 80 per cent.

Lumbar Puncture. Pressure 28 cm; fluid clear; cells 1⅔; protein 72.6 per cent (Kafka). Colloidal gold reaction 56134221000. Mastix test 810 11 12 12 64. Bacteriological culture sterile.

EEG (7 December 1957). Under Somnifen, a picture of barbiturate sleep was obtained. A transient discharge of hypersynchronous potentials was present, sharply confined to the right(!) temporo-occipital region. A further focus showing more extensive spread, and arising closer to the right occipital pole, was demonstrated.

Left Carotid Angiogram (8 December 1957). The internal carotid and anterior and middle cerebral arteries and their branches were normally visualised. In the venous phase, of the serial angiogram, the ascending cortical veins in the occipital part-of the hemisphere failed to fill (Fig. 67).

Pneumoencephalogram (9 December 1957). The ventricular system was normal in size, shape and position.

COURSE. Treatment with antibiotics (penicillin, streptomycin), anticoagulants (Marcumar) and anticonvulsants (somnifene, Mesantoin, Gemonil) produced recovery in the course of 10 days. For the first 3 days, the patient exhibited, in addition to the right-sided attacks, seizures which were predominantly left-sided and generalised. No further attacks occurred until after 11 December 1957. The motor hemiparesis increased until 8 December 1957, and then regressed rapidly, so that by 14 December it was no longer present. Vision also improved rapidly, and on 17 December both eyes were 1.75 (distant vision). The temperature returned to normal on 12 December.

EEG (9 December 1957). A severe generalised

abnormality indicating brain stem damage was demonstrated, in the form of paroxysmal or rhythmical bursts of slow waves; a focus or depression was not present, and no epilepsy potentials were recorded.

EEG (17 December 1957). This disturbance was now only intermittently present.

COURSE. On 23 December 1957, the patient was transferred to the Civil Hospital, Zug, where he was treated until he was discharged, free from symptoms, on 18 January 1958. Follow-up outpatient examinations on 25 February 1958 and 22 February 1961 revealed normal findings. The boy then successfully completed 3 grades of secondary school, before entering a junior technical school.

PROGRESS (until August 1966). The patient has experienced no further complaints. In 1964 he completed his preliminary military training, and in 1965 took a course as a non-commissioned officer. At present he is a farmer.

CASE 54

S.K., born 4 November 1946 (3011, 3252/54).

FAMILY HISTORY. A maternal uncle was mentally defective.

PREVIOUS HISTORY. Nil relevant.

PRESENT ILLNESS. The patient fell ill with an influenzal infection in the middle of February 1954, when he was 7 years old. For a while he complained of earache (? side) but he remained cheerful. On the morning of 25 February 1954, the parents noticed that the boy was holding his head on one side. Two days later, on the morning of 27 February 1954, he exhibited seizures in his left leg, and by the afternoon these had spread to involve the left arm and the left side of the face as well. Despite this, the boy went skiing in the afternoon, and after a slight fall had to be carried home on the suspicion of an injury. The family doctor was called, and he referred the boy to hospital as an emergency because of status epilepticus with severe unilateral clonic seizures; the boy did not lose consciousness.

Admission to the Children's Hospital, Zurich (27 February–10 July 1954), *and to the Department of Neurosurgery, University Hospital. Zurich* (1–29 March 1954).

FINDINGS ON ADMISSION. On admission, clonic seizures each lasting 10-30 seconds were observed occurring at regular intervals of 10-20 seconds; these seizures involved the entire left side of the body and sporadically also the right side. The child did not lose consciousness and denied any pain, but complained only of thirst. The head was rotated constantly to the left side, but could be moved without significant resistance in all directions. The gaze was directed to the right and upwards, punctuated by purposeless roving of the eyes. The fundi and pupils were normal. In the intervals between attacks, the left extremities were spastic; a left Babinski response was present, but the tendon jerks could not be reliably evaluated because of the reflex nature of the seizures. A general physical examination revealed the presence of a systolic cardiac murmur (probably incidental), but otherwise there were no pathological findings; both ear drums were intact and free from infection. Temperature 39.7°C. Blood pressure 100/50 mm Hg. Blood: Hb 97 per cent; leucocytes 13,400, juvenile forms 10 per cent, mature forms 79 per cent; lymphocytes 14.5 per cent; plasmocytes 0.5 per cent. Platelets appeared increased. ESR 40/65 mm. Prothrombin time (Quick) 20.5 seconds; bleeding time (Duke) $2\frac{1}{2}$ minutes; clotting time (Bürker) $5\frac{1}{2}$-$10\frac{1}{2}$ minutes.

Lumbar Puncture. Pressure. 10 cm; fluid slightly xanthrochromic, but clear. Erythrocytes 61, monocytes $4\frac{1}{3}$. Protein 80 mg per cent (Kafka); glucose 94 mg per cent; chloride 503 mg per cent; colloidal gold reaction 1112221111. Bacteriological culture sterile, including tests for tuberculosis. Serological investigations of the CSF for leptospirosis and brucellosis organisms, and of the blood for toxoplasmosis and syphilis proved negative.

EEG (28 February 1954). There was a severe diffuse disturbance, with generalised delta activity, partly polymorphic and partly rhythmic, predominantly over the right hemisphere with a maximum in the posterior region. An extremely active epileptogenic focus was present in the right lateral postcentral region.

Attempted Lumbar Pneumoencephalography failed to visualise the ventricular system.

A Right Parietal Diagnostic Burr-hole (28 February 1954) revealed massive cerebral oedema.

Ventriculogram. The ventricles were markedly reduced in size, but normal in shape and position.

Right Carotid Angiogram (14 April 1954). The common carotid artery was exposed surgically for a contrast injection into it. The arterial tree (internal carotid and anterior and middle cerebral arteries) opacified well and showed normal calibres. Serial angiography revealed stasis of the contrast medium in the arteries and capillaries, so that no venous filling occurred (Fig. 68).

COURSE. Despite massive anticonvulsant drug treatment, the hemistatus epilepticus could be controlled only by general anaesthesia and repeated infusions of 40 per cent glucose, and drug-induced 'hibernation'. The patient returned to complete consciousness following reduction of the drug treatment, and showed a marked flaccid left-sided hemiparesis, mainly in the arm and face. At the same time, clonic left-sided hemiseizures again commenced, which persisted almost continuously for 2 months, despite massive anticonvulsant treatment. The child remained accessible throughout. Antibiotics had little effect on the continuous febrile state, and the septicaemic levels of the temperature. A constant neutrophilic leucocytosis with a mild shift to the left was present, while the ESR was prolonged or showed normal values.

The CSF revealed an increasing content of protein—up to 222 mg per cent, a persistent xanthochromia, often a slight red blood cell content in the presence of a few leucocytes, an increasingly pathological colloidal gold curve, and normal sugar levels.

The carotid angiogram (14 April 1954) led to an increase in the severity and incidence of the hemiseizures, which recurred immediately after contrast injection, even before the general anaesthesia wore off; however, no significant deterioration occurred in the general state of the patient.

At the beginning of May 1954 generalised convulsive seizures commenced. The hemiparesis now involved the right side of the body as well. The child had to be artificially fed, and great difficulty was experienced with the intravenous catheter which became occluded with surprising rapidity. The patient died in extreme cachexia on 10 July 1954.

EEG (5 March 1954). Strong periodic discharges were recorded at 2-3 second intervals in the form of generalised slow solitary waves which were somewhat higher on the right side. There were also episodic short rhythmical bursts of slow waves with phase reversal in the postcentral temporo-occipital region. Over the right hemisphere the bursts were often linked with epilepsy potentials, which were maximal in the occipital region.

EEG (8 March 1954). The recording revealed almost continuous generalised slow wave bursts, which were maximal on the right side. An epileptic focus was present in the right temporal region.

EEG (22 March 1954). The recording revealed continuous 1-1½ second activity, maximal over the right side, which was interrupted by brief generalised seizure complexes.

EEG (8 April 1954). All leads showed rhythmical slow wave activity, which was maximal over the right occipital region. Epilepsy potentials were present in the right temporal region.

EEG (3 June 1954). The picture was dominated by irregular delta and sub-delta waves which were maximal over the right lateral postcentral region, where they were combined with epilepsy potentials.

AUTOPSY FINDINGS (Institute of Pathology, University of Zurich).

There was a thrombotic occlusion in the superior sagittal sinus in its distal two-thirds, as well as in the straight sinus and in the transverse sinus on both sides. Some of the pial veins over the right hemisphere were also involved. Numerous areas of cerebral haemorrhage due to passive congestion were present, as well as oedema and congestive hyperaemia. Internal hydrocephalus and pachymeningosis haemorrhagica interna were found. There was evidence of old and fresh subarachnoid haemorrhage. A recent terminal haemorrhage had occurred on the right side. Both middle ear cavities were purulent.

CASE 55
G.M. born 7 January 1955 (8064/55).

FAMILY HISTORY. Parents and 5 older siblings were healthy.

PREVIOUS HISTORY. Pregnancy, birth and early development normal. Sitting at 6 months, and first attempts to stand up at 10 months. Pneumonia at the age of 2½ months, when radiographic examination raised the suspicion of a congenital cardiac defect. The child made a rapid and good recovery. There were no signs of cardiac insufficiency, and there was no cyanosis.

PRESENT ILLNESS. On 2 December 1955 the child, a healthy 11-month-old girl, suddenly cried out loudly at 7.30 a.m., and her mother found her unconscious in bed with averted eyes and spastic arms.

Emergency Admission to the District Hospital, Affoltern a. A. (2 December 1955).

FINDINGS ON ADMISSION. The child was comatose, with conjugate deviation of the eyes to the right side and fixed pupils. Her extremities were rigid with symmetrical tendon jerks. Other symptoms included marked cyanosis and rapid breathing (60/minute). The girl's temperature was about 38.5-40.1°C. Blood count: leucocytes 29,000, juvenile forms 9 per cent, mature forms 49.5 per cent; eosinophils 1.5 per cent; monocytes 4.5 per cent; lymphocytes 34.5 per cent; plasmocytes 0.5 per cent.

Following oxygen administration, the cyanosis improved, although the child remained febrile despite antibiotic treatment (penicillin, streptomycin, Terramycin).

Admission to the Children's Hospital, Zurich (7 December-9 December 1955).

FINDINGS ON ADMISSION. The patient was not responding to commands, reacted only to pain stimuli, and had severe generalised cyanosis. Recurrent brief tonic and clonic seizures occurred in the right side of the body, particularly in the right arm, accompanied by conjugate deviation of the eyes to the right side. Muscle tone between seizures was increased in the right extremities, and tendon jerks were bilaterally increased. The pupils were reacting to light. The fundi showed sharp margins but the veins were widened, particularly on the right side. Auscultation revealed a loud harsh systolic murmur over the entire praecordium. Chest radiography revealed a heart of normal size with a rounded apex, and an absent pulmonary conus. No hepatomegaly was present, and the chest radiograph also showed no significant increase in broncho-vascular markings. Respirations were rapid and heaving, and the ala nasi was working. The pulse rate was 140/min. Pyodermic foci were found over the buttocks and right thigh (mostly healed), and there was an infiltrated and reddened area of the skin with papules in the vicinity of the right knee. Temperature 38.5°C. Blood: Hb 79 per cent; erythrocytes 6.4 million; reticulocytes 43 per thousand; leucocytes 14,450, juvenile forms 5 per cent, mature forms

62 per cent; basophils 0.5 per cent; monocytes 7.5 per cent; lymphocytes 25 per cent; plasmocytes 0.5 per cent. Micro-ESR 1/2/4 mm. Quick test 18 seconds. Bürker test 5-8 minutes. Duke test 2½ minutes.

Lumbar Puncture. Pressure raised; fluid frankly xanthochromic; 47 monocytes, 7 segmented cells, 83 erythrocytes and 12 foam cells/ml.

EEG (8 December 1955). There was evidence of severe brain damage, most marked over the right hemisphere, in the form of slow polymorphic delta waves which showed a maximum in the temporo-occipital region. In addition, there were rhythmic bursts of delta activity on both sides in the fronto-precentral regions. No epilepsy potentials were present.

Admission to the Department of Neurosurgery, University Hospital, Zurich (9 December 1955).

The patient was admitted on suspicion of cerebral abcess or of cerebral thrombophlebitis. *Right Carotid Angiogram.* The arterial and capillary phases were normal. In the venous phase, there was very defective visualisation of the ascending cortical veins, and defective filling of the superior sagittal sinus. The impression was gained of definite stasis of contrast medium in the parietal and anterior temporal region (Fig. 69).

Ventriculogram. Considerable symmetrical internal hydrocephalus was shown. Ventricular drainage and tracheotomy were carried out.

CSF. Protein 44 mg per cent. Colloidal gold reaction 31000100000.

The patient died in respiratory insufficiency on 11 December 1955.

AUTOPSY FINDINGS (Institute of Pathology, University of Zurich). Thrombosis of the superior sagittal sinus and its tributory veins. Haemorrhagic infarction of both frontal lobes. Severe cerebral oedema. Congenital cardiac disease; tetralogy of Fallot. Muco-purulent tracheobronchitis.

CASE 56

H.F., born 2 April 1953 (3489/54, 7395/55, 4130/58).

FAMILY HISTORY. Nil relevant.

PREVIOUS HISTORY. Pregnancy normal. Spontaneous birth at 8 months; birth weight 970g. Kept for 6 weeks in an incubator (Babies' Hospital, Zurich). 'Spasmophilic seizures' on third and fourth days, a convulsion on sixth day. Psychomotor development retarded (sitting up at 12 months, standing at 21 months, talking at 2 years).

PRESENT ILLNESS. The patient had been prone to upper respiratory infections, sometimes hyperpyrexial, from infancy. The first generalised seizure, which lasted only a short while, occurred during an influenzal infection at the age of 9 months.

First Admission to the Children's Hospital, Zurich.

At the age of thirteen months, the child was admitted to hospital due to recurrent seizures accompanying and following a hyperpyrexial influenzal infection. An EEG, made several days after the symptoms had disappeared, revealed no abnormal findings, and in particular no lateralising differences.

Pneumoencephalogram (12 May 1954). The ventricular system was symmetrically enlarged (Fig. 70a).

The child experienced a generalised seizure of short duration in October 1954, again during a febrile influenzal infection. On 9 September 1955, a right clonic hemistatus epilepticus appeared suddenly without warning, and lasted for 10 hours.

Second Admission to the Children's Hospital, Zurich (9 September-12 October 1955).

FINDINGS ON ADMISSION. The patient was semicomatose, with flaccid right-sided hemiplegia including the face. Reflexes were bilaterally present and symmetrical; a right Babinski response was elicited. No clinical focus of infection was demonstrable. The heart and lungs were normal. Blood pressure 100/65 mm Hg. Shortly after admission, another right hemiconvulsion occurred, and then the child became deeply unconscious. The seizures were controlled with chloral hydrate. Temperature 40.4°C. Leucocytes 25,300, juvenile forms 16.5 per cent, mature forms 55 per cent. Serum calcium, phosphorus and protein levels normal.

Lumbar Puncture. All fluid tests were normal except for a glucose level of 16 mg per cent. In a repeat examination on 21 September all values, including glucose, were normal.

COURSE. After 5 days the child recovered consciousness completely. A complete flaccid right-sided hemiplegia then developed over the course of a few weeks. This gave way to an increasing spastic hemiparesis, in which the right arm was functionally useless, and the gait was markedly disturbed. The facial palsy disappeared completely. After 6 weeks the patient regained normal speech.

Pneumoencephalogram (21 September 1955). There was a massive displacement of the ventricular system to the right of the mid-line, with the body of the left lateral ventricle lying at a lower level (Fig. 70a).

Left Carotid Angiogram (22 September 1955). The anterior cerebral vessels were displaced to the right side. Surprisingly, the ventricular system was now in its normal position (Fig. 70b).

Pneumoencephalogram (23 September 1955). The ventricular system was fairly symmetrically dilatated, but was not displaced (Fig. 70b).

EEG (20 September 1955). A massive depression was recorded over the entire left hemisphere.

EEG (15 November 1955). The depression was virtually unaltered, but there was normal activity over the right hemisphere. No epilepsy potentials were recorded.

Third Admission to the Children's Hospital, Zurich (20 March-3 April 1958).
The patient was referred to hospital because of a febrile upper respiratory tract infection with vomiting. No further epileptic attacks had occurred with regular anti-epileptic treatment.

FINDINGS ON ADMISSION. The patient was suffering from acute rhinopharyngitis. Severe spastic hemiparesis was present, with a functional deficiency of the arm and hand, and a marked disturbance of gait. IQ (Terman-Merrill): 60.

EEG. A marked depression was shown over the entire left hemisphere, with virtually normal right cerebral activity, and no epilepsy potentials.

COURSE (until July 1966). From 1959 to 1961 the child attended a school for children with cerebral palsy, but became unmanageable. With regular anticonvulsant therapy he remained free from attacks until he was admitted to a special children's home. Here treatment was discontinued, and homeopathic remedies were commenced. Thereafter, the child experienced several seizures a day, each of which was usually of short duration. In the Summer of 1966, he became unteachable and increasingly ill-tempered, and had to be admitted to an institution. He was then a complete idiot, and showed severe spastic hemiparesis with a

functionally useless arm, but he was able to walk. Routine anticonvulsant drugs were again commenced, and his attacks ceased. In the summer of 1966 the boy reached puberty.

CASE 57
G.C., born 29 July 1962 (4991/65).
FAMILY HISTORY. Nil relevant.

PREVIOUS HISTORY. Pregnancy normal. Caesarean section at birth for maternal indications. Child healthy; birth weight 3300g. Psychomotor development normal.

PRESENT ILLNESS. On 4 June 1965, an upper respiratory tract infection commenced, with coughing and a sore throat, but no fever. On the morning of 6 June a convulsion occurred which lasted for 10 minutes. At first the seizure was limited to the left side, but then it became generalised. The patient had a temperature of 38°C. In the afternoon she experienced a second attack, which on this occasion was exclusively left-sided. She lost consciousness, and was incontinent of urine and faeces. For the next seven hours rapidly successive left-sided hemiseizures occurred, accompanied by a temperature of 40°C.

Admission to the Children's Hospital, Zurich (7 June-17 July 1965).

FINDINGS ON ADMISSION. The patient was pre-comatose, and reacted to pain. She exhibited a flaccid left-sided hemiplegia and areflexia (but a right ankle jerk and a left Babinski response were present). Her throat was markedly reddened, and pneumococci were cultured from a swab. No enlarged lymph glands were palpable. Temperature 40°C. Leucocytes 10,500, juvenile forms 9 per cent, mature forms 64 per cent. ESR 10/25 mm.

Lumbar Puncture. Fluid normal. It was also normal on repeat examination.

EEG (8 June 1965). A depression was recorded over the entire right hemisphere. There were intermittent epilepsy potentials in the right temporal region.

Pneumoencephalogram (15 June 1965). The ventricular system was slightly displaced to the left side, with depression of the body of the right lateral ventricle.

Repeat Pneumoencephalography (23 June 1965). The displacement of the ventricular system was less pronounced.

COURSE. The fever disappeared in 4 days. For 3 days massive sub-total left-sided hemiplegia was present which completely regressed in the course of a few days. Freedom from attacks followed anti-epileptic medication.

EEG (1 July 1965). A marked disturbance was demonstrated over the right hemisphere, with delta rhythms maximal over the antero-lateral parts. A moderately active epileptogenic focus was present in the right precentral region. The left hemisphere was normal.

COURSE (until August 1966). There was no residual evidence of hemiparesis. The child was very lively. She experienced occasional attacks (nature not defined, but probably generalised seizures), due to irregular administration of anti-epileptic treatment.

CASE 58

P.R., born 26 November 1964 (7273, 7892/66, 784/67).

FAMILY HISTORY. Two older sisters and a paternal uncle suffered from febrile convulsions in infancy.

PREVIOUS HISTORY. Normal pregnancy. Born 2 months after term; normal delivery; birth weight 3300g; child lively. Normal psycho-motor development (first words at 11 months, walking at 13 months). At $4\frac{1}{2}$ months the child experienced recurrent generalised seizures for one hour during a bout of fever (40°C). Otherwise there were no unusual features, and the child was lively. At 9 months, two generalised seizures occurred within 2 hours during a bout of fever of 40°C. Recurrent generalised seizures lasting for four hours occurred at the age of one year, during an influenzal infection, with a fever of 40°C.

PRESENT ILLNESS. On 16 February 1966 at the age of 14 months, the child experienced a bout of acute fever of 39.9°C, but was otherwise lively. On the following day when the temperature was 39.8°C, left-sided hemiconvulsions suddenly commenced with a loss of consciousness and excess salivation. These hemiseizures persisted almost uninterrupted for 12 hours.

Emergency Admission to the Cantonal Hospital, Chur (18 February 1966).

FINDINGS ON ADMISSION. On admission 12 hours after the onset of seizures, the child was still experiencing clonic hemiseizures of the left side of the body including the face; these seizures were brought under control with Luminal. The patient was unconscious; the right pupil was dilated. The left limbs were hypotonic with diminished tendon jerks. Rectal temperature 39.5°C. Pulse 158/min. Heart and lungs normal.

Lumbar Puncture. 3 cells/μl; protein 18 mg per cent; glucose 100 mg per cent. Blood: haematocrit volume 37 per cent; leucocytes 13,800, mature forms 71 per cent, monocytes 7 per cent, lymphocytes 22 per cent. Blood sugar 74 mg per cent. Urine loaded with acetone. Normal serum calcium and chloride levels. The patient recovered consciousness several hours later, and remained apathetic and drowsy. Flaccid left-sided hemiplegia now appeared. Antibiotics (penicillin, chloramphenicol) and corticosteroids (Ultracorten-H) were commenced. After a free interval of 24 hours, severe left-sided convulsions accompanied by a loss of consciousness again occurred at 1-2 hourly intervals for 12 hours. After a second free interval of 24 hours, a third status epilepticus with left hemiseizures, which lasted for many hours, commenced on 21 February 1966, despite anticonvulsant treatment (phenobarbitone, Nembutal).

Admission to the Children's Hospital, Zurich (21 February-29 March 1966).

FINDINGS ON ADMISSION. The patient was unconscious, with complete flaccid weakness of the left extremities, a definite expressive left-sided facial palsy, and a paralysis of conjugate gaze to the left side. There was no evidence of isolated external ocular muscle palsies. The fundi and pupils were normal. Response to brain stimulation over the left side of the body was abnormal. Left tendon jerks were absent, and a left Babinski response was elicited. The child was afebrile. Blood pressure 90/55 mm Hg. Pulse 112/min, fully palpable and regular. A chest radiograph showed a normal heart and lungs, and an electrocardiogram was normal.

EEG (21 February 1966). There was a massive depression of cerebral activity, with continuous polymorphic high amplitude sub-delta and delta activity over the entire right hemisphere. The left hemisphere showed evidence only of a mild disturbance, with polymorphic and sometimes moderate rhythmic theta and delta activity, which was overshadowed by diffuse low beta activity. No epilepsy potentials were observed.

Pneumoencephalogram (22 February 1966). The ventricular system was displaced to the left side. The third ventricle lay 7 mm off centre, the right lateral ventricle appeared narrower than the left one in all regions, and the roof of the left cella media lay 3 mm lower than that of the right lateral ventricle (Fig. 71).

Lumbar Puncture. The fluid was clear and colourless. Cells 1/μl. Protein 27 mg per cent (Biuret method). Glucose 55 mg per cent. Colloidal gold reaction negative.

The blood picture and the ESR were normal. The nasal cavity and fauces showed normal appearances. A detailed clinical examination revealed no foci of infection.

COURSE. Immediately after the pneumoencephalogram an infusion of 30 per cent urea (3 ml/kg body weight) was administered with the object of reducing the cerebral swelling. Clinically, no beneficial effect was observed.

Follow-up Pneumoencephalogram (25 February 1966). The ventricular system was still displaced to the left side, although the displacement was less marked. This finding was confirmed on 4 March 1966. However, repeat examination on 15 March 1966 revealed no trace of ventricular displacement to the side, although the upper limit of the body of the right lateral ventricle was still depressed (Fig. 71).

CSF. Still normal.

Right Carotid Angiogram (8 March 1966). The angiogram was performed by catheterisation of the right brachial artery, and revealed no abnormal findings.

EEG (2 March, 8 March, 25 March 1966). The previous appearances were practically unaltered; there was a depression of the background activity, as well as drug-induced beta activity over the entire right hemisphere. The left side was normal. For the first time, on 25 March 1966, multifocal epilepsy potentials appeared over the right hemisphere.

COURSE. Clinically, the hemiplegia regressed over the course of about three weeks. A definite spasticity now appeared, affecting particularly the arms. At the time of discharge on 29 March 1966, the child had regained, with the aid of regular physiotherapy, moderate movements, and was able to flex and extend the left elbow and wrist. In the leg, only slight differences in power remained, and the facial palsy had

completely disappeared. The spasticity in the arm persisted, but the left tendon reflexes gradually returned to normal. The Babinski response remained positive.

Second Admission to the Children's Hospital, Zurich (25-30 April 1966).

The patient had remained free from attacks with regular anticonvulsant treatment. Moderate to severe spastic hemiparesis had persisted, and hand and finger movements were absent.

EEG. The depression over the right hemisphere was undiminished. Multifocal epilepsy potentials were again demonstrated over the left hemisphere, although they were less marked than previously.

Pneumoencephalogram. There was definite, even moderate enlargement of the right ventricle, with slight displacement of the ventricular system to the left side (Fig. 71).

CSF was normal.

COURSE (until August 1966). Despite regular physiotherapy, a marked spastic hemiparesis remains. The child is sometimes able to grasp toys in the left hand, but then appears unable to release them. His gait is uncertain, and he often falls and limps. He is very emotional and irascible. He has remained free from attacks under anticonvulsant treatment.

CASE 59

W.S., born 2 February 1964 (4437/65).

FAMILY HISTORY. Nil relevant.

PREVIOUS HISTORY. Pregnancy, birth and psycho-motor development normal. No previous illnesses.

PRESENT ILLNESS. The child was healthy and lively until 3 April 1965. On the morning of 4 April she was found lying unconscious in vomitus, experiencing clonic seizures (localisation?); she had a temperature of 40°C. Despite antipyretic treatment, the left-sided seizures continued, and the child remained unconscious. On the next day she was drowsy, with a flaccid left-sided hemiplegia, and a temperature of 40.2°C.

Admission to the Children's Hospital, Zurich (5 April-16 June 1965).

FINDINGS ON ADMISSION. The patient was drowsy, with flaccid left-sided hemiplegia including the face. The right extremities were spastic, with normal spontaneous movements. Tendon jerks were brisker on the left than on the right side. Purulent tonsillopharyngitis was present, due to streptococcus haemolyticus A and pneumococcus. Regional lymph nodes were enlarged on both sides of the neck. Blood culture negative. Temperature 39.3°C. Leucocytes 12,250, juvenile forms 50 per cent, mature forms 31 per cent. ESR 6/23 mm. Cardiovascular system intact. Blood pressure 95/70 mm Hg.

Lumbar Puncture. Fluid normal.

EEG (5 April 1965). Clinically, a hemistatus epilepticus was seen, with extensive epilepsy potentials continuously present over the entire right hemisphere. There was phase reversal in the parietal regions. High amplitude delta activity, partly rhythmical and without epilepsy potentials, was shown over the left hemisphere.

Echoencephalogram (6 April 1965). The septum pellucidum was displaced 5 mm to the left of the mid-line.

Pneumoencephalogram (15 April 1965). Oedema was present in the right hemisphere (Fig. 72*b*).

Right Carotid Angiogram (15 April 1965). The anterior cerebral arteries were displaced to the left side; otherwise appearances were normal (Fig. 72*a*).

Pneumoencephalogram (5 May 1965). The ventricular system was moderately dilated, but now showed no displacement. The right lateral ventricle was more markedly dilated than the left one, and there was considerable enlargement of the third ventricle (Fig. 72*b*).

COURSE. The temperature returned to normal in 3 days following antibiotic medication. The last attack occurred on the day of admission during the EEG examination, and it was controlled by intravenous and intramuscular barbiturates. The child awoke gradually, and regained full consciousness within a week. The flaccid hemiplegia gradually altered into a marked spastic one, with a loss of function of the arm.

EEG (3 March 1966). A persistent massive depression was shown over the entire right hemisphere. The left hemisphere was only slightly abnormal, but bursts of paroxysmal activity were recorded during light sleep.

Final Outpatient Follow-up Examination (25 July 1966). Despite intensive physiotherapy, the severe spastic hemiparesis persisted, with complete loss of function of the hand, mild weakness of the leg, and no facial involvement.

Mentally, the child appeared normal. No further attacks occurred with continuous anti-epileptic treatment.

CASE 60

M.D., born 25 August 1955 (9273/63, 1302/64).

FAMILY HISTORY. Maternal grandfather with encephalitis lethargica in 1914.

PREVIOUS HISTORY. Pregnancy normal. Caesarean section (after induction had failed) 10 days after term. Child healthy; birth weight 3500g. Normal psychomotor development. No illnesses or accidents of importance.

PRESENT ILLNESS. On the morning of 2 August 1963, the boy suddenly felt unwell. A few minutes later he experienced a feeling of pins and needles with itching in the left extremities, followed immediately by the onset of a complete left-sided hemiplegia (? facial palsy as well). He remained fully conscious, and could speak normally. The family doctor was called, and he confirmed these findings and demonstrated an absence of tendon jerks in the left limbs; all reflexes on the right side were preserved. One hour later the child lost consciousness, exhibited tonic convulsions in the left hand and conjugate deviation of the eyes to the left side, and was incontinent of urine. Two hours later, he recovered consciousness. The hemiplegia disappeared completely within 9 hours, and after a brief bout of headache the child again felt quite well. On the same day, 3 hours after the disappearance of the hemi-syndrome, another attack occurred, with clonic seizures of the left arm, conjugate deviation of the eyes to the left side, and urinary incontinence. This attack lasted 30 minutes, and the patient remained conscious throughout. A feeling of tiredness and headache, without paralysis, followed, and thereafter the patient made a rapid recovery. A series of similar attacks, lasting for 2-3 minutes and unaccompanied by pre- or postictal paralysis, occurred during the days that followed. On 3 August 1963, the patient experienced a severe focal clonic attack which lasted for 3 hours. This was followed by a transient clouding of consciousness, and hemiplegia.

Admission to the Children's Hospital, Zurich (8-26 August 1963).

FINDINGS. Between attacks a normal neurological status was preserved (muscle tone, power, reflexes, superficial and deep sensitivity,

272

co-ordination), apart from the bilateral presence of Chvostek's sign.

EEG (9 August 1963). A marked disturbance was shown over the entire right hemisphere; this disturbance was maximal over the post-central region, and took the form of poly-morphic delta activity of medium amplitude. Rhythmic delta activity was also present, and was maximal over the fronto-precentral region. There were only mild disturbances over the left hemisphere, and no epilepsy potentials were demonstrated.

Right Carotid Angiogram (13 August 1963). There was questionable upward displacement of the middle cerebral vessels, and a narrowing of their calibre; no definite abnormality was seen. Permission for a pneumoencephalogram was refused by the parents.

The *CSF* was normal.

Clinical examination revealed no abnormality other than a mild rhinitis and a slightly elevated ESR (10/20 mm) with an otherwise normal blood picture.

EEG (20 August 1963). A massive disturbance was revealed over the right hemisphere, taking the form of high amplitude delta rhythms which were maximal in the fronto-precentral and temporo-occipital regions. No epilepsy poten-tials were demonstrated.

COURSE. Similar attacks lasting only a short time were observed during the patient's stay in hospital; they commenced with conjugate deviation of the eyes to the left side, followed immediately by rhythmic clonic convulsions of the left hand, and a synchronous nystagmus to the left side. The child remained conscious, and was able to move the right extremities and the left leg without difficulty; the left hand showed considerable weakness, particularly in dorsiflexion and finger extension. After 2 minutes, the attack ceased spontaneously, although the patient stated that he still had the feeling of convulsions in the left hand ('ça travaille dedans'). The weakness disappeared very rapidly, and no disturbance of sensation could be demonstrated subsequently. During the attacks, a marked twitching of the entire left arm was present.

With a daily dose of phenobarbitone (75 mg), the patient remained free from attacks. On 9 April 1964, four days after stopping the drug in preparation for follow-up EEG, the patient experienced a clonic left hemiseizure which lasted for 20 minutes and was accompanied by a loss of consciousness. Clinical examination on the following day revealed no abnormal neurological signs. Chvostek's sign and the peroneal nerve phenomenon were present on both sides.

EEG (25 September 1963). As before, there was a focal disturbance in the right hemisphere without epilepsy potentials.

EEG (9 April 1964). Findings virtually un-changed.

EEG (8 January 1965). Findings as before.

Final Follow-up Examination (17 May 1966). Neurological findings were normal. The patient has no complaints and is doing well at school. Serum calcium is within normal limits (8.9 mg per cent), and serum albumin content is normal (7.4 g per cent).

CASE 61

S.M., born 11 May 1962 (8620/63, 968/64, 6103/65).

FAMILY HISTORY. A paternal uncle suffered from post-traumatic epilepsy.

PREVIOUS HISTORY. Mother suffered from oedema in the second half of pregnancy. Birth normal; child healthy; birth weight 4500 g. Psychomotor development retarded (sitting up at 8 months, walking at 2 years, first words spoken at 1½ years).

PRESENT ILLNESS. The child had experienced a few generalised epileptic attacks without after-effects since the 8th month of life.

Admission to the Children's Hospital, Zurich (22 May-13 June 1965).

FINDINGS. The child was physically normal, but showed retarded psychomotor develop-ment. General muscular hypertonia was present, with brisk symmetrical tendon jerks.

COURSE. On 23 May 1963 the child, when attended by the ward sister, appeared quite healthy. A few moments later she was found awake but motionless in her bed. The house physician was called, who examined her and found a complete flaccid left-sided hemiplegia including the face. The right extremity moved normally after light stimulation. The left tendon jerks could not be elicited, but the right ones were normal. Several minutes later, a jerky rhythmical nystagmus to the right side developed. This was followed by clonic seizures of the right hand, which extended to involve both right extremities and finally became a generalised convulsion; the child lapsed into unconsciousness. The attack was brought under control with intravenous amytal. When the child awoke after several hours, the hemiplegia had completely disappeared.

EEG (27 May 1963). A non-specific disturbance was shown over the right hemisphere; this disturbance was maximal over the posterior parts. No epilepsy potentials were present.

Pneumoencephalogram (6 June 1963). Moderate internal hydrocephalus was demonstrated; the anterior parts of the left (!) lateral ventricle were somewhat more dilated than the right side.

CSF. Normal.

COURSE. Despite anticonvulsant treatment, generalised attacks appeared from time to time, usually taking the form of brief clonic seizures accompanied by a loss of consciousness. Repeated following examinations failed to reveal evidence of any weakness.

EEG (6 March 1964). Normal.

EEG (13 October 1965). Bilateral synchronous epilepsy potentials were seen over the posterior parts of both hemispheres.

CASE 62

A.B., born 27 August 1952 (5436/54).

FAMILY HISTORY. Nil relevant.

PREVIOUS HISTORY. The mother had developed toxaemia during the second halves of the previous two pregnancies. Normal birth at term; birth weight 1800g; mild asphyxia at birth, but full recovery after 30 minutes. Psychomotor development was slightly retarded (sitting up at 14 months, walking at 18 months, speech development normal). In the winter of 1953-1954 and in the summer of 1954, she experienced attacks of febrile tonsillitis which lasted for two days.

PRESENT ILLNESS. The child was in good health up to December 1954. On the morning of 18 December 1954, her parents found her experiencing clonic hemiconvulsions of the right side of the body including the face. She was unconscious, with the head turned to the left side, and had been incontinent of urine and faeces. Her temperature was 40°C. The hemiconvulsions continued, with brief intervals, for several minutes. In between seizures, a flaccid

paralysis of the right side of the body was evident.

Admission to the Children's Hospital, Zurich (18 December 1954).

FINDINGS. On admission, 4 hours later, the child exhibited hemistatus epilepticus, with severe right-sided clonic seizures separated by intervals as short as one minute. There was conjugate deviation of the eyes to the left side, but the head was turned to the right. In between seizures, complete flaccid right-sided hemiplegia was observed. Reflexes were absent on both sides, and the patient was deeply unconscious. The pupils were reacting to light, and the fundi were normal. Temperature 41°C. Pulse 180/min. Blood pressure 100/50 mm Hg. Blood culture negative. Leucocytes 12,000, juvenile forms 25 per cent, mature forms 50 per cent; no toxic alterations.

Lumbar Puncture. Fluid clear; one cell/μl; protein 27 mg per cent; glucose 102 mg per cent. Colloidal gold reaction normal. Bacteriological culture sterile. Urine: albumin (+), acetone (+), no sugar; microscopical examination negative. There was slight redness of the left ear drum. There were no signs of a focal infection.

COURSE. Despite chloral hydrate, amytal and phenobarbital medication, severe right-sided focal hemiseizures continued to appear, the first one appearing during sedation with a 'cocktail' medication. The child remained deeply comatose, and died on 20 December 1954 in circulatory failure.

AUTOPSY (Institute of Pathology, University of Zurich). Brain weight 1240g. Otherwise findings were normal, apart from massive oedema. There was severe toxic fatty degeneration of the liver, kidneys and myocardium. Follicular necrosis was seen in the spleen and tonsils, and there was partial oedema, emphysema and atelectasis of the lungs.

Histology. Histological examination showed extensive non-purulent encephalitis of a predominantly periventricular distribution, presenting the picture of inflammatory cerebral oedema.

Opinion. The picture corresponds most closely to that of a virus encephalitis, the aetiology of which cannot be determined from the morphological changes.

CASE 63

B.B. born 4 January 1965 (7580/66).

FAMILY HISTORY. Mother and only maternal uncle suffered from febrile convulsions. Older brother healthy.

PREVIOUS HISTORY. Mother in contact with German measles in 3rd-4th months of pregnancy; gamma globulins increased as a result. No illness, and pregnancy uneventful in all other respects. Birth at term; no complications; birth weight 3550g; child healthy. Normal psychomotor development (laughing at 5 weeks, sitting up at 7 months, standing at 10 months, crawling since about 12 months).

PRESENT ILLNESS. On 9 March 1966, the child was given a smallpox vaccination (scarification on left upper thigh). On 13 March she was miserable, with a temperature of about 39°C. On 15 March she was afebrile and lively. On 16 March she was tearful, with a temperature again of around 39°C. On 17 March she was better again. A routine medical examination on 23 March showed a normal vaccination reaction with vesiculation. On 24 March 1966 her brother fell ill with signs of an influenzal infection with fever and coughing. On 25 March her temperature rose suddenly to 39°C. In the night she cried out twice, although the parents observed nothing untoward. The next morning, she did not wake up normally, and on investigation her right extremities and face were found to be twitching. She was unconscious, with a fixed gaze to the right side and a temperature of 40°C. Severe right-sided clonic seizures continued repeatedly up to the arrival of the family doctor 4½ hours later. The child was given phenobarbitone (200 mg) intramuscularly, and sent to hospital.

Emergency Admission to the Children's Hospital, Zurich.

FINDINGS. The child was unconscious, and exhibited tonic and clonic seizures of the right extremities. The pupils were equal and contracted. The seizures were brought under control with amytal (150 mg intramuscularly) and somnifen (100 mg intravenously). Temperature 39.6°C. Pulse 186/min, full and regular. Heart and lungs normal. Blood: Hb 12.6 g; reticulocytes 7 per thousand, leucocytes 20,900, metamyelocytes 1 per cent, juvenile forms 22 per cent, mature forms 59½ per cent, eosinophils ½ per cent, monocytes 1

per cent, lymphocytes 16 per cent; platelets 267,000. Micro-ESR 1/4/9 mm.

Lumbar Puncture. Fluid clear; total protein 15.5 per cent. Cells normal; glucose 39 mg per cent; colloidal gold reaction negative.

EEG (28 March 1966). There was a severe depression of cerebral activity over the entire left hemisphere, with low and very slow polymorphic activity. Over the right hemisphere, high amplitude polymorphic delta activity was shown, with a marked predominance of low theta waves (Fig. 74a). Clinical examination revealed only a slightly reddened right ear drum; there were no other abnormal findings. The heart and lungs were normal.

Pneumoencephalogram (28 March 1966). The left lateral ventricle was well visualised, and the right one contained only a sliver of air. The ventricular system was shown to be massively displaced to the right of the mid-line, but was not deformed (Fig. 73).

Left Carotid Angiogram (6 April 1966). There was good visualisation of the arterial, capillary and venous phases. Appearances were normal, apart from a displacement of the mid-line vessels to the right side, and a bowed and stretched-looking pericallosal artery.

COURSE. With massive anticonvulsant treatment, the child remained comatose and free from attacks. Consciousness gradually returned, and on 28 March 1966 a flaccid right-sided hemiplegia (including the face) and a paralysis of conjugate gaze to the right side appeared. At the same time the child developed a marked spasticity of the left extremities, holding the arm in a position of flexion (elbow flexed, hand held in a tight fist), and the ankle extended. Tendon jerks were abnormally increased on the right side, and less so on the left side. The persistent lack of affect in the presence of a conscious state was interpreted as evidence of severe mental damage.

At the end of April 1966, the patient presented the following appearances: she showed a lack of affect, did not smile, and allowed herself to be fed with a spoon. Sub-total flaccid right-sided hemiplegia was present, with a pronounced flexion position of the upper extremity and a semi-flexion position of the lower extremity. Talipes equinus, and marked hyper-reflexia with foot clonus were also noted. Markedly positive Babinski and Rossolimo responses were elicited. There were

275

no spontaneous reactions of the right arm, and movements of the right leg were restricted. The left extremities moved spontaneously; the hand was often open, and the talipes equinus position was maintained only intermittently. Definite spasticity during flexion was present in the arm, and during extension in the right leg. The left tendon jerks were markedly increased without clonus; bilateral Babinski and Rossolimo responses were present, less marked on the left than on the right side. Abdominal reflexes were symmetrical. Marked right facial palsy was present. Pupillary movements and the fundi were normal. All extremities were flaccid during sleep.

Follow-up Pneumoencephalogram (5 April 1966). The ventricular system was well visualised, with slight displacement to the right side, compared with the initial appearances. On 19 April, the ventricular system was shown to lie virtually in its normal position, but both lateral ventricles were dilated. On 19 July, severe atrophy of the anterior part of the left cerebral hemisphere was demonstrated (Fig. 73).

CSF examinations were normal throughout.

Follow-up EEG (7 April 1966). A virtually complete depression with very flat cerebral activity was shown over the entire left hemisphere with the exception of the occipital region, over which a marked synchronisation effect appeared with photostimulation. Slight non-specific disturbances were present over the right hemisphere, and marked drug-induced beta activity was observed. On 14 April 1966, repeat examination revealed no change with regard to the left hemisphere depression, but the right hemisphere showed activity compatible with normal for the age of the patient. Similar appearances were shown on 19 July 1966 (Fig. 74c).

TREATMENT. Immediately following pneumoencephalographic demonstration of the left-sided cerebral swelling, the patient was submitted to a course of hyperosmotic treatment with a 30 per cent urea solution (3ml/kg of body weight, daily), without any noticeable benificial effect. Chloramphenicol was given for the febrile condition; the temperature returned to normal within 5 days. During the second week, an intercurrent phlebitis developed at the site of the intravenous catheter in the left arm. Anticonvulsant treatment was commenced with phenobarbitone, initially 120 mg intramuscularly, later 75 mg by mouth.

CASE 64

B.R., born 11 September 1961 (6182/62, 881/64).

FAMILY HISTORY. Nil relevant.

PREVIOUS HISTORY. Pregnancy, birth and development normal. Chickenpox in December 1961. Skin rash after eating raspberries.

PRESENT ILLNESS. On 29 July 1962, when the girl was 10½ months old, she became ill with fever and diarrhoea. Early on the following morning, her mother heard her groan and found her unconscious, lying in vomitus and having a generalised seizure.

Admission to the Children's Hospital, Zurich (30 July-6 November 1962).

FINDINGS. The child was deeply unconscious in status epilepticus, with generalised clonic seizures. There was conjugate deviation, and the pupils were widely dilated and unreactive to light. The fundi were normal. Temperature 40.1°C. ESR 30/65 mm. Blood: Hb 75 per cent; leucocytes 21,550.

Lumbar Puncture. Fluid clear. Protein 26 mg per cent; erythrocytes 260, monocytes 2⅓, segmented cells ⅔. Glucose 149 mg per cent. Colloidal gold reaction 2222211111. Bacteriological culture sterile.

The convulsions could be controlled immediately with intravenous amytal. After an initial improvement, during which the only neurological finding was somnolence, seizures again commenced on 1 August 1962, when the temperature again rose to 40°C; initially these seizures were generalised, but they then developed into clonic attacks confined to the left side of the body. Despite high doses of anticonvulsants (amytal 300 mg, phenobarbitone 340 mg, chloral hydrate 1g in 24 hours) the hemiseizures persisted. An attempt was now made to combat the high fever, which persisted despite chloramphenicol, with therapeutic 'hibernation' (Phenergan, Dolosal); two brief episodes of apnoea were countered without difficulty by artificial respiration. On the morning of 1 August 1962 the child, still unconscious, again showed a flaccid left-sided hemiplegia, with absent reflexes.

EEG (1 August 1962). Recording was commenced in the middle of a generalised attack, which ceased on the left side but continued on the right. Later a fresh attack occurred, which commenced in the right parietal region.

The search for a pathogenic organism produced negative results (blood culture, throat swab, stool examination, and animal inoculation for Echo, Coxsackie and poliomyelitis viruses).

COURSE. On 3 August, the temperature dropped to normal, and the child began slowly to wake up. The flaccid hemiplegia persisted.

EEG (6 August 1962). A massive depression was shown over the right hemisphere (maximally over the postero-lateral parts) with no epilepsy potentials.

On 8 August 1962, the tendon jerks over the paralysed side were shown to be increased, and on 16 August 1962, a left hemianopia was demonstrated (inattention?). The hemiplegia responded slowly to physiotherapy.

Pneumoencephalogram (20 August 1962). Both lateral ventricles and the third ventricle were slightly enlarged, but there was no displacement or deformity of the ventricular system (Fig. 76*a*). The *CSF* was normal.

Follow-up EEGs (6 August, 5 September, 17 October 1962). A gradual improvement was shown, but the depression over the right hemisphere persisted. On 17 October, an epileptogenic focus was demonstrated for the first time in the right temporal region.

IQ (Brunet-Lézine, 3 October 1962): 75.

Upon discharge from hospital on 6 November 1962, a moderately spastic hemiparesis, which was marked in the arm and slight in the leg and face, was still present.

Second Admission to the Children's Hospital, Zurich (24 February-3 March 1964).

With regular anti-epileptic treatment, no further epileptic attacks had been observed. The spastic hemiparesis had regressed further with prolonged physiotherapy over the course of 15 months, but it remained considerable. The left hand was held tightly shut (although with moderate force it could be opened), and fine movements were impossible. During walking, the left leg was circumducted and internally rotated, but the foot was held in a satisfactory position. A facial palsy (seen with expression only) was still present. Only slight atrophy of the left forearm and left calf could be seen, while no radiological differences between the forearm and the hand bones on either side were demonstrable. The child's IQ (Brunet-Lezine) was 77.

EEG (18 February 1964). A marked epileptogenic area was shown in the right central-precentral region.

EEG (25 February 1964). There were no pathological findings, and there was no asymmetry!

Pneumoencephalogram (27 February 1964). The right cerebral hemisphere was extensivley atrophied, with displacement of the ventricular system to the right side, and an enlargement of the right lateral ventricle (Fig. 76*a*).

The *CSF* was normal.

Right Carotid Angiogram (27 February 1964). There was good visualisation of the arterial, capillary and venous phases. No abnormality was demonstrated (Fig. 76*b*).

COURSE (until August 1966). With regular physiotherapy, the hemiparesis further ims proved. The child is now able to use both hand in play, although the left one remains rather clumsy. She has no limp, and has experienced no further attacks with regular anticonvulsant treatment. She can speak clearly, but her speech faculty has diminished.

CASE 65

G.M., born 16 January 1945 (9/53).

FAMILY HISTORY. Mother suffered from eczema, and one older brother from bronchial asthma. The latter and three older sisters were all vaccinated against smallpox between the ages of 4 and 8 years, without incident. Two younger sisters healthy, not yet vaccinated.

PREVIOUS HISTORY. Pregnancy, birth and development normal.

PRESENT ILLNESS. On 1 July 1946, the patient, who was then 1 year 6 months old, was vaccinated against smallpox on the arm. No cutaneous reaction occurred, but on the morning of 11 July 1946 the temperature rose suddenly to 40.5°C, accompanied by headache and exhaustion. A few hours later a status epilepticus suddenly commenced, with tonic and clonic seizures confined strictly to the left side of the body. The seizures lasted 4 hours.

Admission to the Children's Hospital, St. Gallen (11 July 1946 - 12 February 1947).

FINDINGS. The patient's development was normal for her age, and there were no physical findings. She was comatose with a temperature of 40.3°C. Blood: Hb 80 per cent; leucocytes 6850, metamyelocytes 3 per cent, juvenile forms

10 per cent, mature forms 46 per cent, monocytes 8 per cent, lymphocytes 33 per cent.

Lumbar Puncture. Pressure 22 cm; fluid clear; monocytes 5⅓; Pandy reaction negative; bacteriological culture negative.

Mild albuminuria and leucocyturia were present.

COURSE. Consciousness returned on 14 July 1946, and a severe spastic left-sided hemiplegia (including the face) was then present; the temperature fell to normal on the following day. Five months later, specific antibodies against the vaccinia virus to a titre of 1:32 were demonstrated.* Following months of regular physiotherapy, a severe spastic hemiparesis developed, which was maximal in the arms. Initially, the mental development appeared virtually unaffected. Early in 1952, the patient entered grade 1 of the ordinary school, with satisfactory results. In December 1952 she experienced her first attack of left-sided convulsions since the initial acute phase. Despite concentrated drug treatment, the frequency rose within a month to five attacks a day. Apart from the left-sided seizures, occasional generalised convulsions also occurred at a frequency of many dozen a day; these convulsions were accompanied by a brief clouding of consciousness and stereotyped movements of the right arm. Since the onset of these attacks, mental deterioration has increased, and an epileptic personality change has taken place.

Admission to the Children's Hospital, Zurich (31 January - 7 March 1953).

FINDINGS. Severe spastic left-sided hemiparesis was present, with apparently intact tactile and pain sensitivity. The paralysed limbs were markedly hypotrophied, and showed a 3 cm difference in length when compared with the opposite normal extremities. The radiological bone age of the left limbs was retarded by two years. The child was microcephalic (circumference of skull 49.5 cm), with a definite reduction in size of the right side of the cranium. Her IQ was 65. Her memory, including reception and retention, was markedly reduced, and she showed a marked disinhibition and a loss of affect.

EEG (10 February 1953). A severe disturbance was shown in the right hemisphere, with diffuse

*Case previously published in Rehsteiner, R., Weismann, E. (1949) *Ann. paediat. (Basel)*, **172**, 236.

sharp wave formation (which was often rhythmical with a 2.5-3.5/sec frequency) over the whole hemisphere. Isolated unrelated epilepsy potentials were demonstrated over the left hemisphere as well, mainly in the form of bursts of activity, indicating the presence of a subcortical lesion.

Pneumoencephalogram (12 February 1953). The right lateral ventricle was massively enlarged, and the entire ventricular system was displaced to the right side.

The *CSF* was normal.

Admission to the Department of Neurosurgery, University Hospital, Zurich (1-13 December 1954, 10 January - 25 February 1955).

FINDINGS. Neurological examination revealed no change in the patient's condition. There was a suspicion of left homonymous hemianopia. The girl was an imbecile, with an IQ (Biäsch) of 34 (Outpatient Clinic, Department of Child Psychiatry, University of Zurich).

EEG (2 December 1954). Appearances were virtually unchanged, but a constant epileptogenic focus was shown in the right frontal region, with intermittent waves of epilepsy potentials over the left frontal region; compared with the previous recordings, the latter were markedly increased. One attack was recorded which emanated from the left hemisphere!

Pneumoencephalogram (9 December 1954). Appearances were unaltered (Fig. 77).

OPERATION. (Department of Neurosurgery, University Hospital, Zurich; 11 January 1955). Right hemispherectomy, excluding the basal ganglia. The post-operative course was free from complications.

Histological Examination (Research Division, Department of Neurology, University Hospital, Zurich). There was severe hemispherical atrophy, with changes in the cortex including a spongy transformation of the corticomedullary region and isolated perivascular fat granules in the medulla. The choroid plexus was severely atrophied. The aetiology of the atrophy was not identified.

COURSE. The hemispherectomy produced no change in the severe hemiparesis, but the psychical improvement was striking; the patient's personality changes largely disappeared, and her IQ rose to 50 by June 1960. At school she reached the grade 2-3 stage, and learned to read and write, though she failed completely in arithmetic. She also learned to knit and weave. She remained free from attacks with regular anticonvulsant treatment (May 1965).

EEG (24 May 1955). No activity was shown over the right hemisphere; moderate diffuse disturbances were demonstrated over the left hemisphere without epilepsy potentials. There was a tendency to hypersynchrony during photostimulation.

EEG (4 August 1958). There was a marked improvement in the background activity over the left hemisphere. In addition, isolated postcentral epilepsy potentials were demonstrated which showed marked activation during hyperventilation. The right hemisphere leads remained unchanged.

FINAL FOLLOW-UP EXAMINATION (25 April 1964). According to the mother, the girl has been doing the housework since 1962, although not entirely by herself. She can write, read, knit and weave, but she is still unable to caculate. Menarche occurred in February 1960 with regular subsequent menses, accompanied by marked irritability.

Physical Examination. The severe spastic hemiparesis remained with ankylosis of the hand and finger joints, rigidity at the elbow, and extensor spasticity and talipes in the leg. Pain and tactile sensitivity was retained, but movement sensitivity in the left fingers and toes was abnormal. Complete left homonymous hemianopia and residual facial palsy involving the left side of the mouth were also present. The child exhibited generalised obesity.

CASE 66
S.V., born 29 April 1952 (848/64).

FAMILY HISTORY. Mother with migraine and, once, during a severe attack, motor aphasia. Father with a gastric ulcer. A sister with congenital ichthyosis died at the age of 2 years.

PREVIOUS HISTORY. Pregnancy, birth and development normal. The boy suffered from frequent febrile upper respiratory tract infections as a small child. At the age of 10 years, after an evening meal, an episode of expressive dysphasia occurred, which was unaccompanied by receptive dysphasia, headache or vomiting. He was an average scholar in the fifth grade of the primary school.

PRESENT ILLNESS. The boy was completely healthy until the evening of 19 February 1964. After the evening meal, he complained of tiredness, went to bed unusually early, refused to say his prayers, and went to sleep at once. In the night, he woke his mother, unable to speak and vomiting repeatedly. A severe headache then appeared, and the boy held his left forehead. The rectal temperature was 38.2°C.

Admission to the Children's Hospital, Zurich (20 February-21 March 1964).

FINDINGS. The child's level of consciousness varied between waking and severe somnolence. He exhibited a massive expressive and partial receptive dysphasia, and a severe disturbance of writing and calculation. Right homonymous hemianopia and right facial palsy were present. There was a disturbance of fine movements of the right hand, but no weakness. No apraxia was observed. The child was orientated for time and space. He was perseverating. There was a definite disturbance of movement sensitivity, but no other sensory abnormality was observed. His neurological status was otherwise normal. Temperature 38.2°C. Leucocytes 12,850, juvenile forms 9 per cent, mature forms 61½ per cent. ESR 13/2 mm. Heart and lungs normal. Blood pressure 115/55 mm Hg. No lymph node enlargement.

Lumbar Puncture. Fluid clear; cell count normal; protein 30 mg per cent; colloidal gold reaction negative.

EEG. A very marked delta focus with a depression of background activity was demonstrated in the left parieto-temporo-occipital region.

Left Carotid Angiogram (21 February 1964). Stereoscopic six-picture serial angiograms were made, and no abnormality was demonstrated.

Pneumoencephalogram (27 February 1964). The ventricular system was normal in size, shape and position.

Lumbar Puncture (27 February 1964). Slight but definite xanthochromia. Bilirubin 0.1 mg per cent; protein 33 mg per cent; 8⅓ monocytes; colloidal gold reaction negative.

Toxoplasmosis (24 February 1964). Sabin-Feldmann test in blood 1:1024, positive.

COURSE. Within 3 days the neurological deficit had disappeared, and the temperature had returned to normal. The boy continued to complain for several days of headaches of fluctuating severity. In the course of a week noticeable mental slowing occurred.

EEG (22 February 1964). A definite depression was still present over the left hemisphere, accompanied by intermittent polymorphic delta waves in the right occipital region.

EEG (24 February 1964). Slightly depressed cerebral activity was still present in the left parieto-temporo-occipital region. Intermittent bilateral slow wave groups were now demonstrated over the posterior parts of both hemispheres.

EEG (2 March 1964). A deterioration was demonstrated with diffuse delta activity, partly in the form of high amplitude slow-wave complexes over the entire left hemisphere; this activity was maximal in the parieto-occipital region. Mixed theta-delta activity was present on the right side.

EEG (9 March 1964). Definite non-specific disturbances were still present over the left hemisphere, taking the form of diffuse theta-delta activity (which was maximal in the parieto-occipital region) with sporadic rhythmical slow-wave groups.

EEG (7 April 1964). Recordings were now virtually normal, but there was still a suspicious slight diffuse disturbance in the form of scattered theta-delta groups in the background rhythm. No lateralising differences remained.

Toxoplasma Titre (Sabin-Feldmann test) in blood.
(24 February 1964). 1:1024
(10 March 1964). 1:6400
(9 April 1964). 1:1600
(21 July 1966). 1:10

OUTPATIENT FOLLOW-UP EXAMINATION (7 April 1964). The boy was now neurologically normal. His mother was aware of some mental slowing and forgetfulness, which was improving.

FINAL FOLLOW-UP EXAMINATION (11 July 1966). The boy was completely free from complaints, and was neurologically normal. He had been promoted to the second grade in the secondary school, and was experiencing no difficulties.

CASE 67

F.E., born 2 August 1950 (357/63).

FAMILY HISTORY. Nil relevant. In mid-December 1963 the whole family had an influenzal infection.

PREVIOUS HISTORY. Normal development. As a small child, the boy was very prone to upper respiratory tract infections. Tonsillectomy in 1956. 'Pleurisy' (non-tuberculous) in 1962 and 1963.

PRESENT ILLNESS. In mid-December 1963, the child developed a non-febrile unproductive cough. On Christmas Day, he was overcome by a feeling of tiredness which had disappeared by the following morning. In the evening while playing table tennis, he experienced a sudden hot feeling over the right ear, followed by a numb feeling over the entire right side of the body. He was unable to concentrate on the game, and returned to his bedroom. There he experienced a feeling of weakness in the right leg, which disappeared spontaneously after 15-20 minutes. At about midnight his cousin, who was sleeping in the same room, awoke to see the patient writhing on the floor with his left hand to his forehead. On questioning, he gave a confused answer.

Admission to the Children's Hospital, Zurich (27 December 1963-4 January 1964).

FINDINGS. On admission at 2 p.m., the patient was rousable only with difficulty. Complete flaccid right-sided hemiplegia was present, including the face and tongue. There was an absence of reaction to pain over the entire right side of the body. The right pupil was dilated and reacting to light, and there was conjugate deviation to the left side. Slight meningism was present. The fundal veins were dilated, but no papilloedema was observed. There was no clinical evidence of an upper respiratory tract infection. Temperature 38.9°C. Leucocytes 18,300, juvenile forms 14 per cent, mature forms 68.5 per cent. ESR 27/79 mm. Blood pressure 140/55 mm Hg. Pulse 132/min. *Lumbar Puncture.* Pressure above 30 cm. Fluid turbid. 9000 cells, mostly polymorphs. Protein 330 mg per cent. Glucose 102 mg per cent. Culture sterile!

EEG. A depression was shown over the left hemisphere, with a marked delta focus in the left frontal region. There was a moderate diffuse disturbance over the right hemisphere. *Left Carotid Angiogram.* The cerebral circulation was markedly slowed, the veins opacifying only after 10 seconds. Immediately after the angiogram (4 injections, each of 8 ml of 60 per cent Urographin), a respiratory arrest occurred, accompanied by a dilatation of both pupils which failed to react to light. Recovery followed the intravenous injection of 30 mg of 30 per cent urea solution.

COURSE. Deep coma and Cheyne-Stokes breathing with repeated respiratory arrests necessitated tracheotomy and artificial breathing. On 28 December 1963, the patient had bilateral fixed dilated pupils, which were unresponsive to normal stimuli. Cardiac arrest and death followed on 4 January 1964.

AUTOPSY (Institute of Pathology, University of Zurich). Hurst's focal suppurative leucoencephalitis was found, with marked softening of the brain and spinal cord. The left cerebral hemisphere was necrotic. There was marantic thrombosis of the blood vessels. Intense cerebral oedema (weight of brain 1700g) and necrotic mucopurulent tracheobronchitis were also present. There were multiple areas of lung collapse (Fig. 78).

CASE 68

R.C., born 22 February 1956 (9007, 9114/60).

PREVIOUS HISTORY. Pregnancy normal. Caesarean section at term for face presentation. Birth weight 4375g. No asphyxia. Normal development. Otitis media at 2 years. Occasional upper respiratory tract infections.

PRESENT ILLNESS. On 29 December 1959, the child fell off a chair onto his face and slightly injured the upper lip and an upper incisor. There were no signs of cerebral damage. On 4 January 1960, he suddenly developed dysphasia, which was later accompanied by a headache. The next day, the right angle of his mouth was depressed and his speech was indistinct, although it was only slightly dysphasic. The 4-year-old boy was lively and had a good appetite. During the night of 6 January, he was heard to groan and then exhibited twitching of the right side of the face and a severe speech disturbance.

Admission to the Children's Hospital, Schaffhausen (6-11 January 1960).

FINDINGS. The child had expressive dysphasia, but showed no loss of receptive ability. There was intermittent twitching of the right side of the face, and he vomited profusely. His temperature was up to 38°C. Leucocytes 4900. ESR 8 mm in the first hour.

Lumbar Puncture. Markedly increased pressure; no cells; Pandy reaction + +; fluid clear.

Admission to the Children's Hospital, Zurich (11-13 January 1960).

FINDINGS. The patient was fully conscious, but apathetic. He showed complete motor aphasia, but no receptive disability. Central facial palsy was present. There was a flaccid weakness in the right arm with diminished tendon reflexes. An inconstant right Babinski response was elicited. There was no papilloedema, but suture diastasis was found on radiographic examination, and a cracked-pot sound on percussion. A chest radiograph was normal. There were no other relevant clinical findings. Electrocardiogram normal. The patient was afebrile. Leucocytes 10,500, juvenile forms 22 per cent, mature forms 44.5 per cent. Micro-ESR 5/8/16 mm. Macro-ESR 41 mm in the first hour.

EEG. A depression was shown over the left hemisphere, with a delta focus in the left fronto-temporal region. In addition, there was a severe general diffuse disturbance without epilepsy potentials.

Left Carotid Angiogram. A large avascular space-occupying process was demonstrated in the fronto-parietal region (Fig. 79).

Admission to The Department of Neurosurgery, University Hospital, Zurich.

OPERATION (13 January 1960). A radical resection was made of an encapsulated abcess from the left opercular region. Mixed anaerobic and aerobic organisms were isolated from the pus (haemophilus influenzae, streptococcus viridans, fusiform bacilli and streptococci).

COURSE. The neurological signs regressed rapidly, and on 20 January 1960 no deficit could be demonstrated.

EEG (24 February 1960). There was circumscribed slowing in the left fronto-temporal region. There was a suspicion of epilepsy, due to the presence of paroxysmal 3/second rhythms, which were partly generalised and partly over the left hemisphere.

EEG (19 August 1960). A slight diffuse disturbance was present, in that the background rhythm contained slow-wave bursts, some of which were rhythmical. The number of slow waves over the operation site was increased, and there was thus a suggestion of epilepsy potential.

OUTPATIENT FOLLOW-UP EXAMINATION (7 November 1961). The boy appeared to be in excellent condition. Apart from a mild expressive right facial palsy, no neurological deficit could be demonstrated. He remained free from attacks with regular anticonvulsant treatment.

COURSE (until August 1966). The boy continued to remain free from attacks with regular anti-convulsive treatment. There have been no signs of neurological deficit. He is a moderate pupil in the fourth class of the primary school. At times he shows an impairment of concentration.

CASE 69

H.T., born 13 August 1950.

FAMILY HISTORY. Nil relevant.

PREVIOUS HISTORY. Normal development. Pneumonia in 1956, otherwise no illnesses.

PRESENT ILLNESS. The girl was quite well on the morning of 2 April 1958, and participated in a school trip. In the afternoon, she experienced a sudden headache, particularly over the right eye, and vomited. By the following morning she was unable to speak, and presented with a left-sided hemiparesis.

Admission to the Department of Neurosurgery, University Hospital, Zurich (3-9 April 1958).

FINDINGS. On admission at 7 p.m., the patient was sub-comatose and unresponsive to commands, but she reacted to pain stimuli. A partial left-sided hemiparesis and a central left facial palsy were present. Ptosis was seen on the right side. Tendon jerks were symmetrically diminished, and bilateral Babinski responses were elicited. Muscular tone was normal. Right papilloedema was also present.

Right Carotid Angiogram (3 April 1958). There was massive displacement of the blood vessels upwards from the temporal fossa (Fig. 80).

OPERATION. A freshly coagulated haematoma about the size of a hen's egg was evacuated from the right temporal lobe; it had ruptured into the subarachnoid space.

COURSE. The patient made a remarkable recovery. Five days after the operation, she was transferred to another hospital, still with a discrete hemiparesis.

Outpatient Follow-up Examination (22 July 1958). The girl was free from complaints, apart from 'nervousness'. Only a discrete central facial palsy now remained; the limb weakness could no longer be demonstrated. In mid-October 1958, the right temporal craniotomy flap became gradually more prominent, and at the same time the patient began to complain of headache. On the following day she began vomiting.

Second Admission to the Department of Neurosurgery, University Hospital, Zurich (17 October 18 December 1958).

FINDINGS. Afebrile. Leucocytes 3400. ESR 7/17 mm. Blood pressure 120/70 mm Hg. There was a considerable protrusion in the region of the craniotomy flap, and a discrete left central facial palsy was present; there were no other abnormal clinical findings. The girl was mentally alert.

EEG. A severe disturbance was demonstrated over the right hemisphere, particularly in the frontal and postcentral regions. Cerebral activity was virtually normal over the left side.

Right Carotid Angiogram (18 October 1958). There was a massive displacement of the blood vessels from the temporal region (Fig. 80).

OPERATION (19 October 1958). Repeat craniotomy. A solid tumour about the size of a man's fist was radically removed from the tip of the right temporal lobe and the lateral part of the frontal lobe.

Histological Examination (Institute of Pathology, University of Zurich). An ependymoma was discovered.

COURSE. Palliative radiotherapy was commenced. Upon discharge from hospital on 18 December 1958, a moderate spastic hemiparesis remained which was more marked in the arm than in the leg. The right pupil was dilated and reacting to light. A moderate organic psychosyndrome was present.

The patient died at home on 20 June 1959, after outpatient follow-up examination two months previously had shown no change.

CASE 70

W.B., born 10 June 1951 (830, 1170/60).

FAMILY HISTORY. Nil relevant.

PREVIOUS HISTORY. Pregnancy, birth and development normal. In May 1960 the boy injured his head slightly in a bicycle accident. He was 'confused for a moment', but cycled on alone and showed no after effects. He was an average pupil in the third grade at primary school.

PRESENT ILLNESS. At the beginning of August 1960, the patient experienced two episodes of right-sided headache as he was getting up in the morning; these attacks were accompanied by vomiting and a transient feeling of heaviness in the right foot. The boy made a complete recovery, but on the afternoon of 8 August

1960 he suffered a sudden loss of power in the left leg. This was followed immediately by numbness and itchiness of the left arm (which was weak), nausea, and pallor of the face. He recovered in 10 minutes, but continued to drag his left foot on walking. The house doctor was called, and he found an asymmetry of the reflexes but no residual weakness; he referred the boy for specialist investigation.

Admission to the Cantonal Hospital, Lucerne (13 August 1960).

EEG. A delta focus was shown in the right postcentral region, with no epilepsy potentials. *Neurological Examination* performed on the same day revealed no abnormal findings.

For the following 5 weeks the boy attended school normally, except that he appeared to have more difficulty with calculation. During this period, he experienced five more attacks, each of which lasted only a few minutes and was characterised by sudden weakness in the left leg; however, there were no headaches.

Admission to the Children's Hospital, Zurich (12 September-11 October 1960).

FINDINGS. The patient was mentally normal, alert and free from subjective complaints. Apart from a slight difficulty with calculation, his intellectual functions were normal for his age. Muscle tone, power, and superficial and deep sensitivity were symmetrical and intact in all extremities. The only abnormal clinical finding was a slight increase in the reflexes of the left limbs, and a doubtful left Babinski response.

EEG (19 September 1960). A discrete disturbance was shown over the right postcentral region, consisting of low theta-delta waves interspersed in the background rhythm. No epilepsy potentials were demonstrated.

EEG (30 September 1960). Three days after the pneumoencephalogram, a definite intermittently discharging delta focus was demonstrated in the right postcentral region.

Pneumoencephalogram (27 September 1960). The body of the right lateral ventricle was shown to be displaced downwards (Fig. 81). *CSF.* Clear; cells normal; protein 54 mg per cent; colloidal gold reaction: 2222111111.

Right Carotid Angiogram (3 October 1960). There was an abnormal displacement of vessels in the right parietal region.

Admission to the Department of Neurosurgery, University Hospital, Zurich.

OPERATION (17 October 1960). Radical excision of a partly cystic astrocytoma about the size of a tangerine from the paramedian white matter of the right parietal region. *Histological Examination* (Institute of Pathology, University of Zurich). An astrocytoma was confirmed.

COURSE. A mild post-operative left hemiparesis was present, which regressed completely within a few weeks. Upon outpatient follow-up examination in May 1962, no definite neurological deficit could be demonstrated. The child was free from subjective complaints, and was doing well at school.

PROGRESS (up to August 1966). Slight weakness was present in the left extremities, but there was no obvious atrophy. The patient had a slight limp, but did not drag his foot. The weakness was most marked upon climbing. He made good progress at school, and was in the second grade of the secondary school. No attacks were observed, but headaches occurred now and then, especially after mild head injuries (*e.g.* after 'heading the ball' during football).

CASE 71

H.G., born 25 November 1931 (9973/38).

FAMILY HISTORY. Nil relevant.

PREVIOUS HISTORY. Pregnancy, birth and development normal. Frequent attacks of tonsillitis, culminating in tonsillectomy in December 1937.

PRESENT ILLNESS. The patient was well until 17 May 1938, but on the following morning, she experienced a pain in the left axilla followed by a loss of power in the left arm, so that by the time of the mid-day meal she was unable to hold a knife between her fingers. The axillary pain spread into the shoulder and upper arm. On the morning of 19 May 1938, she was free from pain and power had returned to the arm, so she went to school. During the afternoon, she experienced a sensation of formication in the left leg and a transient loss of power which made her fall over.

Admission to the Children's Hospital, Zurich (19 May-4 June 1938).

FINDINGS. The child had a severe flaccid weakness of the left arm, and was only able with great effort to raise the arm briefly to shoulder height, to flex and extend the elbow against light resistance, to dorsiflex the hand, and to make a fist; only minimal finger movements were present. Hyperaesthesia and hyperalgesia were present over the entire left arm. Tendon jerks in both arms were present and normal. Motor power was present, and sensory modalities were intact over both legs. There was a moderate symmetrical increase in knee jerks. No Babinski response was elicited, and abdominal reflexes were present on both sides. There was no meningism.

Lumbar Puncture. 3⅓ monocytes; protein 48 mg per cent; colloidal gold reaction 1223321111. Blood picture normal. The temperature was sub-febrile for several days.

COURSE. On 24 May 1938, the reflexes in the left arm became increased, and the left abdominal reflexes could no longer be elicited. Three days later an inequality of the pupils developed, with the left pupil widely dilated and reacting to light; a left ptosis appeared. All the symptoms disappeared within a few weeks. During the succeeding 17 years the patient enjoyed perfect health. Menarche occurred in the Autumn of 1946.

Early in 1955, when the patient was 23 years old, she experienced a sudden loss of sensation over the entire left leg up to the hip. She made a gradual complete recovery within 3 weeks. Early in 1960, she experienced a sudden loss of sensation and a feeling of coldness in both legs, from the hips to the toes; these symptoms were accompanied by a trembling in both hands, and regressed within 2 months. Early in 1961, she experienced a feeling of itchiness in all the fingers of the right hand. While this disturbance regressed within a week, a sudden numbness appeared in both knee joints and extended within a few days to involve both hips. A simultaneous unsteadiness of gait developed. The symptoms regressed within 3 weeks.

Outpatient Follow-up Examination at the Children's Hospital, Zurich (5 May 1961).

FINDINGS. There was bilateral temporal pallor of the optic fundi. Reflexes were symmetrically increased in all extremities, and a left Babinski response, a right Rossolimo response, and a bilateral Trömner-Hoffman (digital) reflex were all present. The patient also demonstrated dysarthria, left dysdiadochokinesia, and an intention tremor of both hands which was most marked on the left side. Her gait was uncertain, but she showed no tendency to fall.

Abdominal reflexes were absent on both sides, and hyperaesthesia was found in both calves.

CASE 72

C.R. born 4 October 1965 (9832/66).

FAMILY HISTORY. A 26-year-old maternal uncle had diabetes mellitus.

PREVIOUS HISTORY. Pregnancy and birth normal. Birth weight 3300g; child healthy. Psychomotor development normal. Cavernous haemangioma anterior to the hair line of the right temple, cicatrized by superficial irradiation.

PRESENT ILLNESS. The child suffered a mild head injury at the age of 10 months, when she fell 30 cm from the bed onto the carpeted floor. At the age of 11 months she twice bumped her head against the side of a table. There was some question of ill-treatment by her older playmates.

On 11 November 1966, the child was irritable, with a mild catarrhal rhinitis. Two days later she began vomiting, and on 16 November 1966 she became progressively more drowsy and lapsed into a pre-comatose state. Subsequently, it became known that on this day the child had experienced an epileptic attack (generalised, focal or unilateral? duration?).

Admission to the Children's Hospital, Zurich (16 November–20 December 1966).

FINDINGS ON ADMISSION. The patient was very drowsy, with flaccid right hemiparesis, which was more marked in the arm than the leg and involved the face. There was conjugate deviation of the head and eyes to the left side. Tendon reflexes were diminished, and abdominal reflexes were absent on the paralysed side. Several sharp focal haemorrhages were observed in both optic fundi.

Skull Radiographs (antero-posterior and lateral projections). Suture diastasis. No fractures seen.

EEG (17 November 1966). A marked depression of background activity was shown over the left side, with a diffuse non-specific disturbance over the right hemisphere.

Fontanelle Puncture. Bilateral dark, blood-stained effusions were evacuated under pressure from the subdural space.

Lumbar Puncture. The fluid was slightly blood-stained, and was shown after centrifugation to be definitely xanthochromic.

The patient was afebrile. Hb 9.6 g per cent; leucocytes 11,900, with normal differential count.

COURSE. Immediately after the first fontanelle puncture, the conjugate deviation disappeared, and the child regained consciousness. Daily subdural aspirations were carried out for one week. The hemiparesis gradually regressed with physiotherapy, and at the time of discharge on 20 December 1966 only a moderate spastic weakness of the arm remained. Mentally, the girl was normal.

EEG (9 December 1966). A marked, but somewhat reduced, depression was still present over the left hemisphere, particularly over the temporo-parieto-occipital region. There was normal cerebral activity over the right side.

CASE 73

P.B., born 5 November 1962 (8385/56).

FAMILY HISTORY. Mother with migraine and Raynaud's disease. Twin sister a mental defective in a special school.

PREVIOUS HISTORY. Pregnancy, birth and early psychomotor development normal. A regular visitor to the Outpatient Department from infancy (rickets at 4 months; dyspepsia, pharyngitis, impetigo in infancy; forearm fracture at 10 years). Operated on for perforated appendix at the age of 5 years, no complications. Fracture of humerus at 7 years. Transferred to special class at the age of 11 because of backwardness.

PRESENT ILLNESS. From the age of 5 years the boy often complained of headaches, which were frequently accompanied by vomiting. These episodes of headache became somewhat more frequent and severe after he started school at the age of 7 years. In October 1953 (at the age of 11 years), during an errand, he experienced a sudden attack of left-sided headache, followed immediately by a feeling of numbness over the right half of the face and the right arm, and a swollen feeling in the tongue. These symptoms all disappeared after a rest in bed. On 20 November 1953 during school, he suddenly found he could no longer see the blackboard and complained of a stabbing headache (side?), accompanied by a disturbance of sensation in the right arm, and an inability to write. One hour later, when he had been taken home to bed, he cried out and

complained of a numb feeling of the tongue; immediately thereafter he was unable to speak.

Emergency Admission to the Children's Hospital, Zurich (20 November 1953).

FINDINGS. On admission about 3 hours after the onset of the attack, the boy had motor aphasia. analgesia and hypaesthesia over the right half of the face, in the right half of the tongue, and in the right arm; the right leg was not affected. The left pupil was dilated and the left fundal veins were also markedly enlarged (right fundus normal). The patient exhibited areflexia, apart from a normal right ankle jerk; no Babinski response was elicited. Blood pressure 105/60 mm Hg. Pulse about 80/min, regular and full. Apart from an incidental systolic murmur, auscultatory findings of the heart were normal.

EEG (20 November 1953). Immediately after admission to hospital, a marked focal disturbance was demonstrated on the left side, with a maximum in the lateral central-precentral region; this disturbance consisted of rhythmic delta waves. The background rhythm over the left side was irregular and markedly reduced. Cerebral activity over the right hemisphere was normal. There was a normal synchronisation effect with photostimulation (Fig. 82*a*).

COURSE. About 2 hours after admission, the aphasia and the disturbance of sensation disappeared. The boy stated that his vision was no longer blurred, but the headache (left forehead and vertex) and the feeling of nausea were still present. Somewhat later, the patient vomited twice. On 21 November 1953, examination revealed a dilated left pupil, but no other neurological abnormality; the dilated left fundal veins had disappeared. However, the child continued to complain of a left-sided headache. In the course of the following day, he became free from complaints.

EEG (24 November 1953). There was episodic evidence of a very discrete disturbance in the left central region, with accentuated rhythmical delta activity. In addition, the background rhythm over the left hemisphere was on average $\frac{1}{2}$-1 Hertz slower. Hyperventilation accentuated the focal disturbance; photostimulation produced no abnormal effects (Fig. 82*b*).

EEG (30 January 1954). Normal findings.

FURTHER COURSE. On the morning of 26 February 1954, the patient experienced a sudden numbness of the right hand as he was rising. Within minutes, this feeling spread to involve the entire right arm, then the right side of the upper and lower lips, and thereafter the right half of the tongue. Fifteen minutes later, a severe left-sided headache and a feeling of nausea and retching occurred.

Clinical Examination (1 hour later). The child was obviously in pain, with marked expressive dysphasia and a slowness of speech. Definite hypaesthesia and hypalgesia were present in the right thumb and in the right side of the tongue. There was a doubtful disturbance of movement sensitivity in the fingers of the left (!) hand. The left palpebral fissure was more tightly closed than the right one. The left half of the face appeared definitely reddened and bloated. The fundal veins were definitely wider on the left side than on the right. Visual fields and acuity were normal. Cafergot given by mouth at the height of the attack had no effect, but the symptoms disappeared spontaneously in the course of the day. Cafergot appeared to be more useful if given at the onset of an attack of headache.

In May 1955, the patient began complaining every few days of attacks of sharp epigastric pain, which lasted several minutes and usually recurred after an interval of a few minutes. At the same time he experienced a feeling of nausea. Following a particularly severe attack, he was referred to hospital.

Admission to the Department of Surgery, the Children's Hospital, Zurich (7 June 1955).

FINDINGS. A thorough investigation, including gastro-intestinal barium studies, revealed no abnormal findings.

EEG (16 June 1955). Normal.

Detailed psychiatric examination revealed slight mental backwardness, but no evidence of an affective disturbance that could account for the subjective complaints. There were no psychopathological indications to suggest epilepsy.

COURSE. For about 6 months the boy, who was then nearly 13 years old, remained free from complaints. However, on the evening of 22 January 1956 he experienced a sudden attack of headache, which increased on both sides of the forehead, but more so on the right side. He was overcome by a profound sensation of nausea, experienced a numb feeling in the right side of his mouth, and exhibited twitching

movements in all four limbs. Physical examination on admission to hospital one hour later revealed no abnormal neurological findings apart from a slightly dilated left pupil. A sleep EEG (25 January 1956) revealed no abnormality, and repeat EEG examinations (14 February, 28 February 1956) also showed normal appearances.

PROGRESS (until March 1966). Over the years the migraine attacks diminished in frequency and intensity to about four a year. They were triggered off by changes in the weather and by mental tension. In recent years, the attacks have usually been heralded by flickering before the eyes, followed within minutes by unilateral or bilateral frontal headache; they are accompanied by nausea, retching or actual vomiting and anorexia. Only occasionally at present are they accompanied by paraesthesiae in the mouth and hand. On average, they last for one day, and their intensity varies. Treatment consists mainly of 'anti-headache' remedies. After leaving school the boy started an apprenticeship as a central heating mechanic, but he was unable to complete it successfully because of his low intelligence. He now works as a builder's labourer.

CASE 74

D.P., born 20 March 1950 (9501/63).

FAMILY HISTORY. After her first pregnancy the mother suffered from migraine, in the form of hemianopia, unilateral headache and nausea. A sister and maternal aunt had epilepsy. Maternal uncle died of meningitis (tuberculous ?) at the age of 20 years. Father suffered from asthma and eczema.

PREVIOUS HISTORY. Pregnancy, birth and psychomotor development normal. Repeated otitis media as a small child. At the age of $12\frac{1}{2}$ years he suffered mild concussion without losing consciousness, and subsequently he experienced occasional headaches. From early 1963 severe headaches were frequent.

PRESENT ILLNESS. In June 1963 during school classes, the boy experienced an attack of severe headache which followed immediately after a flickering before the eyes; he was unable to write properly or to find the correct words to speak. The dysphasia lasted for several hours.

On 3 September 1963, the boy visited his family doctor for a routine physical examination. In the waiting room he suddenly noticed that he was unable to see out of his right eye. A few minutes later a very severe headache commenced over the left vertex, and at the same time he experienced a numb feeling over the right side of the body, including the arm and the face. A physical examination immediately afterwards revealed an increased sensitivity to percussion over the left parietal region of the head, a marked hypaesthesia and a virtually complete analgesia in the right forearm, diminished tendon jerks in the right arm, and a right dysdiadochokinesia. During the examination, the doctor noted an increasing difficulty with speech, which led to a marked expressive dysphasia. The sensory and speech disturbances disappeared by the end of the morning, while the severe headache lasted for the rest of the day, and then gradually disappeared. The boy was anorexic and irritable, but he experienced no nausea or retching.

Admission to the Children's Hospital, Zurich (5-7 September 1963).

FINDINGS. The boy had no objective complaints, and there were no abnormal findings in the neurological or cardiovascular systems. The blood picture was normal. The pharynx was mildly inflamed. Coagulase positive haemolytic streptococci were isolated. ESR 9/23 mm.

EEG (5 September 1963). An intermittent non-specific disturbance was recorded in the left parietal region, in the form of isolated polymorphic delta waves. Photostimulation revealed only a slight synchronisation effect.

Sleep EEG (18 September 1963). Normal. A slight synchronisation effect was observed.

The field of vision (Goldmann perimeter) was normal in area and boundaries, with no central scotoma.

Skull Radiographs (antero-posterior and lateral projections). Normal.

COURSE. The patient was given Dihydergot (3 x 1 mg, then 3 x 1½ mg per day), and experienced a migraine attack every 1-3 weeks for many months. Only rarely could the attacks be controlled with Cafergot unless this was administered immediately after the onset of the visual disturbances.

PROGRESS (until March 1966). Withdrawal of the Dihydergot in September 1964 made no difference to the frequency of the attacks. On average, an attack occurred every 2-4 weeks, and each possessed a remarkably stereotyped pattern. This pattern was described by the child's teacher as follows: at first flashes occur before the eyes; these flashes are most severe on the side on which the subsequent headache will be most severe. With fixation of gaze, for close rather than for distant vision, a central spot appears which is surrounded by a rim of flashes of light. Following abatement of the visual disturbances after about 15-30 minutes, a unilateral headache commences over the posterior part of the head, usually on the left side and occasionally on the right, but never on both sides; the headache is of increasing intensity, and comes and goes in a rhythm of 2-4 seconds. At the same time a unilateral numbness, usually on the right side, of the mouth, cheek, tongue and fingers sets in; this spreads within seconds or minutes to involve the entire arm, and then passes down the leg to the foot on the ipsilateral side. At this stage, the boy can no longer speak, being unable to find the correct words, but he can indicate with his hands what he wants to say; he cannot read, since he cannot grasp the significance of the written word, and he cannot write since he does not know how to form the characters. These attacks last on average for 10-45 minutes, occasionally longer. When they pass, a very severe headache commences, which forces him to lie motionless, since any movement and particularly shaking of the head is unbearable. After a while, the acute pain changes into a dull and diffuse headache, which is usually still present when the boy awakes on the following day, and only fades away gradually. Retching and vomiting have not been prominent features, but anorexia and fatigue and slight nausea have accompanied the attacks. Trigger factors include all types of mental tension (*e.g.* impending examinations) and occasionally stroboscopic effects (*e.g.* mirror reflections of the sun, and on one occasion a photographic flash exposure). The patient is unable to indicate for certain whether a speech, a reading or a writing disturbance occurs with right-sided hemicranial attacks.

CASE 75

D.P. born 18 February 1951 (5099/65).

FAMILY HISTORY. Paternal aunt with migraine. Mother suffered from periodic headaches without the characteristic features of migraine.

PREVIOUS HISTORY. Pregnancy, birth and psycho-motor development normal. No serious illness or accident.

PRESENT ILLNESS. On 14 June 1965, when the patient was 14 years 4 months old, he suddenly experienced a stabbing pain over the left side of the head, which lasted for several hours; no other symptoms were present. He was given a tablet of Saridone and recovered. When he awoke the following morning, only a mild right-sided headache was present, which disappeared spontaneously in the course of the morning. In the evening, he suddenly developed a painful tingling sensation in the right hand, followed immediately by a complete loss of sensation; the boy appeared unable to resist any pressures on the hand. He had no headache. On the morning of 16 June 1965, he was unable to speak properly, and merely stammered. All sensation was lost from the right side of the tongue ('as after a dental injection'), and there was a tingling sensation over the right half of the tongue and mouth. At the same time, weakness appeared in the right hand *without* any disturbance of sensation. This episode lasted about 5 minutes, and was unaccompanied by headache. On the evening of the same day, he briefly experienced a feeling of numbness in the right thumb.

Admission to the Children's Hospital, Zurich (17-26 June 1965).

FINDINGS ON ADMISSION. The patient stated that he was free from complaints, and his neurological and cardiovascular systems were normal. Blood pressure 120/70 mm Hg. Blood picture normal. ESR 3/8 mm.

EEG (18 June 1965). There was a definite disturbance of function over the left hemisphere; it was maximal in the parieto-temporo-occipital region, and took the form of poly-morphic intermittent delta activity.

Lumbar Puncture. Pressure 8 cm; fluid normal in all respects (protein, cell count, colloidal gold reaction, glucose).

EEG (21 June 1965). An intermittent disturbance of function remained, but it was far less extensive compared with the first recording.

EEG (24 June 1965). The resting curve was normal; however, during hypoventilation a lateralising difference appeared, showing an abnormality in the left hemisphere.

EEG (1 July 1966). Normal findings.

On 20 June 1965, the patient experienced a sensation of formication in the right hand, which lasted only a few seconds and was followed by a mild headache. There were no abnormal physical findings.

COURSE (until July 1966). For 7 months, the patient had been taking dihydroergotamine (3 x 2.5 mg orally per day), and there had been no recurrence of attacks. He was a pupil in the third class of a junior technical school, and was experiencing no difficulty.

CASE 76

D.U., born 24 September 1946 (3930/61).

FAMILY HISTORY. A paternal uncle with cleft palate. No known cases of migraine.

PREVIOUS HISTORY. Pregnancy, birth and psycho-motor development normal. No serious illnesses or injuries before the sixth year when the child started school but was a bad pupil.

PRESENT ILLNESS. One day during school classes, when the patient was 15 years old, she suddenly found that she was unable to hold the pencil she was using, and it slipped out of her right hand. Within a few seconds the paralysis had spread to involve the entire right arm and the right side of the face, and at the same time her speech became indistinct. This hemisyndrome disappeared spontaneously after 10 minutes, and the girl then felt perfectly well. Two months later, on 20 October 1961, she suddenly experienced an attack of nausea and headache. Shortly afterwards a motor weakness of the right arm and the right side of the face occurred, without a disturbance of consciousness. The family doctor was called, although by the time of his arrival 15 minutes later the patient had recovered completely, and a physical examination was negative.

Admission to the Children's Hospital, Zurich (24 October-13 November 1961).

FINDINGS. The patient was mentally normal, and her neurological and cardiovascular systems were normal. Blood pressure 110/55 mm Hg. Pulse 80/min, regular and full. Blood picture normal. Macro-ESR 8/25 mm. There were signs of puberty commencing.

EEG. There were no abnormal findings, either in two routine recordings or in a sleep tracing.

288

Lumbar Puncture. Fluid clear; pressure 14 cm; all values normal (cells, protein, glucose, colloidal gold reaction).

Serum Chemistry. All parameters tested gave normal results (urea, calcium, protein, phosphorus, alkaline phosphatase). Fasting blood sugar normal (3 estimations).

Pneumoencephalogram. All parts of the right (!) lateral ventricles were slightly enlarged, but the remaining ventricles were normal in size, shape and position. There was no displacement of the ventricular system, and the basal cisterns showed normal appearances.

Left Carotid Angiogram. Opacification was good. The sylvian branches of the middle cerebral artery appeared to be rather poorly developed. In all other respects the arterial, capillary and venous phases showed normal appearances.

COURSE (until August 1966). In 1962 the patient experienced a second migraine attack with headache, nausea and sensory disturbances (formication and numbness) in the right arm. She immediately took Cafergot by mouth, and the symptoms cleared up promptly. Since that date, she has experienced an average of one attack of frontal headache a week, unaccompanied by other features. She is accustomed to taking one dragee of Cafergot to make the headache disappear. She works full time as a hairdresser.

CASE 77

E.U., born 30 January 1957 (3815/65).

FAMILY HISTORY. Father gave a history of headaches which had occurred since the age of 15 years, dependent on the weather. Since the age of 25 years they had become more frequent and typically migrainous (predominantly left-sided, inconstantly with fortification spectra, rarely with paraesthesiae of the hand, usually with vomiting at the peak). Paternal grandmother suffered from 'neuralgic headache'.

PREVIOUS HISTORY. Pregnancy, birth and psychomotor development normal. Tonsillectomy at the age of 3 years for frequent attacks of angina. Measles at 7 years, without complications.

PRESENT ILLNESS. On 20 January 1965, when the patient was a healthy 8-year-old girl, she suddenly experienced a tingling sensation in her left hand while writing during school lessons; a few minutes later, this was followed by a weakness in the left hand and a frontal headache (with no definite lateralisation). The headache increased continuously in intensity for several hours, and then receded at about noon. During the afternoon meal she experienced a sudden and severe attack of headache which obliged her to lie down quietly on her bed. She immediately fell deeply asleep. During the course of the afternoon and the night, she vomited once and complained of continuous frontal headache. The rectal temperature was 38.3°C. The frontal headache persisted on the following day, upsetting the child a great deal. The family doctor was called, who noticed a weakness in the left arm. On 22 January 1965, the frontal headache was unchanged and a flaccid left-sided hemiparesis had developed.

Admission to the Children's Hospital, Zurich (22-30 January 1965).

FINDINGS. On questioning, the patient complained of a bilateral frontal headache. She was somewhat apathetic, but gave clear and sensible answers. A flaccid left-sided hemiparesis was present; it was more marked distally, and affected the face only slightly. Tendon jerks were somewhat more brisk on the left side, and Babinski responses were absent. Sensation was not tested in detail, but a gross disturbance was ruled out. No other abnormality was demonstrated on physical examination. The patient was afebrile. Blood pressure 100/65 mm Hg. Pulse about 80/min, regular and full. Heart normal to percussion and auscultation. Leucocytes 6800, juvenile forms 20 per cent, mature forms 43 per cent, differential count otherwise normal.

Lumbar Puncture. Pressure 21 cm; fluid clear; all tests normal (cells, protein, glucose, colloidal gold reaction).

EEG (22 January 1965). A continuous severe disturbance was shown over the right hemisphere in the form of polymorphic slow activity with a widespread absence of normal frequencies; there was a focal maximum in the precentral region. No epilepsy potentials were present (Fig. 83a).

Right Carotid Angiogram. The sylvian branches of the middle cerebral artery appeared stretched and splayed, and at several levels their lumen appeared unusually narrowed. No other abnormality was detected in the arterial, capillary or venous phases.

COURSE. The motor hemiparesis had regressed considerably by the time the patient awoke from the anaesthetic after the carotid angiogram. Within several days, no neurological abnormality remained, and the child felt free from symptoms.

EEG (29 January 1965). A widespread improvement had taken place, although intermittent disturbances remained over the posterior parts of the right hemisphere (Fig. 83*b*). The patient was discharged from hospital on 30 January 1965. In the course of February 1965, two sudden attacks of headache occurred, both of which were frontal in distribution and unaccompanied by other features.

EEG (23 February 1965). Intermittent disturbances were recorded over the right hemisphere, with irregular slow wave groups; the latter were markedly activated by hyperventilation, and showed a parietal maximum.

Outpatient Follow-up Examination (23 February 1965). The neurological system was normal.

EEG (9 February 1966). The recording was normal, even upon hyperventilation and photostimulation.

Follow-up Control Examination (9 February 1966). Again no neurological abnormality was present. Since that date (up to July 1966), the child has remained free from complaints.

CASE 78
M.R., born 13 January 1949 (3501/61).

FAMILY HISTORY. Maternal grandmother and mother suffered from migraine (of variable unilaterality, with vomiting, but with no neurological deficits; in the mother it was usually associated with menstruation). Two older brothers and a younger sister healthy. One paternal aunt died of epilepsy at the age of 21 years.

PREVIOUS HISTORY. Pregnancy, birth and psychomotor development normal. No serious illnesses or injury.

PRESENT ILLNESS. In January 1961, the patient, a 12-year-old boy, awoke from sleep and vomited; he then complained of a severe headache. He went back to sleep, and after several hours awoke again with a persistent frontal headache (side?), followed promptly by a tingling sensation in the right arm, which spread proximally over the limb and the right side of the head (especially the mouth). Meanwhile,

the headache became more severe, and the boy could no longer speak clearly but could only stammer. After a few minutes, the symptoms gradually regressed and he was left in a state of complete exhaustion. He remained free from attacks until 13 June 1961. On this day he was on his way home from a swim when he experienced—immediately after fortification spectra—the sudden onset of a rapidly worsening left frontal headache. Soon after the headache commenced, a tingling sensation appeared in the right hand, and then spread within seconds up the arm until it involved the right half of the face as well. For a few minutes, a speech disturbance was present and he was unable to articulate properly. Then the attack began to fade, until all the symptoms had disappeared. A similar attack occurred a few hours later. On 23 August 1961, a further attack occurred, commencing with fortification spectra, followed by a severe right-sided headache and, after a few minutes, by vomiting. The symptoms regressed completely after 2-3 hours.

Admission to the Children's Hospital, Zurich (28-31 August 1961—during an interval).

FINDINGS. A clinical examination revealed no abnormal findings.

EEG. Normal findings.

CSF. Normal.

Skull Radiographs. Normal findings.

Histamine Stimulation Test. No effect in relation to the attack.

COURSE. In July 1964, when the boy was 15½ years old, he was on his way home from a swimming test when he experienced a sudden fortification spectrum of the right visual field, and could see objects only in the left half. Almost simultaneously tingling developed. It started in the right fingers and then spread up the arm until it involved the right half of the face. The patient continued home and went straight to bed. Apart from a feeling of fullness of the entire right side of the body, a weakness of the right extremities and facial muscles was now present; the patient was almost unable to move his leg, and found it very difficult to move his arm. A speech disturbance was also present, due to an inability to move the tongue. Simultaneously, the boy experienced a fear of death. Two hours later, a severe stabbing headache developed in the frontal region and between the eyes, and at the same time the weakness began to disappear. The boy was nauseated and vomited. All the symptoms regressed completely within half a day. In the Autumn of 1964, he suffered a fresh attack, with fortification spectra, paraesthesiae and unilateral headache, but without motor weakness.

COURSE (until July 1966). At the end of a 3-month course of Dihydergot, the patient experienced on average 1-2 attacks every 3-4 months. These attacks always commenced with fortification spectra, followed by unilateral frontal headache, and often, but not always, were accompanied by a feeling of numbness or tingling on one side in the hand and arm, by nausea and by vomiting. No medical treatment was undertaken. At present the patient is at a trade school, and participates wholeheartedly in sports activities.

CASE 79

R.V., born 9 January 1943 (216/56).

FAMILY HISTORY. Maternal grandmother and brother with epilepsy. No cases of migraine known.

PREVIOUS HISTORY. Birth at eight months gestation (birth weight 2700g). Normal psycho-motor development. No serious illnesses or injuries.

PRESENT ILLNESS. At the beginning of 1956 two attacks occurred. Both these attacks commenced shortly after the child had got up in the morning, and they consisted of a throbbing pain in the left temporal region lasting only a few minutes. On the morning of 18 September 1956 during the first lesson at school, the patient experienced a severe pain in the left temporal region, together with a feeling of giddiness and retching. The complaint was sufficiently severe for the girl to be sent home. On the way, she noticed that vision from her right eye was markedly blurred. At home she vomited, exhibited extreme facial pallor, and was put to bed. Her right extremities now became insensitive—she failed to react to the temperature of the hot water bottle applied close to her—and at the same time her right arm and leg became paralysed. From this point onwards, the patient was unaware of her surroundings until she 'awoke' in hospital with an intravenous drip infusion in her arm. In the afternoon of her attack the family doctor had found her drowsy, disorientated, and dysarthric, with

markedly restricted movements of the tongue; a right central facial palsy was present, with absent right abdominal reflexes, and generalised muscular hypotonia.

Emergency Admission to the Children's Hospital, Zurich (18 September 1956).

CLINICAL FINDINGS. On admission at 3 p.m. the patient was moderately confused, but was able to answer simple questions intelligently and could speak normally. There was a disturbance of swallowing and an abnormal palatal reflex. No weakness was found in the extremities and reflexes were normal. Her complexion was red, without lateralising differences. At 5 p.m. she was dysphasic, had a definite weakness of the right arm, and was no longer able to protrude the tongue. At 6.30 p.m. a definite weakness had also developed in the right leg. Dihydergot was given intravenously.

Lumbar Puncture. The fluid was clear and results were normal in all tests (pressure, cells, and glucose); protein 36 mg per cent (Kafka). Colloidal gold reaction 1223332111.

Blood pressure 105/90 mm Hg; pulse 90/min and regular. Hb 94 per cent; leucocytes 13,200, juvenile forms $\frac{1}{2}$ per cent, mature forms $77\frac{1}{2}$ per cent, basophils $\frac{1}{2}$ per cent, monocytes 11 per cent, lymphocytes 10 per cent, plasmocytes $\frac{1}{2}$ per cent. ESR 10/35 mm. The heart and lungs were normal to percussion and auscultation; radiological examination was also normal. Fasting blood glucose and serum calcium levels were normal. The patient was afebrile.

EEG (at 7 p.m.). A severe widespread disturbance was shown over the left hemisphere, with irregular delta activity which was maximal in the parieto-temporal region. The background rhythm was defective over the left side, and there were intermittent generalised outbursts of solitary slow wave complexes. Only moderate diffuse non-specific disturbances were shown over the right hemisphere, with much theta activity (Fig. 84a).

COURSE. On 19 September 1956, only a mild weakness of the right arm was still present. The patient appeared to be mentally slowed, but she was completely orientated. An EEG on this day revealed a definite lateralising difference, the left hemisphere disturbance being considerably less than on the previous occasion (Fig. 84b). On 22 September 1956, the patient experienced a second attack of severe left-sided headache, which responded to Dihydergot (1 mg intravenously).

Neurological examination revealed no abnormality.

EEGs (21 September 1956, 4 October 1956). Virtually normal (Fig. 84c).

COURSE (until March 1966). The patient continued to have frequent headaches, but they were rarely migrainous, *i.e.* of sudden unilateral onset and associated with visual disturbances. During 1961-1962, in the sixth month of her first pregnancy, she experienced another attack of severe left-sided headache, accompanied on this occasion by a left-sided weakness which lasted for several hours. A medical examination revealed no abnormality. A second pregnancy during 1963-64 passed off free from attacks of migraine.

CASE 80

T.M., born 27 August 1947 (1507/60).

FAMILY HISTORY. No known cases of typical migraine, although the girl's maternal grandmother and mother suffered from frequent severe headaches.

PREVIOUS HISTORY. Pregnancy, birth and psychomotor development normal. Cerebral concussion at the age of 4 years (vomiting, no loss of consciousness, no neurological features). From the age of 6-7 years, severe headaches accompanied each attack of common cold.

PRESENT ILLNESS. On 13 December 1960, when the girl was 13½ years old and in perfect health, she complained at school of a left-sided headache which rapidly increased in intensity and led to vomiting. She was sent home and went to bed. On questioning her, her parents found that she could only say a few words, and was apparently unable to read.

Emergency Admission to the Children's Hospital, Zurich (13 December 1960).

FINDINGS. On admission two hours after the onset of the attack, the patient was conscious and orientated. She was pallid, and had a mild speech disturbance which was more an inability to pronounce syllables correctly than an actual expressive dysphasia. She exhibited tachypnoea, with no spasmophilic symptoms. Her reading ability was severely disturbed. The pupils were unequal, the right one being dilated but reacting to light, and the optic fundi were normal. The visual field was normal to finger

testing. There were no other abnormal neurological findings, and in particular there was no evidence of any motor or sensory deficit. Blood pressure 130/80 mm Hg. The heart was normal to percussion and auscultation, apart from an incidental systolic murmur. Pulse about 80/min, regular and full.

Lumbar Puncture. Fluid clear; pressure 12 cm; total protein 39 mg per cent (Kafka). Normal values for cell count, glucose and colloidal gold reaction.

Hb 98 per cent; leucocytes 6500, with normal differential count. MACRO-ESR 3/7 mm. A routine clinical examination revealed no abnormality.

EEG (14 December 1960). A continuous delta focus was present in the left temporo-occipital region, with a depression of the background rhythm (Fig. 85a).

Left Carotid Angiogram (15 December 1960). A percutaneous puncture under general anaesthesia provided good visualisation of all three phases. No angiographic abnormality was demonstrated.

COURSE. Within a few hours the patient recovered completely.

EEG (16 December 1960). The focal disturbance had regressed considerably, and was now only intermittently present (Fig. 85b).

COURSE (until March 1966). During 1961 and 1962, the patient experienced several attacks of sudden unilateral headache associated with vomiting. Early in 1964, after she had commenced training as a saleswoman, she experienced a sudden attack of very severe left-sided headache preceded by fortification spectra. She became nauseated, and several hours later vomited. The symptoms disappeared in the course of a day, leaving her exhausted. A neurological examination revealed no abnormalities. In the Summer of 1964, she suffered a similar attack, which was successfully controlled by Cafergot. In 1965 she experienced two similar attacks, both preceding menstruation, and both treated successfully with Cafergot. She then remained free from symptoms for 8 months.

CASE 81

Z.P., born 26 November 1950 (4729/65).

FAMILY HISTORY. Father and paternal grandfather both migraine sufferers. Both paternal grandparents died in their sixties from strokes.

PREVIOUS HISTORY. Pregnancy, birth and psychomotor development normal. A middle ear infection, measles, whooping cough and chickenpox all passed without complications. At the age of 5 years, the boy suffered a mild head injury when he struck his head on getting off his bicycle, but he showed no evidence of concussion. During the evening meal a few hours later, he suddenly let a spoon slip from his right hand and at the same time began stammering; his parents noticed an asymmetry of the mouth and a marked redness of the face. All the symptoms disappeared spontaneously within 15 minutes. Upon questioning, the parents could no longer remember whether the child had complained of headache and nausea as well. Since starting school at the age of 7 years, their child has experienced 1-3 attacks of sudden headache a year, but there have been no other neurological disturbances.

PRESENT ILLNESS. On 4 May 1965 the patient, then a 14½-year-old pupil in a grammar school, had to sit a Latin examination which was causing him much anxiety. On arrival at school, he complained of a very severe headache, which was so bad that he was sent home and had to go to bed. After several hours of deep sleep, he was roused only with difficulty and gave monosyllabic, somewhat inadequate answers to questions. During the morning his temperature was normal, but in the evening it was 38°C (axillary). His condition was unaltered on the following day.

Admission to the Children's Hospital, Zurich (5-14 May 1965).

FINDINGS. The boy was drowsy and was unable to give an adequate history. He appeared to understand simple questions incompletely, failed to recognise certain objects, and answered questions in broken sentences that did not always make sense. It appeared that he was no longer familiar with everyday objects. He was unable to read or write. Upon detailed neurological examination, a right hemianopia was demonstrated, but there were no other abnormal findings; the fundi showed normal appearances. The cardiovascular system was normal. Pulse 70/min, regular and full, and palpable at the carotid, radial and dorsalis pedis arteries on both sides. Blood pressure 130/85 mm Hg. No murmurs synchronous with the pulse were heard over the head. The patient was right-handed. His temperature on admission was 38.5°C (axillary), but later he became afebrile. Blood: Hb 15.6 per cent; leucocytes 9500, juvenile forms 18 per cent, mature forms 54 per cent, monocytes 6½ per cent, lymphocytes 21½ per cent. Platelets normal. Macro-ESR 4/10 mm. Blood chemistry: normal values for glucose, urea, protein, calcium, phosphorus, alkaline phosphatase, chloresterol. Routine examination of urine normal.

Lumbar Puncture. Pressure 16 cm; fluid clear; normal values of cells, protein, glucose and colloidal gold reaction.

EEG (6 May 1965). There was a severe disturbance over the left hemisphere in the form of polymorphic, high-amplitude, sub-delta activity, with a definite maximum in the parieto-temporo-occipital region. Background activity was completely absent on this side. Intermittent rhythmic 2/sec wave groups were recorded on the left side, particularly in the frontal region, but were less marked on the right side. In addition, solitary generalised slow wave complexes were present. There was a moderately severe disturbance of cerebral activity over the right hemisphere. No epilepsy potentials were observed (Fig. 86a).

Left Carotid Angiogram (6 May 1965). A percutaneous puncture made under general anaesthesia gave good visualisation in both the antero-posterior and the stereoscopic lateral series. All three vascular phases were well demonstrated. No abnormality was detected.

COURSE. On the evening of 6 May 1965, the patient's condition remained unchanged, and he was given Dihydergot (0.5 mg intravenously). Within 20 minutes a definite improvement had occurred, in that the boy's receptive and expressive speech difficulties improved. However, there remained some disturbance of speech, writing, reading and calculating, as well as an inattention in the right field of vision. A second injection of Dihydergot (0.5 mg) 75 minutes later produced no noticeable effect. The gradual improvement continued throughout the next day. By 8 May 1965 the hemianopia had disappeared, and the boy exhibited mental difficulty only with complicated information. He volunteered that on the first day of the illness he had been seeing close objects at a distance. On 12 May 1965, some forgetfulness and lack of concentration remained present. Upon discharge, the boy was in complete possession of his intellectual faculties, and his neurological system was normal.

EEG (7 May 1965). There had been a gradual improvement, although a severe depression of the background activity of the left hemisphere was still present, and the maximum remained unaltered. A discrete disturbance was still present over the right side. Intermittent rhythmic 2/sec wave groups were recorded in the left frontal region (Fig. 86*b*).

EEG (10 May 1965). A further gradual improvement had taken place, and no other abnormality was detected.

EEG (14 May 1965). Marked intermittent delta rhythms were present over the left parieto-temporo-occipital region. Activity was normal over the right hemisphere (Fig. 86*c*).

EEG (14 June 1965). Intermittent discrete non-specific focal disturbances were recorded over the anterior and middle temporal region on the left side; otherwise cerebral activity was normal.

EEG (30 September 1965). Numerous paroxysmal wave groups were present over the anterior temporal regions of both hemispheres. The previous focal activity had disappeared.

EEG (3 March 1966). Discrete intermittent discharges were recorded over temporal regions of both hemispheres; otherwise all findings were normal.

COURSE. In June 1965, the patient experienced two attacks heralded by fortification spectra, 3 weeks apart, while still under regular treatment with Dihydergot (1 mg, three times per day, by mouth). The visual disturbance disappeared within minutes, and was followed by a throbbing left-sided headache, which was associated with an inability to speak; during one attack there was a 'buzzing' feeling in the right hand. The speech and sensory disturbances disappeared within 30 minutes, while the headache remained present for 3-4 hours on both occasions. No vomiting or nausea occurred. Brief attacks of right-sided headache following preliminary fortification spectra occurred in October and December 1965. In the interval periods between attacks, the patient was completely free from symptoms.

CASE 82

S.S., born 16 November 1959 (9993/66).

FAMILY HISTORY. Mother suffered from severe typical attacks of migraine. Three sisters healthy.

PREVIOUS HISTORY. Difficult pregnancy, but no serious complications. Normal birth one week before term. Birth weight 2700g; child healthy. Slightly delayed physical development (sitting up at 9 months, walking at 18 months). Above normal intelligence.

PRESENT ILLNESS. In November 1966, the child developed an intestinal disease which was initially regarded as Herter's disease, but which was shown upon investigation in the *Children's Hospital, Zurich* (8-26 November 1966) to be cystic fibrosis of the pancreas.

In the course of a pulmonary function test to estimate the level of oxygen saturation in the arterial blood (brachial artery punctured without complication) on 16 November 1966, the patient suddenly complained of dizziness, diminution of vision and flashes of light before the eyes. She appeared to have lost her memory for recent events, including the fact that it was her birthday. She vomited repeatedly, and passed into a state of severe drowsiness.

EEG (about one hour after the onset of the attack—16 November 1966). Bilateral intermittent high-amplitude delta wave groups were present over the parieto-occipital region. Photic stimulation demonstrated evoked responses with poorly differentiated initial components. The patient remained blind for about two hours, before she recovered vision in the left field; she continued to show a complete right hemianopia for a further hour. Repeated fundal examinations failed to show any abnormality. No long-tract signs were observed, although during the hemianopic phase a definite diminution of tactile and pain sensitivity was present over the left half of the body. The drowsiness gradually disappeared, and by the following morning the child had recovered completely.

EEG (17 November 1966). Somewhat less marked but still pronounced, predominantly left-sided, non-specific disturbances persisted with a maximum over the parieto-temporo-occipital regions. Visually evoked responses were now normal.

EEG (21 November 1966). There had been a widespread recovery of normal cerebral activity, and now only mild non-specific disturbances were present over the posterior parts of both hemispheres.

References

Introduction

REFERENCES

Alpers, B. J. (1928) 'The so-called "brain purpura" or "hemorrhagic encephalitis": a clinicopathologic study.' *Arch. Neurol. Psychiat.* (*Chic.*), **20,** 497.

Baker, A. B. (1935) 'Hemorrhagic encephalitis.' *Amer. J. Path.*, **11,** 185.

Benedikt, L. (1868) Elektrotherapie. Wien. (Cited by Freud, S. (1897).)

Cotard, S. (1868) Etude sur l'Atrophie Cérébrale. Paris: thesis. (Cited by Freud, S. (1897).)

Ford, F. R. (1966) Diseases of the Nervous System in Infancy, Childhood and Adolescence, 5th edn. Springfield, Ill.: C. C Thomas.

Ford, F. R., Schaffer, A. J. (1927) 'The etiology of acquired hemiplegia.' *Arch. Neurol. Psychiat.* (*Chic.*), **18,** 323.

Freud, S. (1897) 'Die Infantile Cerebrallähmung', *in* Nothnagel, H., Hölder, A. (Eds.) Specielle Pathologie und Therapie, Theil II, Abt II. Wien: A. Hölder.

Glanzmann, E. (1927) 'Die nervösen Komplikationen der Varizellen, Variola und Vaccine.' *Schweiz. med. Wschr.*, **57,** 145.

Gowers, W. R. (1888) A Manual of Diseases of the Nervous System. London: Churchill, p. 456. (Cited by Freud (1897).).

Grinker, R. R., Stone, T. T. (1928) 'Acute toxic encephalitis in childhood: clinico-pathologic study of 13 cases.' *Arch. Neurol. Psychiat.* (*Chic.*), **20,** 244.

Hurst, E. W. (1941) 'Acute haemorrhagic leucoencephalitis: a previously undefined entity.' *Med. J. Aust.* **2,** 1.

Jendrassik, E., Marie, P. (1885) 'Contribution à l'étude de l'hémiatrophie cérébrale par sclérose lobaire.' *Arch. de Physiol.*, **17,** 51.

Kundrat, H. (1882) Die Porencephalie, eine anatomische Studie. Graz: Leuschner und Lubensky. (Cited by Freud, S. (1897).)

Lovett, R. W. (1888) 'A clinical consideration of sixty cases of cerebral paralysis in children.' *Boston med. surg. J.*, **118,** 641. (Cited by Freud (1897).).

Mac Keith, R. (1962) *in* Bax, M., Mitchell, R. G. (Eds.) Acute Hemiplegia in Childhood. Little Club Clinics in Developmental Medicine, No. 6. London: Spastics Society with Heinemann. Cited in Preliminaries, p. 1.

Moniz, E. (1927) 'L'encéphalographie artérielle, son importance dans la localisation des tumeurs cérébrales.' *Rev. neurol.*, **34,** 72.

Osler, W. (1889) The Cerebral Palsies of Children. Philadelphia: Blakiston. (Cited by Freud (1897).).

Pette, H. (1942) Die akut entzündlichen Erkrankungen des Nervensystems. Leipzig: Thieme.

Scholz, W. (1951) Die Krampfbeschädigungen des Gehirns. Berlin: Springer.

Spielmeyer, W. (1927) 'Die Pathogenese des epileptischen Krampfes.' *Z. ges. Neurol. Psychiat.*, **109,** 501.

Taylor, J. (1905) Paralysis and other Diseases of the Nervous System in Childhood and Early Life. London: J. & A. Churchill. (Cited by Wyllie, W. G. (1948).)

van Bogaert, L. (1932) 'Essai d'interprétation des manifestations nerveuses observées au cours de la vaccination de la maladie sérique et des maladies éruptives.' *Rev. neurol.*, **2,** 1.

von Strümpell, A. (1885) 'Über die akute Encephalitis der Kinder (Polioencephalitis acuta, zerebrale Kinderlähmung).' *Jb. Kinderheilk.* (*Berlin*), **22,** 173.

—— (1890) 'Über primäre akute Encephalitis.' *Dtsch. Arch. klin. Med.*, **47,** 53.

Wernicke, C. (1881) 'Die acute, hämorrhagische Polioencephalitis superior.' *in* Wernicke, C. (Ed.) Lehrbuch des Gehirnkrankheiten für Aerzte und Studirende. Kassel u. Berlin: T. Fischer.

Wyllie, W. G. (1948) 'Acute infantile hemiplegia.' *Proc. roy. Soc. Med.*, **41,** 459.

Zimmerman, H. M. (1938) 'The histopathology of convulsive disorders in children.' *J. Pediat.*, **13,** 859.

ADDITIONAL READING

Leichtenstern, O. (1892) 'Uber primäre acute hämorrhagische Encephalitis.' *Dtsch. med. Wschr.*, **18,** 39.

Spielmeyer, W. (1933) 'Functionelle Kreislaufstörungen und Epilepsie.' *Z. ges. Neurol. Psychiat.*, **148,** 285.

Chapter 1. Arteriovenous Malformations

REFERENCES

Clément, R., Gerbeaux, J., Combes-Hamelle, A., Pertuiset, B., Pétranca, C. (1954) 'Anévrysmes artérioveneux de l'ampoule de Galien chez le nourrisson; leur rôle dans l'hydrocephalie non communicante.' *Presse méd.*, **62,** 658.

Ford, F. R. (1966) Diseases of the Nervous System in Infancy, Childhood and Adolescence. 5th edn. Springfield, Ill.: C. C Thomas.

Hamby, W. B. (1958) 'The pathology of supratentorial angiomas.' *J. Neurosurg.*, **15**, 65.

Harper, W. F., Vyse, H. G. (1953) 'A massive intracranial arteriovenous angioma in an infant.' *W. Indian med. J.*, **2**, 269.

Krayenbühl, H., Yasargil, M. G. (1958) 'Das Hirnaneurysma.' *Docum. Geigy, Ser. chir.*, no. 4.

Litvak, J., Yahr, M. D., Ransohoff, J. (1960) 'Aneurysms of the great vein of Galen and midline cerebral arteriovenous anomalies.' *J. Neurosurg.*, **17**, 945.

Olivecrona, H. (1950) 'Die arteriovenösen Aneurysmen des Gehirns.' *Dtsch. med. Wschr.*, **75**, 1169.

Padget, D. H. (1956) 'Cranial venous system in man in reference to development, adult configuration and relation to arteries.' *Amer. J. Anat.*, **98**, 307.

Poppen, J. L., Avman, N. (1960) 'Aneurysms of the great vein of Galen.' *J. Neurosurg.*, **17**, 238.

Potter, J. M. (1955) 'Angiomatous malformations of the brain; their nature and prognosis.' *Ann. roy. Coll. Surg. Engl.*, **16**, 227.

Russell, D. S., Nevin, S. (1940) 'Aneurysm of the great vein of Galen causing internal hydrocephalus.' *J. Path. Bact.*, **51**, 375.

Schultz, E. C., Huston, W. A. (1956) 'Arteriovenous aneurysm of the posterior fossa in an infant; report of a case.' *J. Neurosurg.*, **13**, 211.

Shealy, C. N., LeMay, M. (1964) 'Unusual vascular malformations and the value of cerebral angiography in patients with mass lesions.' *J. Neurosurg.*, **21**, 461.

Tönnis, W. (1957) 'Symptomatik und Klinik der supratentoriellen arteriovenösen Angiome.' *in* 1. Congrès International de Neurochirurgie, Bruxelles, 1957. Brussels: Acta Medica Belgica.

ADDITIONAL READING

Elkin, D. C., Warren, J. V. (1947) 'Arteriovenous fistulas: their effect on the circulation.' *J. Amer. med. Ass.*, **134**, 1524.

Glatt, B. S., Rowe, R. D. (1960) 'Cerebral arteriovenous fistula associated with congestive heart failure in the newborn.' *Pediatrics*, **26**, 596.

Hamby, W. B. (1957) 'The pathology of supratentorial angiomas.' *in* 1. Congrès International de Neurochirurgie, Bruxelles, 1957. Brussels: Acta Medica Belgica.

Krayenbühl, H., Yasargil, M. G. (1965) Die zerebrale Angiographie. 2nd edn. Stuttgart: Thieme.

Lagos, J. C., Riley, H. D. (1971) 'Congenital intracranial vascular malformations in children'. *Arch. Dis. Childh.*, **46**, 285.

Levine, O. R., Jameson, A. G., Nellhaus, G., Gold, A. P. (1962) 'Cardiac complications of cerebral arteriovenous fistula in infancy.' *Pediatrics*, **30**, 563.

McCormick, W. F. (1966) 'The pathology of vascular ("arteriovenous") malformations.' *J. Neurosurg.*, **24**, 807.

Norman, J. A., Schmidt, K. W., Grow, J. B. (1950) 'Congenital arteriovenous fistula of the cervical vertebral vessels with heart failure in an infant.' *J. Pediat.*, **36**, 598.

Pollock, A. Q., Laslett, P. A. (1958) 'Cerebral arteriovenous fistula producing cardiac failure in the newborn infant.' *J. Pediat.*, **53**, 731.

Pool, J. L., Potts, D. G. (1965) Aneurysms and Arteriovenous Anomalies of the Brain: Diagnosis and Treatment. New York: Hoeber-Harper.

Silverman, B. K., Breckx, T., Craig, J. M., Nadas, A. S. (1955) 'Congestive failure in the newborn caused by cerebral a.-v. fistula.' *Amer. J. Dis. Child.*, **89**, 539.

Tönnis, W., Schiefer, W., Walter, W. (1958) 'Signs and symptoms of supratentorial arterio-venous aneurysms.' *J. Neurosurg.*, **15**, 471.

Walker, W. J., Mullins, C. E., Knovick, G. C. (1964) 'Cyanosis, cardiomegaly and weak pulses. A manifestation of massive congenital systemic arteriovenous fistula.' *Circulation*, **29**, 777.

Chapter 2. Saccular Arterial Aneurysm

REFERENCES

Hofer, S. (1966) 'Unabgeklärte Subarachnoidalblutung.' *Schweiz. Arch. Neurol. Neurochir. Psychiat.*, **97**, 241.

Jane, J. A. (1961) 'A large aneurysm of the posterior inferior cerebellar artery in a one-year-old child.' *J. Neurosurg.*, **18**, 245.

Jones, R. K., Shearburn, E. W. (1961) 'Intracranial aneurysm in a four-week-old infant. Diagnosis by angiography and successful operation.' *J. Neurosurg.*, **18**, 122.

Krayenbühl, H., Yasargil, M. D. (1958) 'Das Hirnaneurysma.' *Docum. Geigy, Ser. chir.*, no. 4.

Laitinen, L. (1964) 'Arteriella aneurysm med subarachnoidalblödning hos barn.' *Nord. Med.*, **71**, 329.

Matson, D. D. (1965) 'Intracranial arterial aneurysms in childhood.' *J. Neurosurg.*, **23**, 578.

McDonald, C. A., Korb, M. (1939) 'Intracranial aneurysms.' *Arch. Neurol. Psychiat. (Chic.)*, **42**, 298.

McKissock, W., Paine, K. W. E. (1959) 'Subarachnoid haemorrhage.' *Brain*, **82,** 356.
Newcomb, A. L., Munns, G. F. (1949) 'Rupture of an aneurysm of the circle of Willis in the newborn.' *Pediatrics*, **3,** 769.

ADDITIONAL READING

Ingraham, F. D., Matson, D. D. (1954) Neurosurgery in Infancy and Childhood. Springfield, Ill.: C. C Thomas.
Kimbell, F. D., Llewellyn, R. C., Kirgis, H. D. (1960) 'Surgical treatment of ruptured aneurysm with intracerebral and subarachnoid hemorrhage in 16-month-old infant.' *J. Neurosurg.*, **17,** 331.
McKissock, W. (1959) 'Some aspects of subarachnoid haemorrhage.' *Brit. J. Radiol.*, **32,** 79.
Poppen, J. L. (1951) 'Specific treatment of intracranial aneurysms. Experiences with 143 surgically treated patients.' *J. Neurosurg.*, **8,** 75.
Ritchie, W. P., Haines, G. L. (1953) 'Spontaneous intracranial hemorrhage in children. Report of eight cases in children fifteen years of age or younger.' *Arch. Surg.*, **66,** 452.

Chapter 3. Cerebral Venous Aneurysm

REFERENCES

Ford, F. R. (1966) Diseases of the Nervous System in Infancy, Childhood and Adolescence. 5th edn. Springfield, Ill.: C. C Thomas.
Lindgren, E. (1939) 'Über corticale Verkalkungen im Gehirn.' *Nervenarzt*, **12,** 138.
Metzger, J. (1950) Les Calcifications Intra-Crâniennes Chez l'Enfant. Paris, thesis.
Poser, C. M., Taveras, J. M. (1957) 'Cerebral angiography in encephalotrigeminal angiomatosis.' *Radiology*, **68,** 327.
Thieffry, S., Arthuis, M., Fauré, C., Lyon, G. (1961) 'L'angiomatose de Sturge-Weber.' *in* XVIIIème Congrès de l'Association des Pédiatres de Langue Francaise. Genève, 1961. Rapports II. Basel: Karger.

ADDITIONAL READING

Di Chiro, G., Lindgren, E. (1951) 'Radiographic findings in 14 cases of Sturge-Weber syndrome.' *Acta radiol. (Stockh.)*, **35,** 387.
Peterman, A. F., Hayles, A. B., Dockerty, M. B., Love, G. J. (1958) 'Encephalotrigeminal angiomatosis (Sturge-Weber disease).' *J. Amer. med. Ass.*, **167,** 2169.
Tönnis, W., Friedmann, G. (1964) 'Röntgenologische und klinische Befunde bei 23 Patienten mit Sturge-Weber-Erkrankung.' *Zbl. Neurochir.*, **25,** 1.

Chapter 4. Dissecting Aneurysm

REFERENCES

Field, C. M., Carson, N. A. J., Cusworth, D. H., Dent, C. E., Neill, D. W. (1962) 'Homocystinuria: a new disorder of metabolism.' *in* Abstracts of 10th International Congress of Pediatrics, Lisbon 1962. Lisbon: Freitas Brito.
Gerritsen, T., Vaughn, J. G., Waisman, H. A. (1962) 'The identification of homocystine in the urine.' *Biochem. biophys. Res. Commun.*, **9,** 493.
Gibson, J. B., Carson, N. A. J., Neill, D. W. (1964) 'Pathological findings in homocystinuria.' *J. clin. Path.*, **17,** 427.
Norman, R. M., Urich, H. (1957) 'Dissecting aneurysm of the middle cerebral artery as a cause of acute infantile hemiplegia.' *J. Path. Bact.*, **73,** 580.
Scott, G. E., Neuberger, K. T., Denst, J. (1960) 'Dissecting aneurysms of intracranial arteries.' *Neurology (Minneap).*, **10,** 22.
Wisoff, H. S., Rothballer, A. B. (1961) 'Cerebral arterial thrombosis in children.' *Arch. Neurol. (Chic.)*, **4,** 258.
Wolman, L. (1959) 'Cerebral dissecting aneurysms.' *Brain*, **82,** 276.

ADDITIONAL READING

Gerritsen, T., Waisman, H. A. (1964) 'Homocystinuria: absence of cystathionine in the brain.' *Science*, **145,** 588.
Isler, W. (1960) 'Aneurysma dissecans und entzündliches Aneurysma mit Angiospasmen bei Kindern.' *Schweiz. Arch. Neurol. Neurochir. Psychiat.*, **85,** 210.
Jacob, J. C., Maroun, F. B., Heneghan, W. B., House, A. M. (1970) 'Uncommon cerebrovascular lesions in children.' *Develop. Med. Child Neurol.*, **12,** 446.
Nelson, J. W., Styri, O. B. (1968) 'Dissecting subintimal hematomas of the intracranial arteries: report of a case (5-year-old boy).' *J. Amer. Osteopath. Ass.*, **67,** 512.

Spudis, E. V., Scharyj, M., Alexander, E., Martin, J. F. (1962) 'Dissecting aneurysms in the head and neck.' *Neurology (Minneap.)*, **12**, 867.

Werder, E. A., Curtius, H. C., Tancredi, F., Anders, P. W., Prader, A. (1966) 'Homocystinuria.' *Helv. paediat. Acta,* **21**, 1.

Chapter 5. Cerebral Microangioma

REFERENCES

Bailey, O. T., Woodard, J. S. (1959) 'Small vascular malformations of the brain: their relationship to unexpected death, hydrocephalus and mental deficiency.' *J. Neuropath. exp. Neurol.*, **18**, 98.

Crawford, J. V., Russell, D. S. (1956) 'Cryptic arteriovenous and venous hamartomas of brain.' *J. Neurol. Neurosurg. Psychiat.*, **19**, 1.

Gerlach, J., Jensen, H. P. (1961) 'Die intrazerebralen Hämatome bei Mikroangiomen.' *Acta neurochir. (Wien)*, Suppl. VII, 367.

Jensen, H. P., Brumlik, J., Boshes, B. (1963) 'The application of serial angiography to diagnosis of the smallest cerebral angiomatous malformations.' *J. nerv. ment. Dis.*, **136**, 1.

Krayenbühl, H., Siebenmann, R. (1965) 'Small vascular malformations as a cause of primary intra-cerebral damage.' *J. Neurosurg.,* **22**, 7.

—— Siegfried, J. (1964) 'Der Neurochirurgische Beitrag zur Behandlung der intrazerebralen Blutung.' *Wien. klin. Wschr.*, **76**, 401.

—— Yasargil, M. G. (1958) 'Das Hirnaneurysms.' *Docum. Geiegy, Ser. chir.*, no. 4.

Lazorthes, G. (1956) L'Hémorragie Cérébrale, Vue par le Neurochirurgien. Paris: Masson.

Margolis, G., Odom, G. L., Woodhall, B., Bloor, B. M. (1951) 'The role of small angiomatous malformations in the production of intracerebral hematomas.' *J. Neurosurg.*, **8**, 564.

—— —— —— (1961) 'Further experiences with small vascular malformations as a cause of massive intracerebral bleeding.' *J. Neuropath. exp. Neurol.*, **20**, 161.

McDonald, J. V. (1959) 'Spontaneous intracerebral bleeding in children from cryptic vascular hamartomas.' *J. Pediat.*, **55**, 200.

Walter, W. (1965) 'Klinik, Diagnostik und operative Behandlung der intrakraniellen Gefässmiss-bildungen und nicht-traumatischen Blutungen. Dissertation: University of Cologne.

—— Schütte, W. (1965) 'Zur Klinik und Pathogenese des spontanen intrazerebralen Hämatoms.' *Dtsch. Z. Nervenheilk.* **187.**, 660.

ADDITIONAL READING

Bailey, O. T. (1961) 'The vascular component of congenital malformations in the central nervous system.' *J. Neuropath. exp. Neurol.*, **20**, 170.

Bell, W. E., Butler, C. (1968) 'Cerebral mycotic aneurysms in children. Two case reports.' *Neurology (Minneap.)*, **18**, 81.

Gerlach, J., Jensen, H. P., (1960) 'Mikroangiome des Gehirns.' *Langenbecks Arch. klin. Chir.*, **293**, 481.

Hassler, O. (1961) 'Morphologic studies on the large cerebral arteries: with reference to aetiology of subarachnoid haemorrhage.' *Acta psychiat. scand.*, Suppl. 154, 36.

Lazorthes, G. (1952) Les Hemorragies Intracrâniennes, Traumatiques, Spontanées et du Premier Age. Paris: Masson.

—— (1959) 'Surgery of cerebral hemorrhage. Report on the results of 52 surgically treated cases.' *J. Neurosurg.*, **16**, 355.

Papatheodorou, C. A., Gross, S. W., Hollin, S. (1961) 'Small arteriovenous malformations of the brain.' *Arch. Neurol. (Chic.)*, **5**, 666.

Chapter 6. Focal Arteritis

REFERENCES

Adler, M. (1965) 'Acute hemiplegia in childhood.' *Brit. med. J.*, **i**, 58.

Bell, W. E., Butler, C. (1968) 'Cerebral mycotic aneurysms in children. Two case reports.' *Neurology (Minneap.)*, **18**, 81.

Bickerstaff, E. R. (1964) 'Aetiology of acute hemiplegia in childhood.' *Brit. med. J.*, **ii**, 82.

Ford, F. R., Schaffer, A. J. (1927) 'The etiology of infantile acquired hemiplegia.' *Arch. Neurol. Psychiat. (Chic.)*, **18**, 323.

Litchfield, H. R. (1938) 'Carotid artery thrombosis complicating retropharyngeal abscess.' *Arch. Pediat.*, **55**, 36.

Pouyanne, H., Arne, L., Loiseau, P., Mouton, L. (1957) 'Considérations sur deux cas de thrombose de la carotide interne chez l'enfant.' *Rev. neurol.*, **97**, 525.

Rocand, J. (1961) Les Thromboses Carotidiennes et Sylviennes de l'Enfant. Paris: thesis.

Shillito, J. (1964) 'Carotid arteritis. A cause of hemiplegia in childhood.' *J. Neurosurg.*, **21**, 540.

ADDITIONAL READING

Garland, H., Pearce, J. (1965) 'Carotid arteritis as a cause of cerebral ischaemia in the adult.'
Lancet, **i**, 993.
Heidelberger, K. P., Layton, W. M., Fisher, R. G. (1968) 'Multiple cerebral mycotic aneurysms complicating post-traumatic pseudomonas meningitis'. *J. Neurosurg.*, **29**, 631.
Isler, W. (1960) 'Aneurysma dissecans und entzündliches Aneurysma mit Angiospasmen bei Kindern.'
Schweiz. Arch. Neurol. Neurochir. Psychiat., **85**, 210.
Keith, H. M., Baggenstoss, A. H. (1941) 'Primary arteritis (peri-arteritis nodosa) among children.'
J. Pediat., **18**, 494.
Malamud, N. (1945) 'A case of periarteritis nodosa with decerebrate rigidity and extensive encephalomalacia in a five-year-old child.' *J. Neuropath. exp. Neurol.*, **4**, 88.
Petit-Dutaillis, D., Janet, H., Thiébaut, F., Guillaumat, L. (1949) 'Les effets d'une inversion circulatoire par anastomose carotido-jugulaire sur une hémiplegie droite avec aphasie, due à une thrombose de la carotide interne d'origine inconnue chez un adolescent.' *Rev. neurol.*, **81**, 997.
Schnüriger, V. (1966) 'Verschlüsse der Arteria carotis interna bei Jungendlichen. Beitrag zur Ätiologie an Hand Zweier Fälle von Arteritis.' *Schweiz. med. Wschr.*, **96**, 615.

Chapter 7. Fibromuscular Hyperplasia

REFERENCES

Connett, M. C., Lansche, J. M. (1965) 'Fibromuscular hyperplasia of the internal carotid artery. Report of a case.' *Ann. Surg*, **162**, 59.
Huber, P., Fuchs, W. A. (1967) 'Gibt es eine fibromuskuläre Hyperplasie zerebraler Arterien?'
Fortschr. Rontgenstr., **107**, 119.
Kincaid, O. W. (1966) Renal Angiography. Chicago: Yearbook Medical Publishers.
McCormack, L. J., Dustan, H. P., Meaney, T. F. (1967) 'Selected pathology of the renal artery.'
Semin. Roentgenol., **2**, 126.
Palubinskas, A. J., Newton, T. H. (1965) 'Fibromuscular hyperplasia of the internal carotid arteries.'
Radiol. clin. biol., **34**, 365.
—— Perloff, J. D., Newton, T. H. (1966) 'Fibromuscular hyperplasia. An arterial dysplasia of increasing clinical importance.' *Amer. J. Roentgenol.*, **98**, 907.

ADDITIONAL READING

Andersen, P. E. (1970) 'Fibromuscular hyperplasia in children.' *Acta Radiol. [Diagn.] (Stockh.)*, **10**, 203.
Baum, S. (1967) 'Renal ischemic lesions.' *Radiol. Clin. N. Amer.*, **5**, 543.
Hunt, J. C., Harrison, E. G., Kincaid, O. W., Bernatz, P. E., Davis, G. D. (1962) 'Idiopathic fibrous and fibromuscular stenoses of the renal arteries associated with hypertension.' *Proc. Mayo Clin.*, **37**, 181.
McCormack, L. J., Poutasse, E. F., Meaney, T. F., Noto, T. J., Dustan, H. P. (1966) 'A pathologic-arteriographic correlation of renal arterial disease.' *Amer. heart J.*, **72**, 188.
Palubinskas, A. J., Wylie, E. J. (1961) 'Roentgen diagnosis of fibromuscular hyperplasia of the renal arteries.' *Radiology*, **76**, 634.
Sandok, B. A., Houser, O. W., Baker, H. L., Holley, K. E. (1971) 'Fibromuscular dysplasia: neurologic disorders associated with disease involving the great vessels in the neck.' *Arch. Neurol. (Chic.)*, **24**, 462.
Wylie, E. J., Wellington, J. S. (1960) 'Hypertension caused by fibromuscular hyperplasia of the renal arteries.' *Amer. J. Surg.*, **100**, 183.

Chapter 8. Multiple Occlusions with Unusual Net-like Collaterals ('Moyamoya Disease')

REFERENCES

Harwood-Nash, D. C., McDonald, P., Argent, W. (1971) 'Cerebral arterial disease in children; an angiographic study of 40 cases.' *Amer. J. Roentgenol.*, **111**, 672.
Kawakita, Y., Abe, K., Miyata, Y., Horiskoshi, S. (1965) 'Spontaneous thrombosis of internal carotid artery in children.' *Folia psychiat. neurol. Jap.*, **19**, 245.
Kudo, T. (1968) 'Spontaneous occlusion of the circle of Willis. A disease apparently confined to Japanese.' *Neurology (Minneap.)*, **18**, 485.
Leeds, N. E., Abbott, K. H. (1965) 'Collateral circulation in cerebrovascular disease in childhood via rete mirabile and perforating branches of anterior choroidal and posterior cerebral arteries.', *Radiology*, **85**, 628.
Maki, Y., Nakata, Y. (1965) 'An autopsy case of hemangiomatous malformation of bilateral internal carotid artery at base of brain.' *Brain Nerve, Tokyo*, **17**, 764.

Nishimoto, A., Takeuchi, S. (1968) 'Abnormal cerebrovascular network related to the internal carotid arteries.' *J. Neurosurg.*, **29**, 255.
Solomon, G. E., Hilal, S. K., Gold, A. P., Carter, S. (1970) 'Natural history of acute hemiplegia of childhood.' *Brain*, **93**, 107.
Suzuki, J., Takaku, A. (1969) 'Cerebrovascular "Moyamoya" disease. Disease showing abnormal net-like vessels in base of brain.' *Arch. Neurol. (Chic.)*, **20**, 288.
—— —— Asahi, M. (1965) 'Diseases showing the 'fibrilla'-like vessels at the base of the brain.' *Brain Nerve, Tokyo*, **17**, 767. (Cited by Suzuki and Takaku (1969).).
Taveras, J. M. (1969) 'Multiple progressive intracranial arterial occlusions: a syndrome of children and young adults.' *Amer. J. Roentgenol.*, **106**, 235.
Weidner, W., Hanafee, W., Markham, C. H. (1965) 'Intracranial collateral circulation via lepto-meningeal and rete mirabile anastomoses.' *Neurology (Minneap.)*, **15**, 39.

ADDITIONAL READING

Busch, H. F. (1969) 'Unusual collateral circulation in a child with cerebral arterial occlusion.' *Psychiat. Neurol. Neurochir. (Amst.)*, **72**, 23.

Chapter 9. Arteriosclerosis

REFERENCES

Andersen, D. H., Schlesinger, E. R. (1942) 'Renal hyperparathyroidism with calcification of the arteries in infancy.' *Amer. J. Dis. Child.*, **63**, 102.
Baker, A. B., Iannone, A. (1959) 'Cerebrovascular disease. I. The large arteries of the circle of Willis. II. The smaller intracerebral arteries. III. The intracerebral arterioles.' *Neurology (Minneap.)*, **9**, 321, 391, 441.
Cochrane, W. A., Bowden, D. H. (1954) 'Calcification of the arteries in infancy and childhood.' *Pediatrics*, **14**, 222.
Duffy, P., Portnoy, B., Mauro, J., Wehrle, P. (1957) 'Acute infantile hemiplegia secondary to spontaneous carotid thrombosis.' *Neurology (Minneap.)*, **7**, 664.
Field, M. H. (1946) 'Medial calcification of the arteries of infants.' *Arch. Path.*, **42**, 607.
Fields, W. S., Edwards, W. H., Crawford, E. S. (1961) 'Bilateral carotid artery thrombosis.' *Arch. Neurol. (Chic.)*, **4**, 369.
Ford, F. R., Schaffer, A. J. (1927) 'The etiology of infantile acquired hemiplegia.' *Arch. Neurol. Psychiat. (Chic.)*, **18**, 323.
Griffioen, H., Pieterse, J. J. (1965) 'Apoplexie bij een twaalfjarige jongen.' *Maandschr. Kindergeneesk.*, **33**, 364.
Holman, R. L. (1961) 'Atherosclerosis—a pediatric nutrition problem?' *Amer. J. clin. Nutr.*, **9**, 565.
Jannsen, W. (1957) 'Zur Frage der kindlichen Arteriosklerose, besonders der Herzkranzgefässe.' *Mschr. Kinderheilk.*, **105**, 361.
Matson, D. D. (1965) 'Intracranial arterial aneurysms in childhood.' *J. Neurosurg.*, **23**, 578.
Mellick, S. A., Phelan, P. D. (1965) 'Internal carotid artery occlusion in a child.' *Arch. Dis. Childh.*, **40**, 224.
Murphey, F., Shillito, J. (1959) 'Avoidance of false angiographic localization of the site of internal carotid occlusion.' *J. Neurosurg.*, **16**, 24.
Prior, J. T., Bergstrom, V. W. (1948) 'General arterial calcifications in infants.' *Amer. J. Dis. Child.*, **76**, 91.
Reisman, M. (1965) 'Atherosclerosis and pediatrics.' *J. Pediat.*, **66**, 1.
Stehbens, W. E. (1960) 'Focal intimal proliferation in the cerebral arteries.' *Amer. J. Path.*, **36**, 289.
Stötzer, H. (1960) 'Beitrag zur Frage der Arteriosklerose des Säuglings- und Kindesalters.' *Zbl. allg. Path. path. Anat.*, **101**, 274.
Stryker, W. S. (1946) 'Arterial calcification in infants, with special reference to the coronary arteries.' *Amer. J. Path.*, **22**, 1007.
van Creveld, S. (1941) 'Coronary calcification and thrombosis in an infant.' *Ann. paediat. (Basel)*, **157**, 84.

ADDITIONAL READING

Clarke, E., Harrison, C. V. (1956) 'Bilateral carotid artery obstruction.' *Neurology (Minneap.)*, **6**, 705.
Hughes, F. W. T., Perry, C. B. (1929) 'Senile arterial changes in a child aged 7 weeks.' *Bristol. med.-chir. J.*, **46**, 219.
Winkelmann, N. W., Eckel, J. L. (1929) 'Endarteritis in the small cortical vessels in severe infarctions and toxemias.' *Arch. Neurol. Psychiat. (Chic.)*, **21**, 863.
—— —— (1935) 'Arterial changes in the brain in childhood.' *Amer. J. Syph. Neurol.*, **19**, 223.

Chapter 10. Hypertension

REFERENCES

Allègre, G., Vigouroux, R. (1957) Traitement Chirurgical des Anévrysmes Intracrâniens du Système Carotidien. Paris: Masson.

Corday, E., Rothenberg, E. S., Irving, D. W. (1963) 'Cerebral angiospasm. A case of the cerebral stroke.' *Amer. J. Cardiol.*, **11**, 66.

Driesen, W. (1962) 'Engstellung (Spasmen?) von Grosshirnarterien im Angiogramm bei Aneurysmen und anderen Schädigungen des Hirns.' *Med. Welt. (Berl.)*, **38**, 1987.

du Boulay, G. (1963) 'Distribution of spasms in the intracranial arteries after subarachnoid hemorrhage.' *Acta radiol. (Stockh.)*, **1**, 257.

Fletcher, T. M., Taveras, J. M., Pool, J. L. (1959) 'Cerebral vasospasm in angiography for intracranial aneurysm. Incidence and significance in 100 consecutive angiograms.' *Arch. Neurol. (Chic.)*, **1**, 38.

Friedenfelt, H., Lundström, R. (1963) 'Local and general spasm in the internal carotid system following trauma.' *Acta radiol. (Stockh.)*, **1**, 278.

Griffioen, H., Pieterse, J. J. (1965) 'Apoplexie bij een twaalfjaige jongen.' *Maandschr. Kindergeneesk.*, **33**, 364.

Haggerty, R. J., Maroney, M. W., Nadas, A. S. (1956) 'Essential hypertension in infancy and childhood.' *Amer. J. Dis. Child.*, **92**, 535.

Johnson, R. J., Potter, J. M., Reid, R. G. (1958) 'Arterial spasm in subarachnoid hemorrhage: mechanical considerations.' *J. Neurol. Neurosurg. Psychiat.(Chic.)*, **21**, 68.

Lende, R. A. (1960) 'Local spasms in cerebral arteries.' *J. Neurosurg.*, **17**, 90.

Maspes, P. E., Marini, G. (1962) 'Intracranial arterial spasm related to supraclinoid ruptured aneurysm.' *Acta neurochir. (Wien)*, **10**, 630.

Mymin, D. (1960) 'Carotid thrombosis in childhood.' *Arch. Dis. Childh.*, **35**, 515.

Nagant de Deuxchaisnes, C., Fanconi, A., Alberto, P., Rudler, J. C., Mach, R. S. (1960) 'Phéochromocytomes extra-surrénaliens multiples avec "dystrophie d'Albright" et hémangiomes cutanés.' *Schweiz. med. Wschr.*, **33**, 886.

Pool, J. L., Jacobson, S., Fletcher, T. A. (1958) 'Cerebral vasospasm—clinical and experimental evidence.' *J. Amer. med. Ass.*, **167**, 1599.

ADDITIONAL READING

Abbott, M. E. (1928) 'Coarctation of the aorta of the adult type. II. A statistical study and historical retrospect of 200 cases with autopsy, of stenosis or obliteration of the descending arch in subjects above the age of two years.' *Amer. heart J.*, **3**, 574.

Baker, T. W., Shelden, W. D. (1936) 'Coarctation of the aorta with intermittent leakage of a congenital cerebral aneurysm.' *Amer. J. med. Sci.*, **191**, 626.

Berthrong, M., Sabiston, D. C. (1951) 'Cerebral lesions in congenital heart disease: a review of autopsies on 162 cases.' *Bull Johns Hopk. Hosp.*, **89**, 384.

Chavany, J. A., Messimy, R., Djiudjian, R., Malo, H. (1955) 'Considérations sur l'arteriographie des oblitérations thrombotiques et emboliques des artères cérébrales.' *Sem. Hôp. Paris*, **29**, 1661.

Davies, J. N. P., Fisher, J. A. (1943) 'Coarctation of the aorta, double mitral a.-v. orifice and leaking cerebral aneurysm.' *Brit.heart J.*, **5**, 197.

Fontana, R. S., Edwards, J. E. (1962) Congenital Cardiac Disease: A Review of 357 Cases Studied Pathologically. Philadelphia: W. B. Saunders.

Forster, F. M., Alpers, B. J. (1943) 'Aneurysm of the circle of Willis associated with congenital polycystic disease of the kidneys.' *Arch. Neurol. Psychiat.(Chic.)*, **50**, 669.

Jacobsen, H. H., Skinhøj, J. E. (1959) 'Occlusion of the middle cerebral artery (an analysis of 56 arteriographed cases).' *Dan. med. Bull.*, **6**, 9.

Lichtenberg, H., Gallagher, H. F. (1933) 'Coarctation of the aorta: anomaly of great vessels of the neck and intermittent leakage of a cerebral aneurysm diagnosed during life.' *Amer.J. Dis. Child.*, **45**, 1253.

Lindseth Ditlefsen, E. M., Tonjum, A. M. (1960) 'Intracranial aneurysms and polycystic kidneys.' *Acta med. scand.*, **168**, 51.

O'Crowley, C. R., Martland, H. S. (1939) 'Association of polycystic disease of kidneys with congenital aneurysms of cerebral arteries.' *Amer. J. Surg.*, **43**, 3.

Peebles Brown, R. A. (1951) 'Polycystic disease of the kidneys and intracranial aneurysms: aetiology and interrelationship of these conditions.' *Glasg. med. J.*, **32**, 333.

Poutasse, E. F., Gardner, W. J., McCormack, L. J. (1954) 'Polycystic kidney disease and intracranial aneurysm.' *J. Amer. med. Ass.*, **154**, 741.

Reifenstein, G. H., Levine, S. A., Gross, R. E. (1947) 'Coarctation of the aorta: a review of 104 autopsied cases of the "adult type" two years of age or older.' *Amer. heart J.*, **33**, 146.

Rocand, J. C. (1961) Les Thromboses Carotidiennes et Sylviennes de l'Enfant. Paris: thesis.

Sachs, A. L., Meyers, R. (1951) 'The coexistence of intracranial aneurysm and polycystic kidney disease.' *Trans. Amer. neurol. Ass.*, **76**, 147.

Suter, W. (1949) 'Das kongenitale Aneurysma der basalen Gehirnarterien und Cystennieren.,
 Schweiz. med. Wschr., **79**, 471.
Weber, F. P. (1927) 'Stenosis (coarctation) of the aortic isthmus, with sudden death from rupture of
 cerebral aneurysm.' *Proc. roy. Soc. Med.*, **20**, 29.
Woltman, H. W., Shelden, H. D. (1927) 'Neurologic complications associated with congenital
 stenosis of the isthmus of the aorta.' *Arch. Neurol. Psychiat. (Chic.)*, **17**, 303.
Wright, C. J. E. (1949) 'Coarctation of the aorta with death from rupture of cerebral aneurysm.'
 Arch. Path., **48**, 382.

Chapter 11. Traumatic Vascular Occlusion

REFERENCES

Boldrey, E., Maass, L., Miller, E. R. (1956) 'The role of atlantoid compression in the etiology of
 internal carotid thrombosis.' *J. Neurosurg.*, **13**, 127.
Boyd-Wilson, J. S. (1962) 'Iatrogenic carotid occlusion, medial dissection complicating arteri-
 ography.' *Wld. Neurol.*, **3**, 507.
Braudo, M. (1956) 'Thrombosis of the internal carotid artery in childhood after injuries in the
 region of the soft palate.' *Brit. med. J.*, **i**, 665.
Caldwell, J. A. (1936) 'Post-traumatic thrombosis of the internal carotid artery. Two cases.' *Amer.
 J. Surg.*, **32**, 522.
Clarke, P. R. R., Dickson, J., Smith, B. J. (1955) 'Traumatic thrombosis of the internal carotid
 artery following a non-penetrating injury and leading to infarction of the brain.' *Brit. J. Surg.*,
 43, 215.
Crawford, T. (1956) 'Pathological effects of cerebral arteriography.' *J. Neurol. Neurosurg. Psychiat.*,
 19, 217.
Duman, S., Stephens, J. W. (1963) 'Post-traumatic middle cerebral artery occlusion.' *Neurology
 (Minneap.)*, **13**, 613.
Fairburn, B. (1957) 'Thrombosis of the internal carotid artery after soft-palate injury.' *Brit. med. J.*,
 ii, 750.
Fleming, J. F. R., Park, A. M. (1959) 'Dissecting aneurysms of the carotid artery following angi-
 ography.' *Neurology (Minneap.)*, **9**, 1.
Frantzen, E., Jacobsen, H. H., Therkelsen, J. (1961) 'Cerebral artery occlusion in children due to
 trauma to the head and neck.' *Neurology (Minneap.)*, **11**, 695.
Idbohrn, H. (1951) 'A complication of percutaneous carotid angiography.' *Acta radiol. (Stockh.)*,
 36, 155.
Jacobsen, H. H., Skinhøj, E. (1959) 'Occlusion of the middle cerebral artery (an analysis of 36 arteriographed cases).' *Dan. med. Bull.*, **26**, 9.
Lepoire, J., Montant, J., Renard, J., Grosdidier, J., Mathieu, P. (1964) 'Anévrysme sacculaire de
 la carotide cervicale. Complication d'une angiographie carotidienne percutanée.' *Neurochirurgie*,
 10, 275.
Leriche, R. (1950) 'Hémiplégie gauche consécutive à une contusion de la carotide interne chez une
 enfant. Traitement par 5 infiltrations stellaires, guérison à peu près complète.' *Lyon. chir.*, **45**, 541.
Liverud, K. (1958) 'Aneurysms as complications of angiography.' *J. Oslo City Hosp.*, **8**, 209.
Murphey, F., Miller, J. H. (1959) 'Carotid insufficiency diagnosis and surgical treatment.' *J. Neuro-
 surg.*, **16**, 1.
Philippides, D., Link, P., Montrieul, B. (1954) 'Thrombose de la carotide interne par contusion
 buccale para-amygdalienne.' *Rev. oto-neurooptal.*, **26**, 39.
Poppen, J. L. (1951) 'Specific treatment of intracranial aneurysms. Experiences with 143 surgically
 treated patients.' *J. Neurosurg.*, **8**, 75.
Rajszys, R., Sabat, E. (1964) 'Valvule de l'artère carotide, provoquée artificiellement.' *Ann. Radiol.*,
 7, 65.
Sedzimir, C. B. (1955) 'Head injury as a cause of internal carotid thrombosis.' *J. Neurol. Neurosurg.
 Psychiat.*, **18**, 293.
Sirois, J., Lapointe, H., Côté, P. E. (1954) 'Unusual local complications of percutaneous cerebral
 angiography.' *J. Neurosurg.*, **11**, 112.
Therkelsen, J., Hornnes, N. (1963) 'Traumatic occlusion of the internal carotid artery in a child.'
 Circulation, **28**, 101.

ADDITIONAL READING

Jacob, J. C., Maroun, F. B., Heneghan, W. B., House, A. M. (1970) 'Uncommon cerebrovascular
 lesions in children.' *Develop. Med. Child Neurol.*, **12**, 446.
Jamieson, K. G. (1965) 'Vertebral arteriovenous fistula caused by an angiography needle. Report
 of a case.' *J. Neurosurg.*, **23**, 620.

Nelson, J. W., Styri, O. B. (1968) 'Dissecting subintimal hematomas of the intracranial arteries.'
 J. Amer. Osteopath. Ass., **67**, 512.
Pitner, S. E. (1966) 'Carotid thrombosis due to intra-oral trauma: an unusual complication of
 a common childhood accident.' *New Engl. J. Med.*, **274**, 764.

Chapter 12. Embolism

REFERENCES

Banker, B. Q. (1961) 'Cerebrovascular disease in infancy and childhood. I. Occlusive vascular disease.'
 J. Neuropath. exp. Neurol., **20**, 127.
Chao, D. H., Henry, M. G., Rosenberg, H. S. (1960) 'Myxoma of the heart with internal carotid
 artery occlusion in a child.' *Neurology (Minneap.)*, **10**, 418.
Dalal, P. M., Shah, P. M., Sheth, S. C., Deshpande, C. K. (1965) 'Cerebral embolism. Angiographic
 observations on spontaneous clot lysis.' *Lancet*, **i**, 61.
—— —— Deshpande, C. K., Sheth, S. C. (1966) 'Recanalisation after cerebral embolism.' *Lancet*,
 ii, 495.
Fisher, C. M. (1959) 'Observations of the fundus oculi in transient monocular blindness.' *Neurology*,
 (Minneap.), **9**, 333.
Geisler, E., Viehweger, G., Schippan, D. (1965) 'Cerebrale Gefässprozesse bei Kindern. Beitrag zur
 Thrombangiitis obliterans cerebri im Kindesalter.' *Helv. paediat. Acta*, **20**, 476.
Gleason, J. O. (1955) 'Primary myxoma of the heart. A case simulating rheumatic and bacterial
 endocarditis.' *Cancer*, **8**, 839.
Paillas, J., Bonnal, J., Payan, H., Bernard-Badier, Mme (1959) 'Thrombose de l'artère carotide
 interne révélatrice d'echinonoccose cardiaque rompue et suivie d'hydatidose intracranio-orbitaire.'
 Rev. neurol., **100**, 166.
Richwien, R., Unger, G. (1966) 'Beobachtung eines Wallenberg-Syndroms im Kindesalter nebst
 Bemerkungen zum kindlichen cerebralen Gefässprozess.' *Mschr. Kinderheilk.*, **114**, 442.
Russell, R. W. R. (1961) 'Observations on the retinal blood vessels in monocular blindness.' *Lancet*,
 ii, 1422.
Schad, N. (1966) Personal communication.

ADDITIONAL READING

Bell, W. E., Butler, C. (1968) 'Cerebral mycotic aneurysms in children. Two case reports.' *Neurology*
 (Minneap.), **18**, 81.
Berthrong, M., Sabiston, D. C. (1951) 'Cerebral lesions in congenital heart disease: review of autopsies
 in 162 cases.' *Bull. Johns Hopk. Hosp.*, **89**, 384.
Fontana, R. S., Edwards, J. E. (1962) Congenital Cardiac Disease. A Review of 357 Cases Studied
 Pathologically. Philadelphia: W. B. Saunders.
Gross, R. E. (1945) 'Arterial embolism and thrombosis in infancy.' *Amer. J. Dis. Child.*, **70**, 61.
Meyer, J. S., Gilroy, J., Barnhart, M. I., Johnson, F. J. (1963) 'Therapeutic thrombolysis in cerebral
 thromboembolism.' *Neurology (Minneap.)*, **13**, 927.
Tyler, H. R., Clark, D. B. (1957) 'Cerebrovascular accidents in patients with congenital heart disease.'
 Arch. Neurol. Psychiat., **77**, 483.

Chapter 13. Spontaneous Cerebral Arterial Occlusion

REFERENCES

Banker, B. Q. (1959) 'Occlusive vascular disease affecting the central nervous system in infancy and
 childhood.' *Trans. Amer. neurol. Ass.*, **84**, 34.
Boldrey, E., Maass, L., Miller, E. R. (1956) 'The role of atlantoid compression in the etiology of
 internal carotid thrombosis.' *J. Neurosurg.*, **13**, 127.
Byers, R. K., McLean, W. T. (1962) 'Etiology and course of certain hemiplegias with aphasia in
 childhood.' *Pediatrics*, **29**, 376.
Bernsmeier, A. (1963) Durchblutung des Gehirns. Physiologie und Pathophysiologie des vegetativen
 Nervensystems. Vol. 2. Stuttgart: Hippokrates.
Dalal, P. M., Shah, P. M., Sheth, S. C., Deshpande, C. K. (1965) 'Cerebral embolism. Angiographic
 observations on spontaneous clot lysis.' *Lancet*, **i**, 61.
—— —— Deshpande, C. K., Sheth, S. C. (1966) 'Recanalisation after cerebral embolism.' *Lancet*,
 ii, 495.
Davie, J. C., Coxe, W. (1967) 'Occlusive disease of the carotid artery in children. Carotid throm-
 bectomy with recovery in a 2-year-old boy.' *Arch. Neurol. (Chic.)*, **17**, 313.
Denny-Brown, D. (1951) 'The treatment of recurrent cerebral vascular symptoms and the question
 of "vasospasm".' *Med. Clin. N. Amer.*, **35**, 1457.

Dooley, J. M., Smith, K. R. (1968) 'Occlusion of the basilar artery in a 6-year-old boy.' *Neurology (Minneap.)*, **18**, 1034.

Faris, A. A., Guth, C., Youmans, R. A., Poser, C. M. (1964) 'Internal carotid artery occlusion in children.' *Amer. J. Dis. Child.*, **107**, 188.

Ford, F. R., Schaffer, A. J. (1927) 'The etiology of infantile acquired hemiplegia.' *Arch. Neurol. Psychiat. (Chic.)*, **18**, 323.

Fowler, M. (1962) 'Two cases of basilar artery occlusion in childhood.' *Arch. Dis. Childh.*, **37**, 78.

Geisler, E., Viehweger, G., Schippans, D. (1965) 'Cerebrale Gefässeprozesse bei Kindern. Beitrag zur Thrombangitis obliterans cerebri im Kindesalter.' *Helv. paediat. Acta.*, **20**, 476.

Harwood-Nash, D. C., McDonald, P., Argent, W. (1971) 'Cerebral arterial disease in children; an angiographic study of 40 cases.' *Amer. J. Roentgenol.*, **111**, 672.

Krayenbühl, H., Yasargil, M. G. (1964) 'Verschluss der Arteria cerebralis media: Ergebnisse der klinischen und katamnetischen Untersuchungen.' *Schweiz. Arch. Neurol. Neurochir. Psychiat.*, **94**, 287.

Lehmann, R., Portsmann, W., Siedschlag, W. D., Müller, K. (1970) 'Akute gefässbedingte Halbseiten-syndrome im Kindesalter.' *Pädiat. Grenzgeb.*, **9**, 1.

Mellick, S., Phelan, P. D. (1965) 'Internal carotid artery occlusion in a child.' *Arch. Dis. Childh.*, **40**, 224.

Meyer, J. S., Denny-Brown, D. (1957) 'The cerebral collateral circulation. I. Factors influencing collateral blood flow. 2. Production of cerebral infarction by ischaemic anoxia and its reversibility in early stages.' *Neurology (Minneap.)*, **7**, 447, 567.

Murphey, F., Shillito, J. (1959) 'Avoidance of false angiographic localization of the site of internal carotid occlusion.' *J.Neurosurg.*, **16**, 24.

Petit-Dutaillis, D., Janet, H., Thiebaut, F., Guillaumat, L. (1949) 'Effets d'une inversion circulatoire par anastomose carotido-jugulaire sur une hémiplégie droite avec aphasie, due à une thrombose de la carotide interne d'origine inconnue chez un adolescent de 13 ans.' *Rev. neurol.*, **81**, 997.

Pouyanne, H., Arné, L., Loiseau, P., Mouton, L. (1957) 'Considérations sur deux cas de thrombose de la carotide interne chez l'enfant.' *Rev. neurol.*, **97**, 525.

Pribram, H. F. W. (1961) 'Angiographic appearances in acute intracranial hypertension.' *Neurology (Minneap.)*, **11**, 10.

Richwien, R., Unger, G. (1966) 'Beobachtung eines Wallenberg-Syndroms im Kindesalter nebst Bemerkungen zum kindlischen cerebralen Gefässprozess.' *Mschr. Kinderheilk.*, **8**, 442.

Rocand, J. C. (1961) Les Thromboses Carotidiennes et Sylviennes de l'Enfant. Paris: thesis.

Rouzaud, M., Gouazé, A., Salles, M. (1962) 'Thrombose primitive de la carotide interne dans sa portion cervicale chez une enfant de 4 ans.' *Rev. neurol.*, **107**, 539.

Sandifer, P. (1962) 'Non-vascular causes of acute hemiplegia in childhood.' *in* Bax, M., Mitchell, R. G. (Eds.) Acute Hemiplegia in Childhood. Clinics in Developmental Medicine, No. 6. London: Spastics Society with Heinemann. p. 17.

Silverstein, A., Hollin, S. (1963) 'Occlusion of the supraclinoid portion of the internal carotid artery.' *Neurology (Minneap.)*, **13**, 679.

Solomon, G. E., Hilal, S. K., Gold, A. P., Carter, S. (1970) 'Natural history of acute hemiplegia in childhood.' *Brain*, **93**, 107.

Stötzer, H. (1960) 'Beitrag zur Frage der Arteriosklerose des Säuglings- und Kindesalters.' *Zbl. allg. Path. path. Anat.*, **101**, 274.

Taveras, J. M., Poser, C. M. (1959) 'Roentgenologic aspects of cerebral angiography in children.' *Amer. J. Roentgen.*, **82**, 371.

Wiesel, J. (1906) Cited by Ford, F. R., Schaffer, A. J. (1927).

Winkelmann, N. W., Eckel, J. L. (1935) 'Arterial changes in the brain in childhood.' *Amer. J. Syph. Neurol.*, **19**, 223.

Wisoff, H. S., Rothballer, A. B. (1961) 'Cerebral arterial thrombosis in children.' *Arch. Neurol. (Chic.)*, **4**, 258.

ADDITIONAL READING

Cabieses, F., Saldias, C. (1956) 'Thrombosis of the internal carotid in a child.' *Neurology (Minneap.)*, **6**, 677.

Cavanagh, J. B. (1962) 'The immediate sequelae of acute cerebral vascular occlusion (acute hemiplegia) in childhood.' *in* Bax, M., Mitchell, R. G. (Eds.) Acute Hemiplegia in Childhood. Clinics in Developmental Medicine, No. 6. London: Spastics Society with Heinemann. p. 49.

Chambers, W. R. (1954) 'Acute occlusion of the internal carotid artery: report of 5 cases.' *Surgery*, **36**, 980.

Davidson, D. T., O'Hara, A. E., Allen, L. W., Kennedy, C. (1957) 'Thrombosis of the internal carotid artery in children.' *Trans. Amer. neurol. Ass.*, **82**, 102.

Duffy, P. E., Portnoy, B., Mauro, J., Wehrle, P. F. (1957) 'Acute infantile hemiplegia secondary to spontaneous carotid thrombosis.' *Neurology (Minneap.)*, **7**, 664.

Fields, W. S., Edwards, W. H., Crawford, E. S. (1961) 'Bilateral carotid artery thrombosis.' *Arch. Neurol. (Chic.),* **4**, 369.

Fisher, R. G., Friedman, K. R. (1959) 'Carotid artery thrombosis in persons 15 years of age or younger.' *J. Amer. med. Ass.,* **170**, 1918.

—— Goran, A. (1961) 'Thrombosis of an intracranial aneurysm and cervical portion of the internal carotid artery in a child.' *J. Neurosurg.,* **18**, 698.

Goldstein, S. L., Burgess, J. P. (1958) 'Spontaneous thrombosis of the internal carotid artery in a seven-year-old girl.' *Amer. J. Dis. Child.,* **95**, 538.

Krayenbühl, H. (1960) 'Beitrag zur Frage des cerebralen angiospastischen Insults.' *Schweiz. med. Wschr.,* **90**, 961.

Lefèvre, J., Lepintre, J., Fauré, C., Perez, J. (1956) 'Résultats de l'angiographie cérébrale au cours des hémiplégies cérébrales infantiles.' *Acta radiol. (Stockh.),* **46**, 456.

Mymin, D. (1960) 'Carotid thrombosis in childhood.' *Arch. Dis. Childh.,* **35**, 515.

Stevens, H. (1959) 'Carotid artery occlusion in childhood. *Pediatrics,* **23**, 699.

Teng, P., Goldenberg, E. D. (1960) 'Thrombosis of the internal carotid artery in a five-year-old child.' *Amer. J. Dis. Child.,* **99**, 228.

Chapter 14. Fetal Cerebral Arterial Occlusion

REFERENCES

Bertrand, J., Bargeton, E. (1955) 'Lésions vasculaires dans l'hémiplégie cérébrale infantile.' *in* Proceedings of the Second International Congress of Neuropathology, London, 1955. Amsterdam: Excerpta Medica.

Burmester, K., Stender, A. (1961) 'Zwei Fälle von einseitiger Aplasie der Arteria carotis interna bei gleichzeitiger Aneurysmabildung im vorderen Anteil des Circulus Willisi. (Zur Frage des Kombination von Sackförmigen Aneurysmen der Hirnarterien mit anderen Fehlbildungen)., *Acta neurochir. (Wien),* **9**, 367.

Clark, R. M., Linell, E. A. (1954) 'Case report: prenatal occlusion of the internal carotid artery.', *J. Neurol. Neurosurg. Psychiat.,* **17**, 295.

Cocker, J., George, S. W., Yates, P. O. (1965) 'Perinatal occlusion of the middle cerebral artery.' *Develop. Med. Child Neurol.,* **7**, 235.

Cotard, S. (1868) Etude sur l'Atrophie Cérébrale. Paris: thesis (Cited by Freud, S. (1897)—*see* Introduction.)

Eicke, W. J. (1947) 'Gefässveränderungen bei Meningitis und ihre Bedeutung für die Pathogenese frühkindlicher Hirnschäden.' *Virchows Arch. path. Anat.,* **314**, 88.

Farber, S., Vawter, G. (1964) 'Clinical pathological conference.' *J. Pediat.,* **65**, 940.

Fisher, C. M. (1959) 'Early-life carotid-artery occlusion associated with late intracranial hemorrhage.' *Lab. Invest.,* **8**, 680.

Hills, J., Sament, S. (1968) 'Bilateral agenesis of the internal carotid artery associated with cardiac and other anomalies. Case Report.' *Neurology (Minneap.),* **18**, 142.

Kundrat, H. (1882) Die Porencephalie, eine anatomische Studie. Graz: Leuschner und Lubensky. (Cited by Freud, S. (1897)—*see* Introduction.)

Lagarde, C., Vigouroux, R., Perrouty, P. (1957) 'Agénésie terminale de la carotide interne et anévrysme de la communicante antérieure. Documents radiologiques.' *J. Radiol. Electrol.,* **38**, 939.

Larroche, J.-C., Amiel, C. (1966) 'Thrombose de l'artère sylvienne à la période neonatale.' *Arch. franç. Pédiat.,* **23**, 257.

Lhermitte, F., Gautier, J.-C., Poirier, J., Tyrer, J. H. (1968) 'Hypoplasia of the internal carotid artery.' *Neurology (Minneap.),* **18**, 439.

Prichard, J. S. (1964) 'The character and significance of epileptic seizures in infancy.' *in* Kellaway, P., Petersen, J. (Eds.) Neurological and Electroencephalographic Correlative Studies in Infancy. New York: Grune & Stratton. p. 273.

Priman, J., Christie, D. H. (1959) 'A case of abnormal internal carotid artery and associated vascular anomalies.' *Anat. Rec.,* **134**, 87.

Tharp, B., Heymann, A., Pfieffer, J. B., Young, W. G. (1965) 'Cerebral ischaemia. Result of hypoplasia of internal carotid artery.' *Arch. Neurol. (Chic.),* **12**, 160.

Töndury, G. (1934) 'Einseitiges Fehlen der A. carotis interna.' *Morph. Jb.,* **74**, 625.

Turnbull, J. (1962) 'Agenesis of the internal carotid artery.' *Neurology (Minneap.),* **12**, 588.

van Creveld, S. (1959) 'Coagulation disorders in the newborn period.' *J. Pediat.,* **54**, 633.

ADDITIONAL READING

Lévin, P. M. (1936) 'Cortical encephalomalacia in infancy.' *Arch. Neurol. Psychiat. (Chic.),* **36**, 264·

Lie, T. A. (1968) Congenital Anomalies of the Carotid Arteries. Amsterdam. Excerpta Medica Foundation.

Chapter 15. Vasospasm

REFERENCES

Allègre, G., de Rougemont, J., Thierry, A. (1963) 'Spasme artériel de la carotide interne dû à un anévrysme rompu du système vertébro-basilaire.' *Neurochirurgie*, **9**, 74.

Bernsmeier, A. (1963) Durchblutung des Gehirns. Physiologie und Pathophysiologie des vegetativen Nervensystems. Vol. II. Stuttgart: Hippokrates.

Buckle, R. M., Du Boulay, G., Smith, B. (1964) 'Death due to cerebral vasospasm.' *J. Neurol. Neurosurg. Psychiat.*, **27**, 440.

Denny-Brown, D. (1951) 'The treatment of recurrent cerebral vascular symptoms and the question of "vasospasm".' *Med. Clin. N. Amer.*, **35**, 147.

Du Boulay, G. (1963) 'Distribution of spasms in the intracranial arteries after subarachnoid hemorrhage.' *Acta radiol. (Stockh.)*, **1**, 257.

Dukes, H. T., Vieth, R. T. (1964) 'Cerebral arteriography during migraine prodrome and headache.' *Neurology (Minneap.)*, **14**, 636.

Fletcher, T. M., Taveras, J. M., Pool, J. L. (1959) 'Cerebral vasospasms in angiography for intracranial aneurysms. Incidence and significance in 100 consecutive angiograms.' *Arch. Neurol. (Chic.)*, **1**, 38.

Friedenfelt, H., Lundström, R. (1963) 'Local and general spasm in the internal carotid system following trauma.' *Acta radiol. (Stockh.)*, **1**, 278.

Krayenbühl, H., Yasargil, M. G. (1965) Die zerebrale Angiographie. 2. Auf. Stuttgart: Thieme.

Lende, R. A. (1960) 'Local spasm in cerebral arteries.' *J. Neurosurg.*, **17**, 90.

Pickering, G. W. (1951) 'Vascular spasm.' *Lancet*, **ii**, 845.

Pool, J. L. (1958) 'Cerebral vasospasm.' *New Engl. J. Med.*, **259**, 1259.

Raynor, R. B., Ross, G. (1960) 'Arteriography and vasospasm. The effects of intracarotid contrast media on vasospasm.' *J. Neurosurg.*, **17**, 1055.

Schneider, M. (1961) 'Zur Pathophysiologie des Gehirnkreislaufs.' *Acta neurochir. (Wien)*, Suppl. 7, 34.

Tönnis, W., Schiefer, W. (1958) Zirkulationsstörungen des Gehirns im Serienangiogramm. Berlin: Springer.

ADDITIONAL READING

Ecker, A., Riemenschneider, P. A. (1951) 'Arteriographic demonstration of spasm of the intracranial arteries with special reference to saccular arterial aneurysms.' *J. Neurosurg.*, **8**, 660.

Huber, P., Handa, J. (1966) 'Der Einfluss von Kontrastmittel auf Hirngefässe und Hirndurchblutung.' *Schweiz. Arch. Neurol. Neurochir. Psychiat.*, **97**, 282.

Krayenbühl, H. (1960) 'Beitrag zur Frage des cerebralen angiospastischen Insults.' *Schweiz. med. Wschr.*, **90**, 961.

Pool, J. L. (1961) 'Cerebral vasospasm associated with ruptured intracranial aneurysms.' *Arch. Neurol. (Chic.)*, **4**, 208.

—— Jacobson, S., Fletcher, T. A. (1958) 'Cerebral vasospasm—clinical and experimental evidence.' *J. Amer. med. Ass.*, **167**, 1599.

Potter, J. (1959) 'Redistribution of blood to the brain due to localized cerebral arterial spasm.' *Brain*, **82**, 367.

Pribram, H. F. W. (1961) 'Angiographic appearances in acute intracranial hypertension.' *Neurology (Minneap.)*, **11**, 10.

Chapter 16. Venous Thrombosis

REFERENCES

Arena, J. M. (1935) 'Vascular accident and hemiplegia in a patient with sickle cell anemia.' *Amer. J. Dis. Child.*, **49**, 722.

Askenasy, H. M., Kosary, I. Z., Braham, J. (1962) 'Thrombosis of the longitudinal sinus. Diagnosis by carotid angiography.' *Neurology (Minneap.)*, **12**, 288.

Ata, M. (1965) 'Cerebral infarction due to intracranial sinus thrombosis.' *J. clin. Path.*, **18**, 636.

Bailey, O. T. (1959) 'Results of long survival after thrombosis of the superior sagittal sinus.' *Neurology (Minneap.)*, **9**, 741.

Barnett, H. J. M., Hyland, H. H. (1953) 'Non-infective intracranial venous thrombosis.' *Brain*, **76**, 36.

Bernheim, M., Larbre, F. (1956) 'Le diagnostique des phlébites cérébrales chez l'enfant.' *Arch. franç. Pédiat.*, **13**, 1021.

Byers, R. K., Hass, G. M. (1933) 'Thrombosis of the dural venous sinuses in infancy and childhood.' *Amer. J. Dis. Child.*, **45**, 1161.

Carels, G., Henneaux, J. (1959) 'Cerebral thrombophlebitis in the child: clinical and electroencephalographic study.' *Acta paediat. belg.*, **13**, 253.

Carrie, A. W., Jaffé, F. A. (1954) 'Thrombosis of the superior sagittal sinus caused by trauma without penetrating injury.' *J. Neurosurg.*, **11**, 173.

Dekaban, A. S., Norman, R. M. (1958) 'Hemiplegia in early life associated with thrombosis of the sagittal sinus and its tributary veins in one hemisphere.' *J. Neuropath. exp. Neurol.*, **17**, 461.

Delille, A., Lhermitte, I., Lesobre, R. (1936) 'Ramollissement hémorrhagique d'origine veineuse chez un enfant atteint de malformations cardiaques.' *Rev. neurol.*, **66**, 754.

Ford, F. R. (1966) Diseases of the Nervous System in Infancy, Childhood and Adolescence. 5th edn. Springfield, Ill.: C. C Thomas.

Girard, P. F., Devic, M. (1954) 'Considérations étiologiques, documents anatomiques et remarques thérapeutiques concernant les phlébites cérébrales.' *Rev. neurol.*, **90**, 863.

Greer, M., Berk, M. S. (1963) 'Lateral sinus obstruction and mastoiditis.' *Pediatrics*, **31**, 840.

Greer, M., Schotland, D. (1962) 'Abnormal hemoglobin as a cause of neurological disease.' *Neurology (Minneap.)*, **12**, 114.

Huhn, A. (1965) Die Thrombosen der intrakraniellen Venen und Sinus. Klinische und pathologisch-anatomische Untersuchungen, Stuttgart: Schattauer.

Krayenbühl, H. (1959) 'Die cerebrale Venenthrombose.' *Schweiz. med. Wschr.*, **89**, 191.

Mitchell, R. G. (1952) 'Venous thrombosis in acute infantile hemiplegia.' *Arch. Dis. Childh.*, **27**, 95.

O'Brien, J. L., Sibley, W. A. (1958) 'Neurologic manifestations of thrombotic thrombocytopenia.' *Neurology (Minneap.)*, **8** 55.

Pollack, R. M. (1956) On the Clinical Aspects of Cerebral Thrombosis. Zurich: dissertation.

Symonds, C. P. (1931) 'Otitic hydrocephalus.' *Brain*, **54**, 55.

—— (1932) 'Otitic hydrocephalus: a report of three cases.' *Brit. med. J.*, **i**, 53.

—— (1937) 'Hydrocephalic and focal cerebral symptoms in relation to thrombophlebitis of the dural sinuses and cerebral veins.' *Brain*, **60**, 531.

—— (1940) 'Cerebral thrombophlebitis.' *Brit. med. J.*, **ii**, 348.

Toomey, J. A., Hutt, B. H. (1949) 'Thrombosis of the dural sinuses.' *Amer. J. Dis. Child.*, **77**, 285.

Walsh, F. B. (1957) Clinical Neuro-ophthalmology. Baltimore: Williams & Wilkins.

Weber, G. (1957) 'Hirnabszesse und zerebrale venöse Thrombosen bei kongenitalen Herzfehlen.' *Schweiz. med. Wschr.*, **87**, 159.

ADDITIONAL READING

Hitzig, W. H. (1964) 'Therapie mit Antikoagulantien in der Pädiatrie.' *Helv. paediat. Acta*, **19**, 213.

Jenkins, M. E., Scott, R. B., Baird, R. L. (1960) 'Studies in sickle cell anemia.' *J. Pediat.*, **56**, 30.

Krayenbühl, H. (1955) 'Cerebral venous thrombosis. The diagnostic value of cerebral angiography.' *Schweiz. Arch. Neurol. Psychiat.*, **74**, 261.

Chapter 17. Postictal Hemiplegia

REFERENCES

Adrian, E. D., Moruzzi, G. (1939) 'High frequency discharges from cerebral neurones.' *J. Physiol. (Lond.)*, **95**, 27P.

Bamberger, Ph., Matthes, A. (1959) Anfälle im Kindesalter. Basel: Karger.

Cavanagh, J. B. (1962) 'The immediate sequelae of acute cerebral vascular occlusion (acute hemiplegia) in childhood.' *in* Bax, M., Mitchell, R. G. (Eds.) Acute Hemiplegia in Childhood. Clinics in Developmental Medicine, No. 6. London: Spastics Society with Heinemann. p. 49.

Earle, K. M., Baldwin, M., Penfield, W. (1953) 'Incisural sclerosis and temporal lobe seizures produced by hippocampal herniation at birth.' *Arch. Neurol. Psychiat.*, (*Chic.*), **69**, 27.

Fowler, M. (1957) 'Brain damage after febrile convulsions.' *Arch. Dis. Childh.*, **32**, 67.

Gastaut, H., Vigouroux, M., Trevisan, C., Regis, H. (1957) 'Le syndrome "hemiconvulsion-hémiplégie-épilepsie" (syndrome H.H.E.).' *Rev. neurol.*, **97**, 37.

Jung, R. (1953) 'Allgemeine Neurophysiologie.' *in* Bergmann, G., Frey, W., Schweigk, H. (Eds.) Handbuch der Inneren Medizin, Bd. V. 4th edn. Berlin: Springer. p. 1.

Lindenberg, G. (1955) 'Compression of brain arteries as pathogenetic factor for tissue necroses and their areas of predilection.' *J. Neuropath. exp. Neurol.*, **14**, 223.

Meyer, A., Beck, E., Shepherd, M. (1955) 'Unusually severe lesions in the brain following status epilepticus.' *J. Neurol. Neurosurg. Psychiat.*, **18**, 24.

Norman, R. M. (1962) 'Neuropathological findings in acute hemiplegia in childhood; with special reference to epilepsy as a pathogenic factor.' *in* Bax, M., Mitchell, R. G. (Eds.) Acute Hemiplegia in Childhood. Clinics in Developmental Medicine, no. 6. London: Spastics Society with Heinemann. p. 37.

Penfield, W., Jasper, H. (1954) Epilepsy and the Functional Anatomy of the Human Brain. Boston: Little, Brown.

Scholz, W. (1951) Die Krampfschädigungen des Gehirns. Berlin: Springer.

Spielmeyer, W. (1927) 'Die Pathogenese des epileptischen Krampfes.' *Z. Neurol.*, **109**, 501.

ADDITIONAL READING

Adrian, E. D., Moruzzi, G. (1939-40) 'Impulses in the pyramidal tract.' *J. Physiol. (Lond.)*, **97**, 153.
Gastaut, H., Poirier, F., Payan, H., Salamon, G., Toga, M., Vigouroux, M. (1959-60) 'H.H.E. syndrome. Hemiconvulsion, hemiplegia, epilepsy.' *Epilepsia*, **1**, 418.
Meyer, A. (1963) 'Epilepsy.' *in* Greenfield's Neuropathology, 2nd edn. London: Edward Arnold. p. 602.
Penfield, W., Erikson, T. C. (1941) Epilepsy and Cerebral Localization. Springfield, Ill.: C. C Thomas.
Schneider, M. (1967) 'Referat am Neurochirurgen-Kongress, Bad Dürkheim; Physiologie und Pathophysiologie der Hirndurch-blutung.' *Acta neurochir. (Wien.)*, **16**, 154.
Scholz, W. (1959) 'The contribution of patho-anatomical research to the problems of epilepsy, *Epilepsia*, **1**, 36.
Zimmermann, H. M. (1938) 'The histopathology of convulsive disorders in children.' *J. Pediat.*, **13**, 859.

Chapter 18. Pre-ictal Hemiplegia

REFERENCE

Penfield, W., Jasper, H. (1954) Epilepsy and the Functional Anatomy of the Human Brain. Boston: Little, Brown.

Chapter 19. Encephalitis: Toxic-infectious and Neuroallergic Encephalopathy

REFERENCES

Bernheim, M., Girard, P. F., Lanternier, Mlle, Larbre, F. (1954) 'Le rôle des thromboses veineuses dans les prétendues encéphalites primitives des enfants.' *Pédiatrie*, **9**, 249.
Fanconi, G. (1955) 'Psychomotorische und Petit-mal-Anfälle als Spätsymptome einer "Masern-encephalitis" der linken Hemisphäre.' *Helv. paediat. Acta*, **10**, 317.
Girard, P. F., Devic, M. (1954) 'Considérations étiologiques, documents anatomiques et remarques thérapeutiques concernant les phlébites cérébrales.' *Rev. neurol.*, **90**, 868.
Gsell, O., Prader, A. (1953) 'Akute Encephalitis durch Leptospira hyos infolge traumatischer Infektion. Postencephalitische Hemiatrophia cerebri bei 3 jährigem Knaben.' *Helv. paediat. Acta*, **8**, 318.
Hedenström, G., Huldt, G., Lagercrantz, R. (1958) 'Toxoplasmosis studies.' *Acta paediat. (Uppsala)*, **47**, 329.
Hurst, E. W. (1941) 'Acute haemorrhagic leucoencephalitis: a previously undefined entity.' *Med. J. Aust.*, **ii**, 1.
Lelong, M., Bernard, J., Desmonts, G., Couvreur, J. (1960) 'La toxoplasmose acquise. Etude de 227 observations.' *Arch. franç. Pédiat.*, **17**, 281.
Sabin, A. B. (1941) 'Toxoplasmic encephalitis in children.' *J. Amer. med. Ass.*, **116**, 801.

ADDITIONAL READING

Appenzeller, K. (1955) 'Die Masernencephalitis im Kinderspital Zürich in den Jahren 1928-1952.' *Helv. paediat. Acta*, **10**, 301.
Baker, A. B. (1962) 'Hemorrhagic encephalitis.' *in* Clinical Neurology, 2nd edn. New York: Hoeber-Harper.
Blackwood, W. W., McMenemy, W. H., Meyer, A., Norman, R. M., Russell, D. S. (1963) Greenfield's Neuropathology. 2nd edn. London: Edward Arnold.
de Vries, E. (1960) Postvaccinal Perivenous Encephalitis. Amsterdam: Elsevier.
Ford, F. R. (1966) Diseases of the Nervous System in Infancy, Childhood and Adolescence. 5th edn. Springfield, Ill.: C. C Thomas.
Hoefnagel, D. (1962) 'Acute transient encephalopathy in young children following smallpox vaccination.' *J. Amer. med. Ass.*, **180**, 525.
Pette, H., Kalm, H. (1953) 'Die entzündlichen Erkrankungen des Gehirns und seiner Häute.' *in* Bergmann, G., Frey, W., Schwiegk, H. (Eds.) Handbuch der Inneren Medizin. Band V, Abt. 3. Berlin: Springer.
Radermecker, J. (1956) 'Systématique et électroencéphalographie des encéphalites et encéphalopathies.' *Electroenceph. clin. Neurophysiol.*, Suppl. 5.
Southcott, R. V., Fowler, M. (1954) 'Further case of hemorrhagic leucoencephalitis (Hurst).' *Med. J. Aust.*, **ii**, 65.
van Bogaert, L., Radermecker, J., Devos, J. (1955) 'Sur une observation mortelle d'encéphalite aiguë nécrosante (sa situation vis-à-vis d'une groupe des encéphalites transmises par arthropods et de l'encéphalite herpétique).' *Rev. neurol.*, **92**, 329.

Chapter 20. Brain Abscess

REFERENCES

Ford, F. R. (1966) Diseases of the Nervous System in Infancy, Childhood and Adolescence. 5th edn. Springfield, Ill.: C. C Thomas.
Gluck, R., Hall, J. W., Stevenson, L. D. (1952) 'Brain abscess associated with congenital heart disease.' *Pediatrics*, **9**, 192.
Keith, J. D., Rowe, R. D., Vlad, P. (1958) Heart Disease in Infancy and Childhood. New York: Macmillan.
McGreal, D. A. (1962) 'Brain abscess in children.' *Canad. med. Ass. J.*, **86**, 261.
Raimondi, A., Matsumoto, J. S., Miller, R. A. (1965) 'Brain abscess in children with congenital heart disease.' *J. Neurosurg.*, **23**, 588.
Weber, G. (1960) 'Traitement et résultats thérapeutiques des abces cérébraux.' *Neurochirurgie*, **6**, 367.

ADDITIONAL READING

Farmer, T. W. (1964) Pediatric Neurology. New York: Hoeber.
Fontana, R. S., Edwards, J. E. (1962) Congenital Cardiac Disease: A Review of 357 Cases Studied Pathologically. Philadelphia: W. B. Saunders.
Ingraham, F. D., Matson, D. D. (1954) Neurosurgery in Infancy and Childhood. Springfield, Ill.: C. C Thomas.
Liske, E., Weikers, N. J. (1964) 'Changing aspects of brain abscesses. Review of cases in Wisconsin, 1940 through 1962.' *Neurology (Minneap.)*, **14**, 294.
Nadas, A. S. (1963) Pediatric Cardiology. 2nd edn. Philadelphia: W. B. Saunders.
Schulze, A., Tucht, W. (1961) 'Hirnabszesse im Säuglingsalter.' *Zbl. Neurochir.*, **21**, 278.
Szenasy, J., Paraicz, E. (1961) 'Beiträge zur Klinik des mit Gehirnabszess einhergehenden Herzfehlers.' *Dtsch. Z. Nervenheilk.*, **183**, 122.
Weber, G. (1957) Der Hirnabszess. Stuttgart: Thieme.
Wright, R. L., Ballantine, H. T. (1967) 'Management of brain abscesses in children and adolescents.' *Amer. J. Dis. Child.*, **114**, 113.

Chapter 21. Intracranial Tumours

REFERENCE

Horster, A., Walter, W. (1961) 'Apoplektiforme Verlaufsformen bei Hirntumoren.' *Dtsch. Z. Nervenheilk.*, **182**, 288.

ADDITIONAL READING

Isler, W. (1965) 'Le diagnostique neurologique et neuroradiologique des tumeurs cérébrales de l'enfant.' *Minerva neurochir.*, **9**, 229.
Matson, D. D. (1964) 'Intracranial tumors.' *in* Farmer, T. W. (Ed.) Pediatric Neurology. New York: Hoeber.
Rath, F. (1965) 'Hirntumoren im Kindesalter.' *Z. Kinderheilk.*, **94**, 148.

Chapter 22. Multiple Sclerosis

REFERENCES

Baasch, E. (1966) 'Theoretische Überlegungen zur Ätiologie der Sclerosis Multiplex.' *Schweiz. Arch. Neurol. Neurochir. Psychiat.*, **98**, 1.
Gall, J. C., Hayles, A. B., Siekert, R. G., Keith, H. M. (1958) 'Multiple sclerosis in children. A clinical study of 40 cases with onset in childhood.' *Pediatrics*, **21**, 703.
Isler, W. (1961) 'Multiple Sklerose im Kindesalter.' *Helv. paediat. Acta*, **16**, 412.
Low, N. L., Carter, S. (1956) 'Multiple sclerosis in children.' *Pediatrics*, **18**, 24.
Palffy, G., Mérei, F. T. (1961) 'The possible role of vaccines and sera in the pathogenesis of multiple sclerosis.' *Wld Neurol.*, **2**, 167.
Sandifer, P. (1962) 'Non-vascular causes of acute hemiplegia in childhood.' *in* Bax, M., Mitchell, R. G. (Eds.) Acute Hemiplegia in Childhood. Clinics in Developmental Medicine, No. 6. London: Spastics Society with Heinemann. p. 17.
Uchimura, Y., Shiraki, H. (1957) 'A contribution to classification and the pathogenesis of demyelinating encephalomyelitis; with special reference to the central nervous system lesions caused by preventitive inoculation against rabies.' *J. Neuropath. exp. Neurol.*, **16**, 139.

Chapter 23. Subdural Haematoma

ADDITIONAL READING

Freundlich, E., Beller, A. J., Berman, S. (1956) 'Subdural hematoma in infancy.' *Amer. J. Dis. Child.*, **91**, 608.

Hollenhorst, R. W., Stein, H. A. (1958) 'Ocular signs and prognosis in subdural and subarachnoid bleeding in young children.' *Arch. Ophthal.*, **60**, 187.

—— —— Keith, H. M., MacCarty, C. S. (1957) 'Subdural hygroma and subarachnoid hemorrhage among infants and children.' *Neurology (Minneap.)*, **7**, 813.

Ingraham, F. D., Matson, D. D. (1954) Neurosurgery of Infancy and Childhood. Springfield, Ill.: C. C Thomas.

Jacobi, G., Kazner, E., Wollensak, J. (1966) 'Subdurale Ergüsse und Hämatome bei Säuglingen und Kindern. Betrachtungen zur Pathogenese, Klinik, Therapie und Prognose.' *Z. Kinderheilk.*, **96**, 199.

Klein, M. R. (1963) 'L'hématome sous-dural du nourrisson.' *Neurochirurgia (Stuttgart)*, **6**, 152.

Krayenbühl, H. (1963) 'Die operative Entfernung des subduralen Hämatoms.' *Wien. klin. Wschr.*, **75**, 494.

Neimann, N., Montaut, J. (1968) Epanchements Sousduraux Chroniques du Nourrisson. Paris: Expansions Scientifiques Françaises.

Töndury, G. D. (1967) 'Das subdurale Hämatom und Hygrom im Kindesalter.' *Schweiz. Arch. Neurol. Neurochir. Psychiat.*, **99**, 299.

Weber, G. (1959) 'Das chronische Subduralhämatom. Eine klinische Übersicht.' *in* Verhandlung der Deutsche Gesellschaft für Pathologie. Vol. 43. Stuttgart: Fischer.

—— Heyser, J., Rosenmund, H., Duckert, F. (1964) 'Subdurale Hämatome.' *Schweiz. med. Wschr.*, **94**, 541, 578.

Chapter 24. Migraine Accompagnée

REFERENCES

Alpers, B. J., Yaskin, H. E. (1951). 'Pathogenesis of ophthalmoplegic migraine.' *Arch. Ophthal.*, **45**, 555. (Cited by Walsh and O'Doherty (1960).).

Balyeat, R. M., Rinkel, H. J. (1931) 'Allergic migraine in children.' *Amer. J. Dis. Child.*, **42**, 1126.

Bickerstaff, E. R. (1961*a*) 'Basilar artery migraine.' *Lancet*, **i**, 15.

—— (1961*b*) 'Impairment of consciousness in migraine.' *Lancet*, **ii**, 1057.

—— (1964) 'Ophthalmoplegic migraine.' *Rev. neurol.*, **110**, 582.

Bille, B. (1962) 'Migraine in schoolchildren.' *Acta paediat. (Uppsala)*, Suppl. 136.

Blau, J. N., Whitty, C. W. M. (1955) 'Familial hemiplegic migraine.' *Lancet*, **ii**, 1115.

Bradshaw, P., Parsons, M. (1965) 'Hemiplegic migraine, a clinical study.' *Quart. J. Med.*, **34**, 65.

Brain, R. (1954) 'Cerebral vascular disorders.' *Lancet*, **ii**, 831.

Buckle, R. M., Du Boulay, G., Smith, B. (1964) 'Death due to cerebral vasospasm.' *J. Neurol. Neurosurg. Psychiat.*, **27**, 440.

Charcot, J.-M. (1892) Hospice de la Salpêtrière. Clinique des Maladies du Système Nerveux. Leçons du Professeur. Paris: F. Alcan. (Cited by Heyck (1956).).

Clarke, J. M. (1910) 'On recurrent motor paralysis in migraine.' *Brit. med. J.*, **i**, 1534.

Connor, R. C. R. (1962) 'Complicated migraine. A study of permanent neurological and visual defects caused by migraine.' *Lancet*, **ii**, 1072.

Dukes, H. T., Vieth, R. G. (1964) 'Cerebral arteriography during migraine prodrome and headache.' *Neurology (Minneap.)*, **14**, 636.

Dynes, J. B. (1939) 'Alternating hemiparetic migraine syndrome.' *Brit. Med. J.*, **ii**, 446.

Ekberg, R., Cronqvist, S., Ingvar, D. H. (1965) 'Regional cerebral blood flow.' *in* Proceedings of an International Symposium, Lund 1965. Copenhagen: Munksgaard.

Ford, F. R. (1966) Diseases of the Nervous System in Infancy, Childhood and Adolescence. 5th edn. Springfield, Ill.: C. C Thomas.

Friedman, A. P., Merritt, H. H. (1959) Headache, Diagnosis and Treatment. Philadelphia: Davis.

—— Harter, D. H., Merritt, H. H. (1962) 'Ophthalmoplegic migraine.' *Arch. Neurol. (Chic.)*, **7**, 320.

Friedman, M. W. (1951) 'Occlusion of central retinal vein in migraine.' *Arch. Ophthalm.*, **45**, 678.

Goltman, A. M. (1936) 'The mechanism of migraine.' *J. Allergy*, **7**, 351. (Cited by Walsh and O'Doherty (1960).).

Graveson, G. S. (1949) 'Retinal artery occlusion in migraine.' *Brit. med. J.*, **ii**, 838.

Guest, I. A., Woolf, A. L. (1964) 'Fatal infarction of brain in migraine.' *Brit. med. J.*, **i**, 225.

Harrington, D. O., Flocks, M. (1953) 'Ophthalmoplegic migraine. A discussion of its pathogenesis with a report of the pathologic findings in a case of recurrent oculomotor palsy.' *Trans. Amer. Acad. Ophthal. Otolaryng.*, **57**, 517.

Heyck, H. (1956) Neue Beiträge zur Klinik und Pathogenese der Migräne. Stuttgart: Thieme.

Lancet, Leading Article (1965) 'Hemiplegic migraine.' *Lancet*, **i**, 896.

Lees, F., Watkins, S. M. (1963) 'Loss of consciousness in migraine.' *Lancet*, ii, 647.
Montgomery, B. M., King, W. W. (1962) 'Hemiplegic migraine. A case with paroxysmal shoulder-hand syndrome.' *Ann. intern. Med.*, **57**, 450.
Naffziger (personal communication). Cited by Harrington and Flocks (1953).
Osler, W. (1909). Cited by Whitty (1953) and by Russell, A. E. (1909) *Clin. J.*, **34**, 414.
Ostfeld, A. M. (1960) 'Migraine headache. Its physiology and biochemistry.' *J. Amer. med. Ass.*, **174**, 1188.
Rosenbaum, H. E. (1960) 'Familial hemiplegic migraine.' *Canad. med. Ass. J.*, **78**, 10.
Ross, R. T. (1958) 'Hemiplegic Migraine.' *Canad. Med. Assoc. J.*, **78**, 10.
Selby, G., Lance, J. W. (1960) 'Observations on 500 cases of migraine and allied vascular headache.' *J. Neurol. Neurosurg. Psychiat.*, **23**, 23.
Symonds, C. (1950-51) 'Migrainous variants'. *Trans. med. Soc. Lond.*, **67**, 237.
Vahlquist, B. (1955) 'Migraine in children.' *Int. Arch. Allergy*, **7**, 348.
—— Hackzell, G. (1949) 'Migraine of early onset. A study of 31 cases in which the disease first appeared between 1-4 years of age.' *Acta paediat. (Uppsala)*, **38**, 622.
ver Brugghen, A. (1955) 'Pathogenesis of ophthalmoplegic migraine.' *Neurology (Minneap.)*, **5**, 311.
Walsh, J. P., O'Doherty, D. S (1960) 'A possible explanation of the mechanism of ophthalmoplegic migraine.' *Neurology (Minneap.)*, **10**, 1079.
Whitty, C. W. M. (1953) 'Familial hemiplegic migraine.' *J. Neurol. Neurosurg. Psychiat.*, **16**, 172.
Wolff, H. G. (1948) Headache and other Head Pain. New York: O.U.P.
—— (1955) 'Headache mechanism.' *Int. Arch. Allergy*, **7**, 210.

ADDITIONAL READING

Barolin, G. S. (1967) 'Familiäre paroxysmale halbseitenausfälle mit und ohne Kopfschmerzattaken.' *Schweiz Arch. Neurol. Neurochir, Psychiat.*, **99**, 15.
Bickerstaff, E. R. (1962) 'The basilar artery and the migraine-epilepsy syndrome.' *Proc. roy. Soc Med.*, **55**, 167.
Chapman, L. F., Ramos, A. D., Goodell, H., Silverman, G., Wolff, H. G. (1960) 'A humoral agent implicated in vascular headache of the migraine type.' *Arch. Neurol. (Chic.)*, **3**, 223.
Friedman, A. P. (1963) 'The pathogenesis of migraine headache.' *Bull. L. A. neurol. Soc.*, **28**, 191.
Heyck, H. (1958) Der Kopfschmerz. Differentialdiagnose und Therapie für die Praxis. Stuttgart: Thieme.
Hinrichs, W. L., Keith, H. M. (1965) 'Migraine in childhood: a follow-up report.' *Proc. Mayo Clin.*, **40**, 593.
Holguin, J., Fenichel, G. (1967) 'Migraine.' *J. Pediat.*, **70**, 290.
Hollenhorst, R. W. (1953) 'Ocular manifestations of migraine: report of four cases of hemianopia.' *Proc. Mayo. Clin*, **28**, 686.
Walsh, F. B. (1951) 'The ocular symptoms of migraine.' *N.C. med. J.*, **12**, 271.
Whitehouse, D., Pappas, A. J., Escala, P. H., Livingston, S. (1967) 'Electroencephalographic changes in children with migraine.' *New Engl. J. Med.*, **276**, 23.
Whitty, C. W. M. (1967) 'Migraine without headache.' *Lancet*, ii, 283.

Conclusions

REFERENCES

Bernsmeier, A. (1963) Durchblutung des Gehirns. Physiologie und Pathophysiologie des vegetativen Nervensystems. Vol. 2. Stuttgart: Hippokrates.
Cavanagh, J. B. (1962) 'The immediate sequelae of acute cerebral vascular occlusion (acute hemi-plegia) in childhood.' *in* Bax, M., Mitchell, R. G. (Eds.) Acute Hemiplegia in Childhood. Clinics in Developmental Medicine, No. 6. London: Spastics Society with Heinemann. p. 49.
Bickerstaff, E. R. (1964) 'Aetiology of acute hemiplegia in childhood.' *Brit. Med. J.*, ii, 82.
Brandt, S. (1962) 'Causes and pathogenic mechanisms of acute hemiplegia in childhood.' *in* Bax, M., Mitchell, R. G. (Eds.) Acute Hemiplegia in Childhood. Clinics in Developmental Medicine, No. 6. London: Spastics Society with Heinemann. p. 7.
Dalal, P. M., Shah, P. M., Sheth, S. C., Deshpande, C. K. (1965) 'Cerebral embolism. Angiographic observations on spontaneous clot lysis.' *Lancet*, i, 61.
—— —— Deshpande, C. K., Sheth, S. C. (1966) 'Recanalisation after cerebral embolism.' *Lancet*, ii, 495.
Denny-Brown, D. (1951) 'The treatment of recurrent cerebral vascular symptoms and the question of "vasospasm".' *Med. Clin. N. Amer.*, **35**, 1457.
Meyer, J. S., Denny-Brown, D. (1957) 'The cerebral collateral circulation. 1. Factors influencing collateral blood flow. 2. Production of cerebral infarction by ischaemic anoxia and its reversibility in early stages.' *Neurology (Minneap.)*, **7**, 447, 567.
Millichap, J. G. (1968) Febrile Convulsions. New York: Macmillan.

General Reading

Bakay, L., Lee, J. C. (1965) Cerebral Edema. Springfield, Ill.: C. C Thomas.

Baker, A. B. (1962) Clinical Neurology, 2nd edn. New York: Hoeber-Harper.

Bax, M., Mitchell, R. G. (Eds.) (1962) Acute Hemiplegia in Childhood. Clinics in Developmental Medicine, No 6 London: Spastics Society with Heinemann.

Bergmann, G., Frey, W., Schweigk, H. (Eds.) (1953) Handbuch der Inneren Medizin, Band V, Abt. 1-3. Berlin: Springer.

Blackwood, W., McMenemey, W. H., Meyer, A., Norman, R. M., Russell, D. S. (1963) Greenfield's Neuropathology, 2nd edn. London: Edward Arnold.

Carter, S., Gold, A. P. (1967) 'Acute infantile hemiplegia.' *Pediat. Clin. N. Amer.*, **14**, 851.

Farmer, T. W. (1964) Pediatric Neurology. New York: Hoeber.

Finney, L. A., Walker, A. E. (1962) Transtentorial Herniation. Springfield, Ill.: C. C Thomas.

Ford, F. R. (1966) Diseases of the Nervous System in Infancy, Childhood and Adolescence, 5th edn. Springfield, Ill.: C. C Thomas.

Ingvar, D. H., Lassen, N. A. (1965) 'Regional cerebral blood flow.' *in* Proceedings of an International Symposium, Lund, 1955. Copenhagen: Munksgaard.

Jabbour, J. T., Lundervold, A. (1963) 'Hemiplegia: a clinical and electroencephalographic study in childhood.' *Develop. Med. Child Neurol.*, **5**, 24.

Sarkari, N. B. S., Holmes, J. M., Bickerstaff, E. R. (1970) 'Neurological manifestations associated with internal carotid loops and kinks in children.' *J. Neurol. Neurosurg. Psychiat.*, **33**, 194.

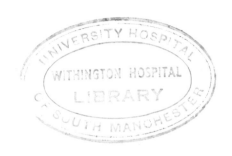

314